The Pharmacology of Alcohol
and Drugs of Abuse and Addiction

Norman S. Miller

The Pharmacology of Alcohol and Drugs of Abuse and Addiction

Springer-Verlag
New York Berlin Heidelberg London
Paris Tokyo Hong Kong Barcelona

Norman S. Miller, M.D.
Cornell University Medical College
New York Hospital–Cornell Medical Center
21 Bloomingdale Road
White Plains, New York 10605
USA

With 3 illustrations.

Library of Congress Cataloging-in-Publication Data
Miller, Norman S.
    The pharmacology of alcohol and drugs of abuse and addiction /
Norman S. Miller.
        p. cm.
    Includes bibliographical references.
    Includes index.
    ISBN-13: 978-1-4612-7774-3   e-ISBN-13: 978-1-4612-3044-1
    DOI: 10.1007/978-1-4612-3044-1

    1. Alcoholism – Physiological aspects.   2. Substance abuse –
Physiological aspects.   3. Alcohol – Physiological effect.
4. Psychotropic drugs – Physiological effect.
5. Neuropsychopharmacology.   I. Title.
    [DNLM: 1. Alcohol, Ethyl – pharmacology.   2. Narcotics –
pharmacology.   3. Street Drugs – pharmacology.   4. Substance Abuse.
5. Substance Dependence.   QV 84 M649p]
RC565.M444   1990
615′.78 – dc20
DNLM/DLC
for Library of Congress   90-10046

Printed on acid-free paper.

© 1991 Springer-Verlag New York Inc.

Softcover reprint of the hardcover 1st edition 1991

Typeset by Bytheway Typesetting Services, Norwich, NY.

9 8 7 6 5 4 3 2 1

To my wife Nicole, and my daughters Mia and Natasha.
Persistent partisans who generously devoted their time
for this book.

Preface

This volume is intended for clinicians, researchers, residents, and students. The range is wide and the depth considerable for all the topics covered in the treatment of this timely and relevant subject. This book may serve equally well as a general introduction and a scholarly reference. Ultimately, it is designed to serve those patients suffering from abuse of and addiction to drugs and alcohol.

The content and organization of the book flow from general concepts of abuse and addiction to specific details of the pharmacology of alcohol and drugs. Special chapters on topics not found in most other books, such as pharmacology of drug–drug interactions, abstinence, and prevention, are included.

This book is written especially for the clinician interested in the *pharmacology* of alcohol and drugs of abuse and addiction. The pharmacology is integrated into a conceptual approach to diagnosis and treatment of alcohol and drug abuse and addiction.

The form and style are didactic, critical as well as straightforward in presentation. Literature references from recent clinical research and basic research provide the foundation for the chapters throughout the book. Because the book is written by a clinician–researcher, the information is readily adaptable to clinical problems and research ideas.

I would like to express my deep appreciation to Susan Newsom and Darlene Tucci for their invaluable technical assistance.

Norman S. Miller

Contents

Introduction to the Pharmacological Effects of Alcohol and Drugs and Addiction on the Brain and Behavior

History

The course of one drug addiction is significantly affected by the addiction to another drug or alcohol. It is clinically acknowledged that the course of alcoholism is often significantly altered by the addiction to another drug. From the histories of many alcoholics, interestingly, comes the comment that the course of the alcoholism could have continued if addiction to cocaine or opiates or sedatives had not developed. Review of the histories and clinical presentations strongly suggests that this is likely the case, as in many instances the development of an addiction to another drug motivated an earlier seeking of treatment in spite of a substantial, standing addiction to alcohol that had already existed with significant consequences.

Prevalence and Patterns of Use

The identification of multiple drug addictions is critical to clinical diagnosis, prognosis, and treatment, as well as formulation of research models for the etiology, of abuse and addiction to alcohol and drugs. The theoretical implications for the genetic vulnerability and transmission of both alcoholism and drug addiction are interesting and far reaching. The traditional understanding of the neurobiology of addiction to individual drugs is challenged by the concept of multiple addiction, which suggests a universal susceptibility to alcohol and drug addictions.

The contemporary alcoholic usually becomes addicted to alcohol as the first drug, but progresses to other drug addictions at a rapid rate and to a significant degree. Most alcoholics under the age of 30 years are addicted to at least one other and more often to many drugs. The addiction to the other drugs is frequently followed by consequences similar to those of the alcohol addiction. Furthermore, the multiplicity of drugs to which addiction develops is not limited to the alcoholic, that is, most drug addicts who first become addicted to a drug later develop alcohol addiction, or alcohol may

1

be the first drug used addictively for many drug addicts. Moreover, although alcohol is not usually the drug of choice for the drug addict it is used addictively as an adjunct with a drug or in substitution of a drug (1).

The number and variety of drugs that the multiple addicted seek has become increasingly extensive. In addition, the traditional boundaries of addictive use of illicit drugs and the therapeutic use of prescribed medications are considerably less distinct. The nonmedical use of medical drugs such as benzodiazepines and amphetamines by drug addicts is widespread. The pure drug addict who is addicted to only one drug is a rare species; it is difficult to find a heroin addict who is not or has not also been addicted to marijuana and/or alcohol, and more recently to cocaine. The common practice of adulteration (mixing during preparation) of one illicit drug with another drug makes it difficult and at times impossible for the addict to determine and maintain a monodrug addiction, particularly when the drugs are obtained "on the street."

The effect on personality development and on the manifestation of psychiatric symptoms in the personality by the use of multiple drugs is a poorly documented area of research. Although it is a frequent clinical observation that the multiple drug addict has greater personality disturbances than the monodrug addict, the impact on the personality by alcohol and multiple drugs has not been measured by any standardized method. The contemporary alcoholic and drug addict becomes addicted usually sometime in adolescence when the personality is developing and when no definite stability or maturity has been established. The result is often a mixture of alcoholism, drug addiction, and an immature personality. The salient clinical observation is that the personality undergoes an arrest of maturation in personality with the onset of addiction.

A source of the manifestations of the personality disturbances is the pharmacological effects of drugs on the brain and behavior. Alcohol, marijuana, cocaine, opiates, sedative/hypnotics, and other drugs produce signs and symptoms of drug intoxication and withdrawal that include disturbances in mood, cognition, and vegetative states. These psychoactive effects on the brain and behavior are often chronic and cumulative in the multiple addicted. The degree of personality disorganization is sometimes marked in the multiple addicted because of the chronic addiction to multiple drugs (2,3).

Diagnosis

Because denial is a part of the addictive process, an underreporting and underestimation of drug use are to be expected in a clinical interview, especially if only the alcoholic is interviewed. Corroborative sources increase the likelihood of obtaining a more accurate history but still may not reveal the total pattern and amount of alcohol and drug use. These sources may include family, employer, legal agencies, and urine and blood testing for drugs (4).

The criteria for addiction that include a preoccupation with compulsive use or relapse to alcohol and drugs are candidly denied by many alcoholics and drug addicts who are actively using the alcohol and drugs. Questions regarding the development of tolerance and dependence to alcohol and drugs are equally difficult to have adequately answered. Persistent pursuit of the patient in subsequent interviews, and a knowledge of the natural history of alcohol and drug use and addiction, particularly in the multiple addicted, will often yield rewarding results (5).

Intoxication

Alcohol produces significant depression that is distinguishable from major depression as defined in the Diagnostic and Statistical Manual of Medical Disorders, Third Edition–Revised (DSM-III-R). The severe disturbance in mood and affect can be associated with mood-congruent psychotic delusions, psychomotor retardation, vegetative symptoms, and suicidal actions. Alcohol withdrawal with its hyperexcitable and hyperaroused state, and alcohol intoxication with its episodes of euphoria, poor judgment, and poor insight with consequent behaviors, have been confused with mania. Alcohol hallucinosis with auditory and sometimes visual hallucinations is to be differentiated from schizophrenia. The anxiety produced by repeated stimulation of the sympathetic nervous system in alcohol intoxication and withdrawal is distinguishable from the anxiety disorders or generalized anxiety, panic attacks, and phobias. Phobias such as agoraphobia are quite common in alcoholics as a result of chronic alcohol consumption. The older terminology of "alcoholic paranoia" described a syndrome that fits well into the criteria for agoraphobia, only caused by alcohol.

Cocaine and other stimulant intoxication produce effects that fulfill the criteria for mania; that is, the triad in mania of euphoria, hyperactivity, and distorted self-image are principal pharmacological effects of cocaine intoxication. The withdrawal from cocaine, particularly in chronic use, is characterized by severe depression with the attendant signs and symptoms that fulfill criteria for major depression. The chronic effects of cocaine are delusions, particularly paranoid, and hallucinations, both visual and auditory, which are indistinguishable from schizophrenia. Furthermore, the anxiety generated from the pharmacological effects of addictive chronic cocaine use is in the form of generalized anxiety, panic attacks, and intense agoraphobia.

Marijuana, phencyclidine, and other hallucinogens are drugs that produce intense distortions of mood, affect thinking, and perceptions with the development of depression, mania, delusions, and hallucinations. The chronic effects of marijuana are similar to both alcohol and cocaine, as

marijuana appears to have psychopharmacological effects somewhere between sedative and stimulant properties. Other hallucinogens such as lysergic acid diethylamide (LSD), methamphetamine, and psilocybin share
properties with marijuana.

All these drugs have the aforementioned effects on personality when used
chronically in an addictive mode. The deterioration in personality and the
delay in maturation in personality are produced by all the drugs, including
alcohol. The multiple addicted is more severely affected and experiences a
more pronounced effect on the personality.

The combined effects of the multiple addiction of the drugs and alcohol
are commonly seen in the contemporary drug addict. The penchant to become addicted to multiple drugs and alcohol is clearly established in the
contemporary drug addict and alcoholic. The difficulty in sorting out and
the attributing various drug effects to the correct drug or a combination of
drugs is significant and at times impossible. The differentiation of the effect
of acute and chronic drug use and addiction from that of other psychiatric
disorders is important to distinguish a psychiatric disorder from a drug-
induced state.

An important aspect is to maintain a differential diagnosis and not be
compelled to make a single, final diagnosis. Furthermore, it is essential to
keep in mind that alcohol and drug addiction are primary disorders that
produce symptoms and syndromes. The treatment of the multiple addiction
with detoxification and abstinence will frequently be sufficient to establish
the definitive diagnosis. However, occasionally the drug effects, particularly
in the multiple addicted, will persist for protracted periods so that prolonged
observation may be necessary before the effect of alcohol and drugs can be
reliably ruled out. The mood disturbances and anxiety production from
alcohol, cocaine, and marijuana may endure although lessening with passing weeks and months. The delusions and hallucinations may continue in
the various drug states for prolonged periods. Finally, the deterioration in
personality may take years to reverse, although a substantial beginning is
made with abstinence and commitment to a treatment program.

Neurochemistry

Twin, adoption, familial, and high-risk studies have demonstrated a significant genetic predisposition to alcoholism (6–10). Identical twins are more
concordant for alcoholism than fraternal twins. The biological parent of an
adoptee is a more important determinant of alcoholism than the foster
parent who reared the adoptee. More than 50% of the alcoholics have a
family history positive for alcoholism. A child of an alcoholic is more likely
to have certain neurophysiological and behavioral manifestations in common with other offspring of alcoholics than with matched controls without
an alcoholic parent (11–14).

Corresponding studies for the prevalence of alcohol dependence in the family history of cocaine and opiate addicts and other drug users have been performed. In one study, the rate of the diagnosis of alcohol dependence in first- or second-degree relatives in the families of 263 cocaine addicts was greater than 50%; in other words 132 cocaine addicts had at least one relative with alcohol dependence by DSM-III-R criteria (15).

Opiate addicts with a parental history of alcoholism were more frequently diagnosed with concurrent alcoholism. In one study, opiate addicts ($N =$ 638) had at least one parent with alcohol dependence in 21.3% of families. Opiate addicts with the diagnosis of alcohol dependence ($N = 422$) without parental alcohol dependence had a 12.5% rate of alcohol dependence in their families. Among the opiate addicts with alcohol dependence, those with parental alcoholism had more severe problems with alcohol (16).

A study of young alcohol users in their twenties revealed a higher rate of alcohol-related problems and drug use if a family history of alcoholism was present in first- and second-degree relatives. Young alcohol users without, or with fewer, relatives with alcoholism had a lower rate of alcohol-related problems and drug use (11).

These findings compare favorably with the familial studies of alcoholism in which alcoholics have at least a 50% probability for a positive family history of alcoholism. The high rate of alcohol dependence among cocaine and opiate addicts and drug users and their families suggests a generalized vulnerability of alcohol and drugs that may have a genetic contribution. The genetic predisposition to alcoholism may overlap or share transmission with the tendency to cocaine, opiate, and other drug addictions (17).

Tolerance and Dependence

Alcoholism may predispose individuals to cocaine dependence by genetic determination or by the induced vulnerability to an additional drug dependence when one already exists. Drug effects, particularly in the "dependent state," are more similar than different or multiple drugs such as alcohol, marijuana, cocaine, and others that share pharmacological properties. Alcohol is a depressant that produces depressant effects during intoxication and stimulant effects during withdrawal with discharging of the sympathetic nervous system. Alcohol alters the membrane fluidity of the neuronal membrane by a disordering effect on the phospholipids contained in the membranes. The neuronal membrane becomes more ordered or rigid as a homeostatic response to the disordering effect of alcohol, which correlates with the development of tolerance. The disordering effect reflects the depressant effects of alcohol, and the compensatory ordering effect reflects the stimulatory effects (18).

Cocaine, a stimulant during intoxication, becomes a depressant during withdrawal as a manifestation of the exhaustion of the sympathetic nervous system, which has been discharging excessively under the effect of cocaine. Cocaine exerts its pharmacological effects by blocking the reuptake of the catecholamines norepinephrine, epinephrine, and dopamine by the presynaptic neurons. The reuptake blockade promotes an enhanced effect of the neurotransmitter at the postsynaptic site. Following chronic stimulation, the presynaptic site becomes depleted of catecholamines because the reuptake mechanism is responsible for replenishing the presynaptic neuron with catecholamines. Clinically, the enhanced state with excess neurotransmitter correlates with the stimulation and the exhausted state with depleted neurotransmitter correlates with depression (19).

Marijuana may act by disordering the neuronal membrane to produce depression and enhancing catecholamine transmission to produce stimulation. Marijuana appears to possess both depressant and stimulatory properties that are similar to those of alcohol and cocaine. Marijuana is also strongly attracted to fat deposits and consequently is stored in large amounts, particularly with chronic use. The drug is then slowly released back into circulation as the equilibrium shifts from the lipid compartment to the blood compartment (20).

Alcohol's drug effect is to induce euphoria and a sense of exhilaration in low doses, depression in moderate to high doses, and increasing anxiety during the withdrawal period as the chronicity and severity of the alcohol consumption increases. Cocaine induces euphoria at any dose but tends to induce depression during withdrawal, increasing as the dose escalates. Marijuana is similar to cocaine in inducing stimulation in lower doses but is clearly depressing in high doses. The similarities in the effect on mood become increasingly stronger with more chronic and heavy use as is seen with addictive use.

Other consequent effects on cognition, psychomotor abilities and coordination, and psychological parameters such as blood pressure and pulse also become more common with chronic, higher, and frequent doses. Acute and particularly chronic alcohol consumption is associated with elevated blood pressure and pulse during the inevitable withdrawal state. In contrast, acute and chronic cocaine consumption is associated with elevated blood pressure and pulse rate during the intoxicated state.

That alcohol and drug addiction so commonly occur together provides theoretical implications for a neurobiological basis for multiple addicted. The loss of control that underlies all the criteria for addictive behavior is manifested by a drive to pursue, use, and resort to alcohol and drugs repetitively and spontaneously. The substrate for the mechanism for the drive in addiction resides in the limbic system. The limbic structures include the amygdala and septal area for mood, the hippocampi for memory association, and the hypothalamus for the drive states of hunger, libido, and thirst. The reward center is also represented among the limbic structures in the lateral hypothalamus and ventral tegmental area (18,19).

The distinguishing features of addiction are subserved by the functions in the limbic system. Alcohol and drugs profoundly alter mood and drive states. An association between alcohol and drugs and the drive states may be reinforced by the reward center and recorded in memory by the hippocampi. The drive states may entrain the use of alcohol and drugs in a fashion similar to their autonomous control over their other functions. The pursuit and uncontrolled use of alcohol and drugs become as easily stimulated and spontaneous as eating, drinking, and sexual behavior.

As an example, cocaine may activate the limbic system through stimulation of the dopamine transmissions. The reward system consists of neurons located in the lateral hypothalamus that traverse the median forebrain bundle to synapse on dopamine-containing neurons in the ventral tegmentum. The dopamine neurons send fibers into the nucleus accumbens (mesolimbic pathway) and the limbic cortex (mesocortical pathway). These dopamine-containing neurons possess opiate receptors for endorphins and enkephalins.

The limbic system may provide a final common pathway for the addictive process to occur without regard to the particular drug. Alcohol appears to have a widespread effect on many of the neurotransmitter systems in the limbic system and reward system. All the drugs of addiction, including alcohol, affect mood, libido, memory, and appetite. These drugs may also stimulate the mesolimbic areas that are responsible for the symptoms of hallucinations and delusions. Finally, all the drugs, especially alcohol, suppress frontal lobe function to produce the impairment in judgment and insight that is characteristic of alcohol and drug addiction (18).

References

1. Galizio M, Maisto SA (1985). Determinants of substance abuse relapse. In *Determinants of Substance Abuse*, Tucker JA, Vuchinich RB, Harris CV, eds., New York: Plenum, pp. 383–424.
2. Miller NS (1987). A primer of the treatment process for alcoholism and drug addiction. *Psychiatry Lett* 5(7):30–37.
3. Hoffman FG (1983). *A Handbook on Drug and Alcohol Abuse,* 2d ed. New York: Oxford University Press.
4. Miller NS, Gold MS, Cocores JA, Pottash AC (1988). Alcohol dependence and its medical consequences. *NY State J Med* 88:476–481.
5. Miller NS, Gold MS (1989). Suggestions for changes in DSM-III-R criteria for substance use disorders. *Am J Drug Alcohol Abuse* 15(2):223–230.
6. Kaij L (1960). *Studies on the Etiology and Sequels of Abuse of Alcohol.* Lund, Sweden: University of Lund.
7. Partanen J, Bruun K, Markkanen T (1977). Inheritance of drinking behavior: A study on intelligence, personality and use of alcohol of adult twins. In *Emergency Concepts of Alcohol Dependence*, Pattisn RM, Sobel MB, Sobel LC, eds., New York: Springer-Verlag.
8. Murray RM, Clifford C, Gurlin HM (1983). Twin and alcoholism studies. In *Recent Developments in Alcoholism*, Galanter M, ed. New York: Gardner Press.
9. Roe A (1944). The adult adjustment of children of alcoholic parents raised in foster homes. *Q J Stud Alcohol* 5:378–393.

10. Frances R, Timm S, Bucky S (1980). Studies of familial and nonfamilial alcoholism. I. Demographic studies. *Arch Gen Psychiatry* 37:564–566.
11. Schuckit MA, Goodwin DW, Winokur G (1972). A half-sibling study of alcoholism. *Am J Psychiatry* 128:1132–1136.
12. Tarter R (1981). Minimal brain dysfunction as an etiological predisposition to alcoholism. In *Evaluation of the alcoholic: Implications for research, theory and practice*, Meyer R, et al., eds., pp. 167–191. Rockville, MD: US DHHS.
13. Pollack VE, Volavka J, Goodwin DW, et al. (1983). The EEG after school in men at risk for alcoholism. *Arch Gen Psychiatry* 40:857–861.
14. Beglieter J, Porjesz B, Kissin B (1982). Brain dysfunction in alcoholics with and without a family history of alcoholism. *Alcohol Clin Exp Res* 6:36.
15. Miller NS, Gold MS, Belkin B, Klahr AL. Family history of alcohol dependence in cocaine dependence. *Psychiatr Res* 29:113–121.
16. Kosten TR, Rounsaville BJ, Babor TF, Spitzer RL, Williams JBW (1987). Substance use disorders in DSM-III-R: Evidence for the dependence syndrome across different psychoactive substance. *Br J Psychiatry* 151:834–843.
17. Miller NS, Gold MS (1988). Cocaine and alcoholism: Distinct or part of a spectrum. *Psychiatr Ann* 18:9.
18. Miller, Dackis CA, Gold MS (1987). The relationship of addiction, tolerance and dependence: A neurochemical approach. *J Subst Abuse Treat* 4:197–207.
19. Wise RA (1981). Brain dopamine and reward. In *Progress in Psychopharmacology*, Cooper SJ, ed., pp. 165–196. New York: Academic Press.
20. Miller NS, Gold MS (1989). The diagnosis of marijuana (cannabis) dependence. *J Subst Abuse Treat* 6:183–192.

CHAPTER 2

The Behavioral Concepts of Abuse and Addiction in Diagnosis

History

The DSM-III-R criteria for substance-dependence disorders represent significantly favorable revisions toward a valid and reliable diagnostic description (1,2). However, further improvements may be indicated. The following discussion attempts to critically review the validity and utility of the DSM-III-R for clinicians and researchers and to provide suggestions for consideration of further changes in the diagnostic categories (*see Appendices I and II*).

Nosology for the substance-abuse disorders is a constant source of confusion for both clinicians and researchers. Several errors in basic definitions are responsible for some of the abstruseness in clinical concepts and research criteria. The class name of "dependence" is misleading and inaccurate, and the use of the term "abuse" for pathological use is unscientific. The effort to disguise an old disease in a more fashionable and less offensive name of "dependence" instead of "addiction" is avoiding the truth in definition. Future research, particularly biological investigations of neurochemical correlates, and clinical accuracy both depend on valid definitions.

The criteria themselves are not clear statements of addictive behavior and are written in a cumbersome style that is not easily appreciated by nonspecialists. Furthermore, there is no simplified scheme to direct the clinicians to search for a diagnosis and provide the researcher with operational constructs.

Special considerations in diagnoses that are important and not addressed by the DSM-III-R include denial of drug use by the addict and by those surrounding him, polysubstance use, and psychological states affected by drug addiction such as personality, mood, cognition, and attitudes. Areas for future research to test the diagnostic criteria in substance dependence (addiction) may include natural history, relationship between other psychiatric disorders and substance dependence, symptoms and dynamics of drug addiction, biological markers, and neurochemical correlates of drug addiction.

Nosology

Class Name

The replacement of the word "drug" for "substance" as used in the DSM-III-R diagnosis of "substance-use disorders" may provide a more definitive term. A valid and contemporary "class name" might be "drug-use disorder." The term substance is overly inclusive and not specific enough to denote important characteristics peculiar to drugs. Substance is a generic word that is defined as an essence, spirit, form, or property, physical or otherwise (3). The term drug is a species-specific designation for pharmacologically active substances that are chemical agents affecting living processes (3). Other agents such as vapors, solvents, and residues are clearly chemicals that would qualify for the definition of a drug. Alcohol (ethanol) is a chemical agent that fits easily into the terminology of drug.

Disorders that arise from the use of drugs may be defined as "drug-use disorders" (1). Significant confusion may arise from the modern usage of the term "drug" to refer to medications only misleads and restricts important implications. Abuse, addiction, tolerance, and dependence do occur to a variety of medications, and to emphasize these aspects of drugs is to encourage a more complete understanding and knowledge of the assets and liabilities of the usage of medications (4,5). Furthermore, many of the drugs of abuse and addictive potential are pharmacologically and neurochemically similar to the drugs used for medicinal and therapeutic purposes. Some antidepressants affect the same neurotransmitter systems in the brain as does cocaine, because both drugs block the reuptake mechanism in the presynaptic neuron for the termination of the neurotransmitters dopamine and norepinephrine (6). The neuropharmacological similarities do not necessarily imply that all or most therapeutic drugs have significant abuse and addictive potential. The use of the term drug will only emphasize the commonality between drugs of abuse and medication effects, rather than create artificial and confusing differences by the use of the term substance.

The term "substance" allows for the inclusion of a wide variety of disorders that have similarities and often overlap with drug-use disorders but are not states of intoxication that pharmacologically affect the brain as do drugs. Food is a substance that is not foreign biochemically but can be used in a nonpharmacological fashion resulting a variety of addictive behaviors. Drug-use disorders possess important psychological, social, medical, and cultural differences from these other nondrug disorders. Although addictions to substances such as food may share with drugs a correspondingly common underlying neurophysiological and neurochemical basis that is located as such in the limbic system, risk of diluting the importance of foreign, pharmacological effects on the brain and behavior by drugs in drug addiction or dependence should be avoided. Drug and brain-receptor interactions represent distinct neurochemical processes that produce stereotypic and predictable responses in mood, cognition, and behavior (4,7).

Abuse versus Dependence

The term abuse as originally defined for pharmacological and behavioral purposes differs from the various popular meanings it has acquired. The term abuse means improper use or misuse outside the norm or standard for a given social structure in which the drug is used (8). The term implies voluntary use, that is unethical and morally wrong. Abuse as used frequently *but not necessarily* implies unfavorable or untoward consequences to drug use.

The diagnosis of "abuse" as presented in DSM-III and DSM-III-R contains definitions that are really not different from the diagnostic category of dependence as is described in DSM-III-R. "A pattern of pathological use" is required for the diagnosis of abuse and implicit in this definition is "loss of control," that is, an inability to cut down or stop drinking that is clearly outside the original intent of the term abuse and more in the domain of addiction and dependence as defined in DSM-III-R (9). Other definitions of abuse stated in the diagnostic criteria in DSM-III imply tolerance and dependence, that is, "need for daily use of alcohol for adequate functioning," that again are not usually contained in the meaning of abuse. The term abuse cannot correctly indicate, without confusion, a description of an entire medical/psychiatric disorder for which a diagnosis, treatment, and clinical course exist (4,8).

The differentiation between abuse and dependence on physiological grounds as operationally defined in DSM-III was eventually eliminated in DSM-III-R. The difference between abuse and dependence based on tolerance and withdrawal (dependence) does not appear to be clinically relevant. Schuckit concluded that there was no pronostic implication for the division between alcohol abuse and dependence in 403 male primary alcoholic patients. The two diagnostic groups differed in that subjects with alcohol dependence drank more per day, but did not differ in the number of days spent drinking, compared to the patients with alcohol abuse. The two groups were demographically virtually identical, and this similarity extended to presence of early life antisocial problems, drug-use patterns, psychiatric histories, and family histories of psychiatric disorder (10).

The term abuse was retained as a diagnostic category in DSM-III-R (*see Appendix II*) (2). The intention was to preserve a diagnostic category for milder and recent-onset cases of substance abuse. However, "loss of control" was pervasive in the criteria for abuse: (1) continued use despite a persistent (preoccupation) social, occupational, psychological, or physical problem that is caused or exacerbated by use of the substance (compulsive use), and (2) recurrent use (relapse) in situations when use is hazardous (e.g., driving while intoxicated). Abuse differs from dependence in DSM-III-R by the inclusion of the physiological states of tolerance and dependence in the latter diagnostic category. Most if not all the individuals who demonstrate "loss of control" as in alcohol abuse will qualify for the diagnosis of "dependence" by DSM-III-R criteria. The loss of control in "dependence syndrome" implies an involuntary state consistent with a primary addictive disorder. The criteria 1, 2, 5, 6, and 9 in the diagnosis of dependence in DSM-III-R are found in the diagnosis of abuse in DSM-III-R. Inaccurately, abuse is defined as "mild dependence" without a clear distinction in definition between abuse and dependence in DSM-III-R. The remaining criteria, 3, 4, 7, and 8 for "substance dependence," are largely physiological, and the old DSM-III distinction between pattern of pathological use (abuse) and tolerance (dependence) is actually retained.

Addiction versus Dependence

The broadening of the definition of "dependence" to include clinically relevant behaviors, cognitions, and symptoms that indicate a significant degree of involvement with a psychoactive substance, as done in DSM-III-R, does not serve to clarify diagnostic terminology. The diagnostic designation of "clinical dependence syndrome" to describe pathological drug use with characteristic symptoms and course is to overstate the original pharmacological meaning of dependence and to further add to the accumulated confusion (1,8,11). The pharmacological definition of dependence is the onset of a predictable, stereotypic set of signs and symptoms on the cessation of the use of a drug and the suppression of those signs and symptoms by further drug use. In short, definition of the term addiction includes behaviors, cognitions, and symptoms that indicate a significant degree of involvement with a psychoactive substance whereas the term dependence does not.

The use of the diagnosis addiction instead of dependence disorder is operationally valid and less ambiguous. The term dependence because of historical import presents too much confusion to many diagnosticians. The term suffers from too many derivations and connotations for uniform acceptance. In clinical practice, the term dependence has evolved to denote a variety of conditions that have little theoretical and empirical basis.

The term dependence represents many of the current concepts contained within the medical model of "substance abuse and dependence" that may be overstated or in error. The following points discuss some of these concepts.

1. The need to self-medicate with a drug to relieve symptoms of an underlying psychiatric or medical disorder will lead to compulsive use is a pervasive concept. Individuals may use a drug because of distressing symptoms but not necessarily addictively. The reverse may be true as studies indicate that alcoholics use alcohol in spite of depression because continued alcohol use worsens rather than lessens depression. The depression that results from cocaine use is frequently worse than any depression that may promote its use.

2. The concept of hedonism as a goal of drug use may be outdated. Pleasure may be a factor for early drug use, but subsequent drug use frequently leads to adversive symptoms such as anxiety and depression that more than neutralize any pleasure derived originally. Evidence for this line of reasoning can be obtained from clinical histories from addicts and inferred from high suicide rates among addicts.

3. The severity of withdrawal symptoms correlated with relative addictive liability of drugs ishmisleading. Cocaine and marijuana are two of the most addicting drugs known, yet neither produces a "dramatic and physiologically evident withdrawal" such as can be seen with morphine and alcohol.

4. Dependence or withdrawal symptoms as an explanation for compulsive use is a common misconception. Addiction frequently occurs in the absence of measurable "withdrawal symptoms." Severe dependence may in fact motivate discontinuation of the drug because further use only worsens the withdrawal symptoms and abstinence will alleviate them eventually. Compulsive use appears to occur in spite of the severity of dependence.

5. Dependence or withdrawal symptoms do not account for relapse or reinstatement of addiction in detoxified or abstinent individuals.

6. Several drugs that cause physical dependence are refused in self-administration experiments in animals despite the ability of the drugs to relieve withdrawal.

7. The "need" to use or to be dependent on a drug is an erroneous use of the term dependence (withdrawal). To be dependent on a drug in the sense of "needs" is not the same as to be addicted to a drug. An example of being "dependent on a drug" in the sense of need is digitalis in the treatment of congestive heart failure. An individual who discontinues digitalis will suffer from a relapse of the symptoms of congestive heart failure. A usual situation of an addiction to digitalis would suppose that the individual uses digitalis with loss of control that results in toxicity. An addiction to a drug is the use of the drug to the point of development of toxicity, particularly with chronic use. The reasons for including "craving" or a "drive to use a drug" as seen in addictive use in the jargon of dependence as a need is unclear. Addiction to drugs and alcohol is a primary disorder that is positive, self-sustaining, self-perpetuating, and automatic, and probably is not dependent on negative withdrawal effects for its expression.

Addiction is a descriptive and behavioral term that possesses inherently the meaning of "pattern of pathological use." Addictive behavior is illustrated by a pattern of pathological use that implies a pervasive "loss of control" of the use of drugs. Addictive behavior regarding the use of drugs can be defined as preoccupation with the acquisition of a particular drug, compulsivity manifested by continued use in spite of adverse consequences of the drug, and relapse or return of the use of the drug (8,11). Addiction is an empirical term that does not require physiological criteria, although it does have a neurochemical basis and is accompanied by physiological changes. The term may have acquired unfavorable stigmata with usage, but remains a clinically useful and accurate definition.

Many of the criteria in DSM-III-R (five) actually describe addictive behavior to substances. Those criteria in DSM-III-R that illustrate preoccupation are experiencing frequent preoccupation with seeking or taking the substance, and having given up some important social, occupations, or recreational activity to see or take the substance. Criteria that illustrate compulsivity are often being intoxicated or impaired by substance use when expected to fulfill social or occupational obligations, or when the substance use is a hazard (e.g., the person does not go to work because of being hung over or high, goes to work high, drives when drunk), and continuing substance use despite a physical or mental disorder or a significant social or legal problem that the individual knows is exacerbated by the use of the substance. A criterion that illustrates relapse is repeated effort or persistent desire to cut down or control substance use (*see Appendix I*). The remaining four criteria describe tolerance and dependence (withdrawal) to drugs: *tolerance*, need for increased amounts of substance to achieve intoxication or desired effect, or diminished effect with continued use of same amount; and *withdrawal*, substance-specific syndrome following cessation or reduction of intake of substance. The person often uses a psychoactive substance to relieve or avoid withdrawal symptoms (e.g., takes a drink or diazepam to relieve morning shakes), or often takes the substance in larger doses or over a longer period than he or she intended.

The DSM-III-R Criteria for Substance Dependence

Simplification of Addiction Criteria

A convenient approach to understanding the criteria for substance-dependence disorder is to group them according to the three principles of addiction as suggested by Jaffe (8). Preoccupation, compulsive use, and relapse constitute a behavioral strategy for identifying addictive behavior. The criteria themselves are perhaps difficult to discriminate from each other because of the similarity and overlap and the ultimate adverse consequences attendant on any of them. All indicate loss of control with a substance that is clearly evident in a pattern of use in which the substance or drug occupies a high priority in the individual's repertoire of choices. The distinguishing feature of these criteria of addiction is the pursuit of the substance or drug. The substance or drug is the object of the pathological use. The antecedent condition is drug-seeking behavior from which consequences, positive or negative, may follow. The reverse in which the consequences are given an etiological placement is often an incorrect interpretation of addictive use, that is, the addict uses *addictively* because of depression whereas depression is more likely to be a consequence of addictive use. The confusion in the sequence of cause and effect is important in determining the presence of addictive behavior.

Preoccupation with the acquisition is illustrated by criteria 5 and 6 (*see Appendix I*). These criteria require a judgment as to what is meant by preoccupation with acquisition. In simple terms, the addict clearly assigns a high priority to acquiring the substance, for example, he frequently chooses recreational and social activities in which alcohol is present or spends hundreds of dollars to purchase cocaine on a salary that does not support that cost. Family or occupational considerations are sacrificed for the time and energy to use substances, such as choosing to be with drinking friends rather than with the wife or children, or consistently working at a job with a hangover or actually missing time by arriving late or leaving early.

Compulsive use is a misunderstood and misapplied concept. By compulsivity is meant continued use of a substance in spite of (not because of) adverse consequences. Regular or frequent use is implied but not necessarily required. Episodic or binge drinking or drug use may involve a few hours or days, but if repeated in a pattern of pathological use over time will constitute addictive use by virtue of recurrent loss of control (*see Appendix I*). The major difficulties with these criteria are similar to those discussed with criteria for preoccupation that pertain to social or occupational consequences. Again, the emphasis should be placed on the compulsive drug use despite the adverse social or occupational consequences. The antecedent position of drug use that results in adverse consequences must be identified. Too often other consequences of drug use are attributed the causal role incorrectly; that is, someone is drinking abnormally because of employment problems, whereas the reverse may be more likely to be true. A rule of thumb in clinical practice is that if drugs or alcohol are abnormally used (i.e., with consequences), then an addiction is responsible for adverse consequences. It is important to remember is that the addict will frequently deny unconsciously or consciously that substances are causing physical, mental, legal, or employment problems.

Relapse is the sine qua non of diagnosing addictive behavior. An individual may have one or a few bad experiences with alcohol and drugs. A few instances of loss of control with a substance that may lead to adverse consequences over time, especially in a relapsing fashion is confirmatory. It is a misconception that addicts cannot stop drug use, because many do but not indefinitely; the addict returns to abnormal use. Again denial and faulty recollection make obtaining a true history of relapse difficult, so that corroborative history by others who observe the addict is often necessary. Even then denial may be present in some who know the addict. The antecedent condition of drug seeking must be established because often a "reason" other than drugs is given for the return to their use, such as depression, anxiety, and interpersonal difficulties, whereas the reverse is often the actual sequence. The addict will frequently deny "loss of control" unconsciously or consciously so that it must be inferred at times.

The message is clear that alcohol or drugs have assumed a central position in the addict's life and the expense to the addict to acquire substances may be great as measured by time, interpersonal relationships, and money. These social and occupational consequences may vary and because of denial may be difficult to assess.

A reduction in the primary emphasis in these important areas was made in DSM-III-R because the emphasis is on the drug-seeking behavior and not the consequences in determining whether a given criterion is met. The criteria required for social and occupational impairment may be subject to changing laws, social customs, and practices, and therefore be difficult to judge in a universal way. However, addiction by its definition is difficult to judge in a universal way. Addiction by its definition is difficult to conceive without envisioning some degree of impairment in social or occupational functioning (12). The critical and fundamental component of a drug addiction is "loss of control," which would appear to inevitably result in social and occupational consequences depending on the definition, disclosure, and measurement of impairment. More sensitive indicators for consequences should be developed for accurate identification of social and occupational impairment. The emphasis by DSM-III-R criteria on the drug seeking behavior is refreshing and needed, nonetheless.

Tolerance and Dependence (Withdrawal) as Required Criteria for "Dependence Syndrome" or Addiction

Tolerance and dependence (withdrawal) are important but may be confusing and misleading concepts to use as criteria for "dependence syndrome" or "addiction." Tolerance and dependence do accompany addiction although their presence depends on definition. Tolerance and dependence also can occur in the absence of a "loss of control" of the use of a drug. Frequently, potent analgesics that are prescribed for legitimate indications for pain produce tolerance and dependence without a concurrent or consequent pattern of pathological use. The many forms of tolerance include dispositional, pharmacodynamic, behavioral, and genetic mechanisms. The presence or absence of any of these forms does not necessarily confirm or refute the diagnosis of addiction to a drug; for example, a large individual who has increased tolerance for an addiction or dependence. Nor does a college student who has increased his/her capacity for alcohol by regular use without developing ostensible signs of addiction meet the criteria for a drug-use disorder. Because tolerance develops at different rates and degrees to various classes of drugs—for example, dramatically to opiates and subtly to alcohol (ethanol) and THC (marijuana)—the addiction to the drug may or may not be obvious before the onset of definable and measurable tolerance. Individual differences can pose problems in interpreting a given case (4,8). Tolerance to certain drugs such as alcohol may be more inherited than acquired. Early increased tolerance may be indicative of a predisposition to alcohol addiction.

The criteria for tolerance in DSM-III-R are these: develops a need for increased amounts of substance to achieve intoxication or desired effect or diminished effect with continued use of same amount; often takes the substance in larger doses or over a longer period than person intended. The criteria for dependence: substance-specific syndrome following cessation or reduction of intake of substance; often uses a psychoactive substance to relieve or avoid withdrawal symptoms (e.g., takes a drink or diazepam to relieve morning shakes) (see Appendix I). Generally, tolerance and dependence often accompany chronic and regular use of many drugs so that the effect is less on a constant dose or increasing amounts of a drug are required to achieve the same desired effect or to offset incipient withdrawal symptoms (4).

Development of tolerance and dependence may be considered expected pharmacological accompaniments of drug use as a general physiological adaptation by the cellular components of the body, whether or not addiction occurs. The development of tolerance and dependence occurs with continued use of either cocaine or antidepressants regardless of the addictive potential, which is clearly different for these two drugs. Tolerance to the sedative effect and perhaps even the antidepressant effect may develop with continued use of antidepressants (6). A dependence syndrome (withdrawal symptoms) may develop to antidepressants as manifested by anxiety, malaise, bradycardia, and restlessness (6). The addictive potential to these therapeutic drugs is considered low. Tolerance to euphoria, alertness, hypertension, and tachycardia and a dependence syndrome (withdrawal) of intense depression, somnolence, and hyperphagia may occur in response to repeated cocaine use (13,14). The addictive potential to the drug cocaine is very high.

Time-honored concepts that long and heavy or even regular use are necessary for the development of tolerance and dependence may also be inaccurate. Tolerance to alcohol and opiates may develop to a single dose (15). Also, dependence or withdrawal symptoms may occur after a single dose of alcohol or opiates (4,15). A common hangover from alcohol is a form of dependence yet does not necessarily imply addiction. The criteria specified for dependence will determine their presence or absence. For instance, if depression, hyperphagia, hypersomnolence, and delusions are not attributed to a physiological basis (as they should be), then the symptoms of cocaine withdrawal will be considered psychological and not physiological or pharmacological. The use of only the "gold standard" of alcohol and morphine withdrawal for physiological dependence is outdated and exclusive. There are many valid symptoms of dependence that indicate physiological changes in addition to the traditional criteria of changes in vital signs and occurrence of seizures. Delirium tremens includes hallucinations, delusion, anxiety, agitation, and hypervigilance, which are psychological manifestations of underlying neurophysiological aberrations (16). The most striking feature of opiate withdrawal is the "craving" and drug-seeking behavior. Physiological symptoms of nausea, vomiting, cramps, and piloerection, although significant, are subjective and sometimes barely behavioral manifestations.

Perhaps the concepts of tolerance and dependence should be deemphasized as criteria for "drug-use disorder" because of these various problems, such as greater correlations with drug use than with addictive behavior and frequent misattributions and misconceptions of the significance of tolerance and dependence to addiction. Inclusion of these physiological markers may still be useful if the implication was restricted to use, or regular use, of the drug. The nonspecific symptoms of tolerance and dependence and their lack of close relationship with a time course for all drugs suggest an accurate and chronic generalized neurochemical adaptation of the brain to the pharmacological effects of drug use (17). Nausea, malaise, anxiety, depression, irritability, and tremor occur as withdrawal symptoms from acute or chronic use of a wide variety of drugs, both stimulants and depressants, and often differ quantitatively and not qualitatively (17).

Special Considerations in Diagnosis

Research Areas

Research investigations are urgently needed in many areas of substance-abuse disorders, particularly in diagnosis. The magnitude and severity of drug and alcohol use cannot be accurately assessed without proper criteria for incidence and prevalence estimation. The underlying neurochemical correlates will not be definitely identified without a clear diagnostic formulation. Other psychiatric disorders that are often confused with addiction cannot be separated from addiction without correct assignment of symptoms to diagnostic categories.

The natural history of drug-use disorders is virtually unknown for many drugs. Important epidemiological, psychiatric, and biological studies depend heavily on some agreement of diagnostic criteria that are valid and reliable. More emphasis might be placed on the commonalities than differences of drug (alcohol) addictions to arrive at more generalized concepts that fit today's practices.

Both longitudinal and cross-sectional studies need to be done to test the validity and reliability of these criteria for diagnosis of substance-use disorders (addictions). Basic assumptions regarding addiction and traditional psychiatry can be challenged. Presently, an opposing "philosophy" exists between the two. Traditional psychiatry requires a reason or etiology for a secondarily derived substance-dependence syndrome. Also, concepts of abnormal drug use based on antiquated notions of dependence or need should be reexamined. New investigations in addiction as a primary disorder aided by neurochemical formulations may provide a clearer understanding for treatments to be developed and applied (18).

Denial of Substance Use

Denial regarding drug use and consequences from drugs (alcohol) is undoubtedly a common and prevalent problem that is inherent in a drug use disorder. Because of the denial that is imminent in the addiction process, self-report by an addict is often unsatisfactory and misleading, and makes obtaining a history of a drug use difficult. The denial that is both intentional and unintentional is present in the user and often in those persons associated with the user. The denial may be severe enough to persist in spite of overwhelming medical, psychiatric, social, and occupational evidence in support of a drug-use disorder. The network of denial is pervasive, firmly rooted, and resistant to confrontation with facts in a manner similar to that of a delusion. Recognition of these rather critical obstacles is important to making a clinical diagnosis that is dependent on available clinical data. A diagnosis based on empirical observations of addictive behavior such as preoccupation, compulsive use and relapse can be made without full cooperation of the addict, and other corroborative historical sources can be used. The power of the denial can be of delusional proportions and not responsive to persuasive logic.

Laboratory testing can be an important method to detect drug use, especially in the drug-use disorders in which loss of control of drug use is operative. Drugs may be found in a variety of "body fluids" even in the presence of emphatic and unequivocal denial of actual drug use. Conversely, a positive test for the presence of drugs does not confirm a drug-use disorder but only suggests or supports the diagnosis. The danger of accepting a false sense of security by a negative result in drug testing is important. For a variety of reasons, a negative result for drugs can occur in the presence of a highly active addiction. Many drugs of addiction have short half-lives, some routinely used instruments to measure drugs have low sensitivities, and close observations must be made in the specimen collections to avoid deceptive exchanges (19). Finally, the addict may not be using the drug(s) at the particular time of laboratory testing.

The Duration Criteria

Once the pattern of pathological use has been established and the criteria for addiction have been identified, the duration is essentially irrelevant for the purpose of establishing a diagnosis. The underlying assumption is that addiction to drugs and alcohol is a primary disorder that does not depend on time or other factors for expression. For example, once an infiltrate is identified in the lungs, the diagnosis of pneumonia can be made without requiring a duration of symptoms. Each class of drugs has a predictable constellation of signs and symptoms to make it possible to identify a general course and prognosis for that class (4,20). Each individual has a characteristic pattern of addiction to drugs, contributing personality factors, life stressors, and biophysiological predispositions to the addiction. The properties of the drug and characteristics of the individual in concert will determine the time required to develop an active addiction. Considerable variability exists across classes of drugs and types of individuals; that is, cocaine addiction may take weeks and alcohol addiction may take months or years to develop. The diagnosis of a drug use disorder may be made by recognizing the essential core of addiction that is "loss of control" manifested by preoccupation, compulsivity, and relapse to any drug, in any individual, and in any time course.

Polysubstance Diagnosis

The use of more than one drug simultaneously or at least regularly and interchangeably by those who have a drug-use disorder is more the rule than the exception. Eighty percent of those under the age of 30 years who qualify for the diagnosis of alcohol dependence have an addiction to an another drug in addition to alcohol (21). The possible clusters of drugs are numerous, and to assign diagnostic categories that are meaningful and valid to cover all combinations is difficult. This multiple drug use implies a commonality of vulnerability to drugs across classes of drugs by those who are addicted. Although a drug addict may often have a priority or hierarchy of drugs used, addiction to a large number of drugs may often exist. The era of the monodrug user is rapidly passing. This increasingly common fact necessitates use of the more diagnostic category such as drug-use disorder that includes the polydrug user and the alcoholic.

Other States Affected by Drug Addiction (Consequences)

Other possible additions, clarifications or revisions to the DSM-III-R criteria might include states such as mood, affect, cognition, interpersonal relationships, attitudes, values (individuals), and standards (social). Because denial is so pervasive and central to a drug addiction, many of the criteria listed in DSM-III-R are often difficult to ascertain. Often the addicted individual presents initially with complaints regarding mood, affect, interpersonal relationships, and attitude before the addiction is apparent and detected. Moreover, these states suffer substantial deterioration as a result of a drug addiction and should be considered in the evaluation of a drug-use disorder. Because alcohol and drugs have profound neurochemical effects on the brain that are translated into subjective and behavior manifestations, an aid to identifying alcohol and drugs as an etiology is to understand the derivation of disturbances in these functions.

Anxiety and depression are frequent consequences of chronic drug use that may motivate the user to seek treatments for these symptoms but not for the original addiction (3, 22). The presence of these symptoms may suggest further investigation for drug and alcohol use and an addiction. Alcohol is a significant depressant on mood, and withdrawal from alcohol is often associated with anxiety (15). Cocaine intoxication elevates mood and produces anxiety, and withdrawal from cocaine often produces depression and agitation (10,13). A common error is to attribute addictive drug use as contingent on disturbances in mood states such as anxiety and depression and to treat these symptoms without addressing the addiction, which is self-perpetuating and automatic.

Furthermore, symptoms such as mood disturbances occur as part of and originate from the addictive process in the abstinent state. Treatment of only the symptoms often will not alleviate the anxiety and depression because the addiction is allowed to continue unabated (23). The hopelessness, pathos, and worthlessness felt by the addict are a product of the mood disturbances derived from the addiction; treatment will correct these other symptoms of anxiety and depression. The basis for this contention is the common location of mood disturbance and addiction that may be in the limbic system (18).

As previously noted, interpersonal relationships are often affected by abnormal drug use. Eventually some disturbance with either family, friends, employer, or the legal system is present in virtually all drug disorders as preoccupation and compulsive drug use leads to adversely altered interpersonal relationships. Finally, attitudes, values, and standards often become distorted and sacrificed in a drug addiction. Addicts will resort to crime, prostitution, and other acts of poor judgment to support acquisition of expensive drugs and to compensate for the financially costly consequences of drug use and addiction. Although these subjective and personal entities are difficult to measure and assess, some consideration and enumeration of the impact by the addiction by other than an intitutive basis may be desirable (24).

Summary

The specific suggestions for further revisions to the DSM-III are listed here for convenience.

1. Redefine confusing terminologies of "abuse" and "dependence." Retain them as descriptive terms for drug use but not as diagnostic categories.
2. Adopt the term "addiction" as the major diagnostic category in lieu of "dependence syndrome."

3. Use the class name "drug" instead of "substance" to denote pharmacological importance in addiction to drugs and alcohol.
4. Clarify tolerance and dependence as pharmacological criteria for drug use and eliminate them as the sine qua non for drug and alcohol addiction.
5. Emphasize essential characteristics that are key to understanding addiction to alcohol and drugs such as loss of control, denial, preoccupation, compulsivity, and relapse.
6. Acknowledge the primary nature of addiction as the origin of psychiatric symptoms.
7. Understand the commonalities of the vulnerability to alcohol and drugs; that the similarities between drugs (alcohol) of addiction may be greater than the differences.
8. Direct new research for diagnosis and treatment at the neurochemical basis of the components of addiction such as preoccupation, compulsivity, and relapse.
9. Emphasize influence of drug addiction on mood, cognition, attitude, values, and personality.
10. Suspect and confirm addictive use once a consequence has been identified in the presence of drug or alcohol use.

Appendix I: DSM-III-R Criteria for Diagnosis of Substance-Dependence Disorders

1. Repeated effort or persistent desire to cut down or control substance use.
2. Often intoxicated or impaired by substance use when expected to fulfill social or occupational obligations when substance use is a hazard (e.g., does not go to work because hung over or high, goes to work high, drives when drunk).
3. *Tolerance*: need for increased amounts of substance to achieve intoxication or desired effect, or diminished effect with continued use of same amount.
4. *Withdrawal*: substance-specific syndrome following cessation or reduction of intake of substance.
5. Frequent *preoccupation* with seeking or taking the substance.
6. Has given up some important soicial, occupational, or recreational activity to see or take the substance.
7. Often uses a psychoactive substance to relieve or avoid withdrawal symptoms (e.g., takes a drink or diazepam to relieve morning shakes).
8. Often takes the substance in larger doses or over a longer period than he or she intended.
9. Continuation of substance use despite a physical or mental disorder or a significant social or legal problem that the individual knows to be exacerbated by the use of the substance.

Appendix II: DSM-III-R Criteria for Diagnosis of Substance-Abuse Disorders

A. A maladaptive pattern of substance use is indicated by at least one of the following:

   1. *Continued use* despite a persistent social, occupational, psychological, or physical problem that is caused or exacerbated by use of the substance

   2. *Recurrent use* in situations in which use is hazardous (e.g., driving while intoxicated).

B. Some symptoms of disturbance have persisted for at least 1 month or have occurred repeated over a longer period of time.

C. Patient has never met the criteria for psychoactive substance dependent for this substance.

References

1. Rounsaville BJ, Spitzer RL, Williams JBW (1986). Proposed changes in DSM-III substance abuse disorders: description and rationale. *Am J Psychiatry* 143:463–468.

2. Rounsaville BJ, Kosten TR, Williams JBW, Spitzer RI (1987). A field trial of DSM-III-R psychoactive substance dependence disorders. *Am J Psychiatry* 144:3.

3. Benet LZ, Sheiner LB (1985). Introduction. In *The Pharmacological Basis of Therapeutics*, 7th Ed., Gilman AG, Goodman LS, Rall TW, Murad, F, eds., pp. 1–2. New York: Macmillan.

4. Hoffman FG (1983). *A Handbook on Drug and Alcohol Abuse*, 2d ed. New York: Oxford University Press.

5. Schuckit MA (1984). *Drugs and Alcohol Abuse*. New York: Plenum.

6. Baldessarini RJ (1985). *Chemotherapy in Psychiatry*. Cambridge: Harvard University Press.

7. Dackis CA, Gold MS (1985). Pharmacological approaches to cocaine addiction. *J Subst Abuse Treat* 2:139–145.

8. Jaffe JH (1983). Drug addiction and drug abuse. In *The Pharmacological Basis of Therapeutics*, 6th Ed., Gilman AG, Goodman LS, Rall TW, Murad F, eds. New York: Macmillan.

9. Robins LD (1984). The diagnosis of alcoholism after DSM-III. In *Psychiatry Update. The American Psychiatric Association Annual Review, Vol. III*, Grinspoon L, ed. Washington, D.C.: American Psychiatric Press.

10. Schuckit MA, Zisook S, Mortola J (1985). Clinical implications of DSM-III diagnosis of alcohol abuse and alcohol dependence. *Am J Psychiatry* 142:12.

11. Edwards G, Arif A, Hodgson R (1981). Nomenclature and classification of drug and alcohol related problems. *Bull WHO* 59:225–242.

12. Milam JR, Ketchum K (1981). *Under the Influence*. Kirkland, WA: Madrona Publishers.

13. Gold MS, Vereby K (1984). The psychopharmacology of cocaine. *Psychiat Ann* 14(10):714–723.

14. Mule SJ (1984). The pharmacodynamics of cocaine. *Psychiatr Ann* 14(10):724–727.
15. Ritchie JM (1985). The aliphatic alcohols. In *The Pharmacological Basis of Therapeutics*, Gilman AG, Goodman LS, Rall TW, Murad F, eds. New York: Macmillan.
16. Lieber CS (1982). *Medical Disorders of Alcoholism: Pathogenesis and Treatment*. Philadelphia: W.B. Saunders.
17. Hill MA, Bangham AD (1975). General depressant drug dependency: A biophysical hypothesis. *Adv Exp Med Biol* 59:1–9.
18. Miller NS, Dackis CA, Gold MS (1987). The neurochemistry of addiction, tolerance and dependence. *J Subst Abuse Treat* (in press).
19. Gold MS, Dackis CA (1986). Role of the laboratory in the evaluation of suspected drug abuse. *J Clin Psychiatry* 47:1 (Suppl.).
20. Gilman AG, Goodman LS, Rall TW, Murad F, eds. (1985). *The Pharmacological Basis of Therapeutics*, 7th ed., pp. 532–581. New York: Macmillan.
21. Galizio M, Maish SA (1985). *Determinants of Substance Abuse*, pp. 383–424. New York: Plenum.
22. Miller NS, Gold MS (1987). The medical diagnosis and treatment of alcohol dependence. *Medical Times* 115(9):109–12.
23. Miller NS (1987). A primer of a treatment process for alcoholism and drug abuse. *Psychiatry Lett* 5(7):30–37.
24. Vaillant GE (1983). *The Natural History of Alcoholism*. Cambridge: Harvard University Press.

CHAPTER 3

The Neurochemistry of Tolerance, Dependence, and Addiction

History: A Confusion in Terms

Confusion surrounds the definitions and uses of the concepts of tolerance, dependence, and addiction to alcohol and drugs. Although in standard medical texts the definitions appear relatively straightforward, the relationship between them is not nearly as clear (1,2).

This confusion is a result of a number of factors. The first factor is a lack of definitive knowledge regarding alcohol and drug addiction. Addiction is largely a descriptive term, whereas tolerance and dependence have firm physiological foundations. The second is that personalized usage, additions, and subtractions by both specialists and laymen have led to misleading alterations and misconceptions for these terms.

The third factor is that various disciplines have different criteria for establishing tolerance and dependence and defining addiction. Psychologists and behavioralists describe these phenomena as certain observable behaviors. Physiologists record measurable variables such as blood pressure, pulse, and brain-wave activity. Clinicians determine the meaning of these terms through the acquisition of historical information, and the clinical relevance is judged. A fourth factor is that the relevance of tolerance and dependence to the clinical course and prognosis of drug addiction is not well understood (2).

A neurochemical approach for defining addiction, tolerance, and dependence may be helpful in clarifying the confusion. The following discussion attempts to provide a model or models for a uniform basis for considering neurochemical addiction, tolerance, and dependence to alcohol and drugs. The models are in part speculative and derived from the available, current neuroanatomical and neurochemical concepts underlying brain function.

Diagnosis

Definition of Alcohol and Drug Addiction

Alcohol or drug addiction may be defined by three major behavioral characteristics: (i) preoccupation with the acquisition of alcohol or a drug, (ii) compulsive use, and (iii) relapse (1,3). Pervasive to the three requisites is the phenomena of "loss of control." The World Health Organization concludes that the cardinal manifestation of addiction is "loss of control" of the use of a particular substance. The WHO proposed definition of a drug-dependence syndrome is a cluster of cognitive, behavioral, and physiological phenomena that include a compulsion, the desire to stop, a stereotypical drug-taking habit, evidence of tolerance and withdrawal, use of the drug to alleviate withdrawal symptoms, high priority of drug-seeking behavior, and rapid reinstatement of the syndrome after a period of abstinence. These criteria are essentially similar to the definition of drug addiction. Tolerance and dependence are additional concepts that may or may not be important in drug-seeking behavior (4). These behaviors of addiction probably, but not necessarily, imply a physiological basis. Our inadequate methods of measurement and disagreement regarding what to measure make elucidation of the neurochemical variables difficult (2).

Preoccupation

Preoccupation with the acquisition of a drug suggests that the drug has a high priority in the user's mental and affective states (5). The drug occupies a central importance in the addict's life; in a hierarchy of priorities, the acquisition of the drug ranks at or near the zenith. Even drive states such as hunger, sex, and survival may become subordinated and sacrificed for the pursuit of the drug or alcohol.

Compulsion

Compulsivity is often, but not always, indicated by regular and frequent use. More significant is that the use of a particular drug continues in the presence of the untoward consequences. Compulsivity is dramatically illustrated when the addict uses a drug in spite of compelling reasons to abstain. It is critical to recognize that the individual is using a drug because of its addictive nature, and not because of its consequences. The consequences are the result of and not the cause of the compulsive use (5). The consequences are often psychological, such as anxiety, depression, and disturbed interpersonal relationships. The major areas of the addict's interpersonal life that are affected adversely as a result of the addiction include family, friends, employment, and legal issues.

Relapse

Relapse is an informative criterion, as addicts can and often do discontinue their drug use for varying periods of time. The rule, and not the exception, is that there are periods of abstinence intermingled with prolonged abnormal drug use. If an accurate corroborative history can be obtained, the time for drug use will often be greater than is admitted by the addicts. The true episodic, or binge, user is not as common as may appear by clinical histories for the same reasons of denial. Relapse is a state in which there is a voluntary return to drug and alcohol use, or when regardless of conscious resolve and apparent commitment to abstain, the addict inexplicably returns to the use of alcohol or drugs. This relapse often occurs without apparent recollection, or at least with defiant disregard of the aversive consequences of the drug use in the past (6).

Physiological Basis for Tolerance and Dependence to Alcohol and Drugs

Alcohol

Although a physiological basis for addiction to drugs and alcohol almost certainly exists, the underlying neurochemical events have not been fully elucidated. Alcohol and drugs clearly do initiate addictive behavior. The interaction between the drug and brain is most likely responsible for initiating the addictive process (7). Subsequent and sequential neurochemical communications and changes ensue for the development of the actual addictive process. The mechanism of action for alcohol is to disturb the membrane fluidity of the cells. Ethanol acutely disorders the membranes to make them more fluid (8,9). The development of tolerance is manifested by changes in the brain neuronal membranes to a less fluid or more rigid form (10–18). This adaptive change in membrane fluidity is to maintain homeostasis for normal physiological functioning in the presence of the drug. Behavioral tolerance correlates with the development of the adaptive change in membrane fluidity (13).

Cocaine

Cocaine addiction may serve as a model for neurotransmitter changes in the development of addiction. A major pharmacodynamic effect of cocaine is to block the reuptake of dopamine into the presynaptic neuron (19). Reuptake is a major mechanism for termination of dopamine action. Degradation by intraneuronal enzymes and uptake into storage vessels are the subsequent routes of elimination for dopamine. If reuptake is prevented, then greater concentrations of dopamine remain in the synaptic cleft, and more dopamine is available at the postsynaptic site for stimulation of specific receptors in the cell membrane. Many of the signs and symptoms produced by cocaine can be attributed to the enhanced dopaminergic activity that results from the increased dopamine–receptor interaction. Mood, appetite, thought (delusions) and perceptual disturbances (hallucinations), and increased mental and motor activity are subserved by dopamine neurons (20).

Tolerance that develops to the signs and symptoms produced by cocaine in the intoxicated state is accompanied by these adaptive changes in the neurons in the central nervous system. Dependence is manifested by signs and symptoms opposite to those to which tolerance is developed to the presence of cocaine and a reversal of the neuroadaptive changes. Cocaine can produce euphoria, insomnia, anorexia, delusions, hallucinations, and increased mental and motor activity to which tolerance develops. Withdrawal from cocaine is marked by depression, hypersomnolence, hyperphagia, and slowness of mental and motor activity (21,22). Depletion of dopamine from storage sites and a reduction in subsequent release from presynaptic neurons may occur in the development of tolerance during chronic cocaine usage. The dopamine agonist, bromocriptine, can reverse or prevent the onset of these withdrawal syndromes that result from development of cocaine dependence (23). The suppression of withdrawal symptoms by bromocriptine suggests that dopamine depletion is operative in the development of dependence.

Tolerance and Dependence as Criteria for Alcohol and Drug Addiction

Connection

The connection between tolerance and dependence and addiction is controversial. Tolerance and dependence to narcotics, and even to alcohol, can occur without developing addictive behavior. Larger doses may be required to achieve the same effect, and a predictable withdrawal syndrome on cessation of the drug may ensue without a demonstrable preoccupation with acquisition, compulsive use, and relapse to the drugs. Examples are abundant in patients who receive potent analgesics such as morphine and meperidine in hospitals for pain. Most patients do not continue to seek these drugs even though they have become tolerant and dependent pharmacologically. Addiction, on the other hand, may recur in the absence of the development of tolerance and dependence. Finally, addiction, tolerance, and dependence coexist frequently, although the causal temporal relationship between them is not clear.

Definitions

There are many drugs that produce addiction, although the development of tolerance and dependence is not clinically obvious and easily measurable. Examples of this phenomenon are alcohol and marijuana. The popular conception is that tolerance and dependence do not develop to marijuana use. This is also the current claim for cocaine (24). This lack of acceptance for marijuana and cocaine in producing tolerance and dependence may be a problem of definition and accurate measurement and observation. Addiction to alcohol frequently occurs in the absence of significant tolerance and dependence if the criteria are measured by changes in vital signs. The chief manifestations of cocaine and amphetamine intoxication are mood elevation, hyperactivity, anorexia, hallucinations, delusions, and increased blood pressure (25,26). Increasing doses are required to maintain these effects as tolerance to cocaine and amphetamines occurs regularly. Doses of amphetamines up to 30,000 mg intravenously per day have been reported, and cocaine addicts regularly report the development of tolerance (2). Marijuana intoxication leads to a distortion of perceptions, particularly of time and space, mood fluctuations, decreased motor activity, and increased appetite. Tolerance to these effects of marijuana and cocaine may be difficult to measure and quantitate clinically and experimentally.

The withdrawal from cocaine and amphetamines can be dramatic and is manifested by severe depression, decreased motor activity, increased appetite, intense craving for more drug, disordered thinking, and delusions of persecution (27). Blood pressure and other vital signs are usually normal. This withdrawal syndrome is distinct, although not unique in the symptomatology; variations of these withdrawal symptoms can be seen in a number of other drugs, such as alcohol (27). The withdrawal from marijuana is subtle and marked by restlessness, intense craving for more drug, mood changes, malaise, and nausea. There are nonspecific symptoms that are present in other drug withdrawals as well.

Prototypes

The prototypes for tolerance and dependence are alcohol and morphine. These drugs have been used as a gold standard for unclear reasons (2). Curiously, morphine withdrawal is most remarkable for the craving that is more behavioral than any observable physiological measurements. Nausea, vomiting, myalgias, and piloerection may be present, but otherwise the physical signs and symptoms of withdrawal are uncomplicated and benign (28). Morphine, however, is accepted without question as producing physical dependence.

Alcohol dependence is marked by a spectrum of signs and symptoms. All, or more often only a part, of the spectrum is evident in the withdrawal period. This spectrum of signs and symptoms includes anxiety, depressions, insomnia, tremors, malaise, hallucinations, disordered thinking, delusions, seizures, hypertension, fever, and tachycardia.

The more common symptoms in alcohol withdrawal of anxiety and depression are not used as "hard" criteria for dependence. For unclear reasons, dependence as a deadaptation to alcohol by the body is determined by only hypertension and tachycardia, and only of a severe and abnormal degree. If careful measurements are made during withdrawal in regular users of alcohol, a transient elevation of blood pressure and pulse rate over baseline frequently occurs to both acute and chronic alcohol administration. These elevations may or may not be in the abnormal range. The vascular changes are attributable to the sympathetic nervous system discharge that occurs during the deadaptation of the body from alcohol during the acute onset of abstinence. Anxiety is now accepted as a manifestation of the sympathetic nervous system function. The same autonomic nervous system response underlies the symptoms of anxiety from different states including withdrawal from alcohol and drugs or an apparently spontaneous or provoked mood change.

Addiction

Tolerance and dependence probably occur regularly in alcohol and drug addiction. Our operational definitions may not include sufficient criteria to describe the manifestations of tolerance and dependence in addiction. There is a need to redefine the criteria for tolerance and dependence to include more manifestations of the adaptation and deadaptation by the body to the presence and absence of a drug. More signs and symptoms are needed to be inclusive of the abstinence syndrome. More commonality than difference will then be found for various drugs; cross-tolerance, dependence, and addiction will be more fully explained. The central nervous system response to drug intoxication and withdrawal may be less specific than our theories and suppositions suggest. Development of tolerance and dependence by the central nervous system may be nonspecific with only clusters of variations that are secondary and determined by each drug.

Tolerance and Dependence

Definition of Tolerance and Dependence to Alcohol and Drugs

The pharmacological and physiological definitions of tolerance to alcohol or a drug specify that an increasing dose is necessary to maintain the same effect or the effect is less at a particular dose. Tolerance may develop to the hypothermic effect of alcohol after repeated exposure, such that a particular dose fails to lower temperature and a larger dose is needed to produce hypothermia. A behavioral definition of tolerance is an observable adaptation of a particular behavior to a specific dose of drug. Tolerance to a drug has developed if more drug is needed than previously to reach the same expected state of intoxication or impairment in a behavior (2).

The definition of dependence is the onset of a predictable and stereotypic set of signs and symptoms on the cessation of the use of a particular drug. The continued use of the drug is necessary to suppress the development of those signs and symptoms that tend to be constant and specific for a given drug. For instance, alcohol has a predictable array of signs and symptoms as part of the abstinence withdrawal syndrome (29). The withdrawal syndrome is a spectrum that includes anxiety, insomnia, tremor, headache, nausea, seizures, and other objective and subjective parameters. Not all components need be present, and frequently are not, to confirm withdrawal from alcohol or other drugs.

Relationship Between Tolerance and Dependence
to Alcohol and Drugs

The relationship between tolerance and dependence is controversial, although there are empirical evidence and theoretical considerations to support the view that the two form one entity on a continuum.

Tolerance

Tolerance is an expression of adaptation of a particular organism or cell to a continued presence of a foreign substance such as a drug. This homeostatic response represents the body's (the cells') adjustment to maintain a normal physiological function (30). The cellular membrane's response to alcohol can be measured on a biochemical level (13). An increase in order (or a decrease in fluidity) of the bilipid layer of the cell membrane in the continued presence of ethanol occurs during the development of tolerance (31,32). The greater rigidity of the cell membrane is a homeostatic response to the persistent disordering or fluidizing effect of alcohol. Tolerance to cocaine may involve changes in dopamine presynaptic terminals may occur as a result of chronic blockade of reuptake. A supersensitivity of the dopamine postsynaptic receptor may result from an upregulation in response to low dopamine release. Presynaptic depletion and postsynaptic supersensitivity of dopamine neurons may represent the adaptive changes that occur during the development of tolerance.

Dependence

Dependence, on the other hand, is an expression of the deadaptation of the organism or cell to the absence of a drug. Symptoms accompany the movement from the "adaptive" pharmacodynamic set point in the presence of alcohol to the original pharmacodynamic set point in the absence of alcohol (30). The final effect is to maintain homeostasis for normal physiological functioning. The fluidity or order parameters of cell membranes and dopamine stores and receptor sensitivity may return from the tolerant state to normal baseline values during withdrawal from alcohol and cocaine (20,23,33).

Relationship

Tolerance and dependence appear to be inversely related in the clinical setting. The greater the tolerance is to a drug, the less severe is the dependence syndrome. Conversely, the less the tolerance, the more severe the signs and symptoms of dependence. Alcoholics with increased tolerance to alcohol have milder withdrawal symptoms. As alcoholics progressively lose tolerance to alcohol, the severity of the dependence syndrome increases. This loss of tolerance is also seen in the effect of aging on the response to alcohol.

Tolerance to alcohol decreases with increasing age in animals and humans. The severity of the dependence or withdrawal signs and symptoms also increases correspondingly with increasing ages (34).

Dependence alternatively may be viewed as a failure of the homeostatic mechanisms of adaptation to a drug. The signs and symptoms of withdrawal may represent the lack of the organism or cell to change further or reach a maximum point of adaptation in response to the presence of a drug. The pharmacodynamic set point is not at a state for normal functioning. Dependence may be an expression of a physiologically abnormal set point for functioning (30).

Neurochemistry

Neurochemistry of Alcohol and Drug Addiction

Preoccupation

Cocaine Model

Preoccupation, compulsivity, and relapse have an identifiable neurochemical basis, and a more correct description of an addiction may be psychological and behavioral manifestations that are drug induced and drug sustained.

The addict often appears preoccupied with the drug even after prolonged periods of abstinence. This recall, or recurrence of obsessional thoughts about the drug, probably has a neurosubstrate that is located in the hippocampus of the limbic system. The hippocampi are responsible for registration and recall of recent experiences; the left hippocampus stores verbal memory, and the right hippocampus stores nonverbal memory. Deficits in neuronal discharging in the hippocampus result in disturbances in the acquisition and storage of new information or memories. An enhancement of neuronal discharges in these same areas of the limbic system might lead to excessive or obsessional recall of previously registered experiences, particularly those associated with drug use. Stimulation of depth electrodes placed in the hippocampus or temporal lobe in humans results in recall of a series of "forgotten" or stored experiences. Addicts appear to have an increased amount of obsessional thinking regarding a variety of mental and physical experiences, including those pertaining to drugs.

A change in presynaptic or postsynaptic function might account for involuntary recall present in the preoccupation. A supersensitivity of the postsynaptic receptors with increased neuronal firing in the hippocampus could lead to spontaneous and enhanced recall of events. Dopamine binding sites are increased after chronic exposure to cocaine. Dopamine toxins such as 6-hydroxydopamine that destroy presynaptic neurons lead to increased postsynaptic dopamine (DA) binding sites. This type of "denervation supersensitivity" appears to represent a compensatory response to the destruction of DA neurons by 6-hydroxydopamine and subsequent reduction of presynaptic release of dopamine (20).

The development of persistent alteration in the postsynaptic receptor activity in cocaine stimulation may be similar to what is observed in tardive dyskinesia. Neuroleptic blockade of dopamine postsynaptic receptors apparently leads to a supersensitivity of dopamine-related function. Dopamine is a major neurotransmitter responsible for motor activity that is controlled by the basal ganglia. The supersensitivity of the dopamine receptors leads to spontaneous and enhanced activity of the neurons in the substantia nigra. Overactivity of basal ganglia function is manifested by hyperkinetic motor behavior such as orolingual buccal dyskinesias. Cocaine addicts can be extremely sensitive to extrapyramidal side effects from neuroleptic blockade in early withdrawal from cocaine. The increased reactivity to neuroleptics indicates a postsynaptic supersensitivity caused by the presynaptic dopamine deficiency (23).

A "dyskinetic" recall may occur in the hippocampus as a result of chronic depletion of dopamine by cocaine that is in effect a "functional or chemical blockade." Dopamine postsynaptic receptors in the hippocampus may be hypersensitive analogously to that which recurs in the basal ganglia. An increased recall may produce recurrent or obsessional thoughts about drug use. This recall may be more sensitive to environmental cues or simply arise spontaneously as impulses motivating drug use from the reverberating circuits in the hippocampus. The recall from supersensitive postsynaptic dopamine neurons in the hippocampus may underlie relapse that appears to occur with or without external stimuli and cues.

Compulsivity

Cocaine Model

Dopamine Reward System. The dopamine reward system may play a role in the neurochemical basis of compulsive use of drugs. The endogenous reward system has a neuroanatomical location. Olds discovered discrete brain regions in the hypothalamus that he termed "pleasure centers" (23). Electrical stimulation of these "pleasure centers" in animals lead to reward-like behavior. The circuit of the reward system includes descending fibers from the lateral hypothalamus that project to the ventral tegmentum via the medial forebrain bundle. The ventral tegmental area is the location of major dopamine neurons. Interruption of dopamine neurotransmission decreases the reward behavior produced by electrical stimulation of the lateral hypothalamus.

Central stimulants that are readily self-administered appear to activate dopamine neurons in the reward center. The ventral tegmentum projects to several other dopamine areas in the striatum, limbic system, and cerebral cortex. Lesions in the nucleus accumbens located in the limbic system, results in a decrease in the self-administration of cocaine in animals (20,23).

Limbic System. Electrodes implanted in the septal area of the limbic system in humans have provoked subjective sensations of intense pleasure similar to orgasm (35,36). The subjects continue to ask for repeated stimulation because of the unusually strong, positive, reward-like reinforcement received.

Cocaine is considered to be an extremely reinforcing drug that is used compulsively; a monkey, if given an unlimited supply of cocaine, will continue to press the bar until the point of self-destruction (1). Cocaine may act on the dopaminergic nerve endings in the reward center to produce dramatic enhancement in the reward states and reward behavior.

Dopamine Antagonists. Dopamine agonists, such as apomorphine and piribedil, have amphetamine-like reward-reinforcing properties. Selective dopamine antagonists reduce both electrical and central stimulant self-administration by animals. Noradrenergic receptor antagonists have no such effect. In humans, amphetamine-induced euphoria is blocked by dopamine-receptor antagonists. Acute administration of cocaine induces euphoria that appears to result from increased dopamine neurotransmission. Chronic cocaine administration may lead to a depletion of neuronal dopamine in the brain and an inhibition of dopamine function. Reuptake blockade prevents the recycling and reuse of dopamine in the presynaptic sites, resulting in brain dopamine levels falling after repeated administrations of cocaine. In humans, dopamine inhibits prolactin secretion, and the hyperprolactinemia that occurs in a number of chronic cocaine addicts may be an expression of dopamine depletion. The hyperprolactinemia peaks about 10 days after the cessation of cocaine use and thereafter gradually returns to normal over 2 weeks (20,23).

The intense depression that occurs with cocaine use may also be related to the chronic dopamine depletion. Decreased dopamine activity may be the neuronal basis for the subjective experience of drug craving. Administration of the dopamine agonist bromocriptine may ameliorate the intense craving that occurs in acute withdrawal from cocaine. Cocaine addicts report increased craving after administration of dopamine antagonists. Neuroleptic treatment may increase drug craving in cocaine addicts (20,23).

Alcohol Model

Dopamine System. The dopamine reward system may play a role in the neurochemical basis of addiction to alcohol. Rats that are implanted with slow-release pellets containing the stimulants amphetamine or nicotine show a dramatic increase in ethanol self-selection. This appears to represent a self-medication effect, because it does not occur with a variety of other drugs (hallucinogens, depressants) (37).

The administration of thioridazine and dihydroergotoxine (DHET) in combination reduced ethanol intake in rats. Either chemical alone did not significantly reduce ethanol intake. DHET counteracts the activation of dopamine neurons by the postsynaptic blockade of thioridazine. This suggests that the drug combination exerts a synergistic effect on reducing dopaminergic transmission in the central nervous system. These results support an important role of dopaminergic transmission in the rewarding effect of ethanol (38).

Intravenous ethanol preferentially stimulated the firing rate of dopamine neurons in the ventral tegmental area that project to limbic and cortical areas of the forebrain over that of dopamine neurons in the substantia nigra. The intravenous ethanol was more effective in stimulating the firing rate of dopamine neurons in the ventral tegmental area in high- than low-ethanol-preferring rats. Also, under the same conditions the dopamine content was decreased and the Dihydroxyphenylacetic acid (DOPAC) content increased in the prefrontal cortex of the high-, but not low-, ethanol-preferring rats (39).

GABA System. Other neurotransmitters play a role in the compulsive use of alcohol. The neurotransmitter gamma-aminobutyric acid (GABA) has been implicated in alcohol use in humans and animals. Stimulation of GABA-B main receptors by calcium bis-acetylhomotaurine (Ca AOTA) or of noradrenergic receptors by metapromine reduces the voluntary intake of ethanol in rats. The effect of metapromine was opposed by a treatment with (+)-bicuculline and not by a treatment with bicuculline metobromide (does not cross the blood–brain barrier). Baclofen, a GABA-B agonist, reduces voluntary intake of ethanol (40).

Serotonin System. Clinical and animal studies suggest that ethanol consumption is influenced by 5-hydroxytryptamine (5-HT, serotonin) transmission. The treatment with a selective 5-HT receptor agonist, 8-OH DPAT, caused a significant reduction in ethanol consumption in high-ethanol-preference rats. This finding suggests that activation of the central 5-HT system reduces ethanol intake. Neurochemical studies have shown that ethanol-preferring rats have lower levels of serotonin (5-HT) in cerebral cortex and hippocampus and higher levels of norepinephrine in cerebral cortex in comparison to ethanol-nonpreferring rats. Additionally, significantly higher receptor numbers for 5-HT in frontal cortex and hippocampus of ethanol-preferring rats have been found. No difference in receptor numbers for α_1, and α_2, and adrenergic receptors in cortical membranes between preferring and nonpreferring rats was observed (41).

In severe, dependent alcoholics abstinent from alcohol for 2 to 20 days, [³H]serotonin uptake loss was significantly lower than in nonalcoholic controls and in former dependent alcoholics (1–12 years).

Human and animal studies suggest a role for neurotransmitters in alcohol preference. Dopamine appears to play a role in enhancing or rewarding compulsive alcohol consumption. GABA, serotonin, and norepinephrine appear to decrease compulsivity of alcohol intake.

Relapse

Current Research

The literature regarding relapse is quite diverse. A variety of personality, demographic, cognitive, physiological, environmental, and behavioral variables have been investigated, and many different conceptual systems have been employed to explain relapse. The majority of studies fall within one of two general classes: (i) studies that attempt to identify predictors of relapse over time or that assess variables between groups of relapsed and nonrelapsed subjects; and (ii) studies that investigate specific events surrounding discrete relapse episodes. The available evidence suggests that studies of the latter type are more likely to yield informative generalizations about the determinants of relapse (42–49).

Neurochemical Model

A neurochemical model does not fully explain why some individuals may relapse while others may not. A variety of personality, demographic, cognitive, environmental, and behavioral factors play important roles in determining relapse.

Relapse is perhaps more difficult to understand on a neurochemical basis than preoccupation and relapse. Preoccupation with the acquisition of a drug, especially while the addiction is active, and compulsive use during the time of the development of tolerance and dependence to a drug may be evident because of concurrent drug–brain interactions. A motivation for drug acquisition and use may be to offset the onset of incipient withdrawal symptoms, which can be unpleasant. The mood of depression that immediately follows cocaine use, especially chronic use, is described as very intense and severe by users; more cocaine will temporarily relieve the depression, however. The anxiety and depression that accompany acute alcohol withdrawal appear to be motivating factors for repeated alcohol consumption, because alcohol can be an antidote for these aversive mood states.

The self-treatment or self-administration of drugs for the withdrawal symptoms with more drugs is not always a sufficient explanation for repetitive and compulsive use because the addict is aware that these aversive effects from chronic drug use will subside spontaneously with abstinence. The distress and discomfort of enduring the short-term unpleasant withdrawal symptoms may be preferable to "medicating" symptoms that only worsen with repeated use. Also, relapse must explain why an addict returns to drug use after long periods of abstinence during which symptoms of withdrawal have subsided.

Craving

Craving is a term that has been used to describe the intense desire to use more drug. Craving is a drive that appears to supersede the anguish of the adverse symptoms of intoxication and withdrawal that inevitably follow the return to drug use. The craving occupies a preeminent position in the acute and prolonged periods of withdrawal in alcohol and drug addiction. The basis of the craving in cocaine addiction may be crucial in the reward pathways. Decreased dopamine availability at the synapse or supersensitivity of the dopamine postsynaptic neurons may be experienced as craving by the cocaine addict. The dopamine neurons in the reward system may be set in an undercompensated state that signals an increased need for reward sensation (20,23).

Alcohol may produce persistent changes in membrane fluidity that result in craving. A more ordered neuronal membrane may lead to subjective experiences that create a drive state for more alcohol use. The altered cellular membrane fluidity may affect dopamine presynaptic or postsynaptic function in the reward area. Acute alcohol administration enhances dopamine transmission similarly to cocaine (37,39). Chronic alcohol use may result in a persistent decrease in dopamine activity similarly to cocaine by producing a more rigid membrane (13).

Dopamine Deficiency

The addict's return to the use of alcohol or a drug after weeks or perhaps months and years of abstinence may be explained in part by a persisting physical alteration in brain neuronal membranes. The clinical effect of dopamine deficiency may remain because of a relatively permanent exhaustion of presynaptic dopamine stores or a supersensitivity of postsynaptic receptor sites. This relative neuronal dopamine lack may manifest itself in a psychological state manifested by craving that may signal a relapse (23). The postsynaptic dopamine-deficient neurons in the hippocampus may be supersensitive and fire spontaneously at low levels of stimulation similarly to that which occurs in tardive dyskinesia to provoke relapse to alcohol and drugs.

Hippocampus

The hippocampus in the limbic system contains the memory function of recall. Drive states located in the limbic system such as sex, hunger, or mood may be associated directly with recall mechanisms, so that recall is linked to the instincts. The effect of the drug on the instincts becomes a stored memory that can be recalled such that the drive states become permanently associated with the drug. Persistent neurotransmitter changes such as supersensitivity may underlie these larger and more functional alterations in the drive states. The reward and the memory centers in the limbic system may become associated with the drive states that were provoked by the drug alterations in dopamine function. Relapse may involve spontaneous firing of dopamine neurons in the hippocampus that serves recall of the drive states that become linked to the drug and alcohol. Alcohol and drugs are then used in response to the stimulus from the drive states that are augmented by the reward center. The alcohol and drug use become entrained by the drives for survival, sex, food, and mood.

Frontal Lobe

Drugs have effects on the brain that enhance the uninhibited expression of the instincts. Alcohol and cocaine affect important frontal lobe functions that ordinarily inhibit the drive states in the limbic system. The frontal lobe subserves psychological and behavioral functions such as judgment, motivation, ethical conduct, propriety, impulse control, planning, and initiation that are significantly affected by alcohol and drugs. Behaviorally and neurophysiologically there is a suppression or slowing of these important functions, and subsequently the instincts are allowed uninhibited, freer, and more complete expression. Individuals with frontal lobe impairment frequently show persistent, repetitive, perseverating behavior similar to that present in the automatic and stereotypic behavior of an addiction. The powerful motivation to use alcohol and drugs associated with the drive states reinforced by the reward center is relatively unabated and uninhibited by the higher cortical centers such as the frontal lobe.

Drive States and Addiction to Alcohol and Drugs

Instincts

Mood, appetite, survival, and sexual reproduction are drive states that are located in the limbic system (50). Relatively discrete neuroanatomical designations exist for each of the drives. Electrode stimulation experiments in these various areas have demonstrated that a particular sensation in humans and a behavior in animals reflecting these drive states can be provoked. Electrodes implanted in the septal area of the limbic system in humans have aroused subjective sensations of intense pleasure similar to sexual orgasm. The subjects vigorously seek repeated stimulation because of the apparently strong positive reinforcement received (51). These sensations and pleasure-seeking behaviors are similar to those described by cocaine users (2).

Drug Effects

These drive states, particularly sex and hunger, are understandably enormously potent and are responsible for the survival of a species. Any alteration or provocation of these drive states can result in powerful and incorrigible behavior such as is manifested in an addiction. A persistent association may develop between the drive states, which are essentially instincts, and the alcohol and drug that stimulated them (50). Drugs such as alcohol and cocaine may be altering and redirecting the instincts; in a sense, the alcohol and drugs are overtaken and orchestrated by the drive states. These changes in the instincts by the drugs are subserved by the neurotransmitter systems in the brain. Dopamine, GABA, serotonin, and norepinephrine may undergo alterations in synaptic function to enhance or diminish the neurochemical functions underlying the behavioral changes that result from the addiction to alcohol and drugs.

Other Addictions

Other nonchemical addictions such as gambling, sex, and eating may share common underlying neuroanatomical and neurochemical mechanisms. The same drive states and instincts may form the bases of all the addictions. Eating disorders, particularly bulimia, and gambling disorders are associated with a particularly high prevalence of alcohol and drug addictions.

Psychological and behavioral phenomena are similar in all of these disorders. Bulimics and gamblers are preoccupied with the acquisition and compulsive use, and frequently relapse to stereotypic food behaviors and to risk-taking, respectively. The obvious difference is that an exogenous drug–brain interaction occurs with alcohol and drug addiction to initiate addictive behavior. In regards to eating and gambling, other endogenous interactions appear to take place to initiate the additive behavior.

Genetics

The reasons that some individuals become addicted to alcohol and drugs and others do not have received considerable attention in research in the past 10 to 20 years. Genetic research, namely adoption, twin, familial, and high-risk studies, has demonstrated that a predisposition to alcoholism may be inherited. The children of alcoholics may carry an increased risk of becoming alcoholic, whether or not they are raised by the alcoholic. Environmental factors appear to play a secondary role if the genetic predisposition is present.

A neurochemical explanation for this inherited vulnerability has not been confirmed, although one probably exists in the form of genetic alterations. The genetic basis for nonalcohol drug addiction has not been as discretely and specifically studied as it has been for alcoholism. Drugs appear to have common characteristics with alcohol as presented in the neurochemical models. The susceptibility to develop an addiction to drugs appears to overlap significantly with that of alcohol. More than 50% of alcoholics under the age of 30 have an addiction to at least one additional drug. Increased exposure through availability may be only a partial explanation. The genetic neurochemical predisposition may be similar for alcohol and drugs.

Higher and Lower Brain Function

An addiction may have neuroanatomical and neurophysiological bases. The preoccupation with alcohol and drugs may be attributed to memory changes produced in the hippocampus. Compulsive use may result from an interaction of stimulation of the reward center, suppression of physiological function to inhibit the drive states by the frontal lobe and recruitment by the drug, and association with the drive states in the limbic system. Relapse can be attributed to a combination of poor planning and impulse control from frontal lobe damage and provoked or spontaneous recall of the drug-stimulated instincts within the hippocampus, underlying and compelling the addict to seek and use more of the drug. New or short circuits have formed with the instincts that are ultimately counterproductive to the user, and are in control and redirect their perpetuation through drugs. The higher brain centers no longer exert final control over the powerful and automatic expression by the instincts reinforced by the reward center of the drug-induced changes.

Basis of Addiction

The basis of alcohol and drug addiction may involve distortion and redirection of drive states by the drug. The preoccupation, compulsive use, and relapse in behavioral terms are descriptive and confirmatory. Tolerance and dependence may only be incidentally associated with addiction as a result of a nonspecific adaptation to the drug by the body. The cellular adaptation by the body to the drug may be similar in all organs, including the neurons in the brain.

Tolerance and dependence may have no specific relationship to alcohol and drug addiction. Tolerance and dependence can occur in the absence of observable addiction. Addiction is probably more complex than tolerance and dependence, because it may involve the lower brainstem and higher cortical functions. Tolerance and dependence may be largely limited to universal cellular alterations. Addiction is difficult to study because of the variability of behavioral phenomena and the underlying intricacies of the neurosubstrates.

Tolerance and dependence are still useful as they are indicators of alcohol and drug use. However, it is a misconception that long-term chronic use is necessary for tolerance and dependence to develop (2,1). Some studies have shown that tolerance can develop within hours and days to a single dose of alcohol or a drug (52,53). It is known that anxiety, depression, and insomnia can occur after a single dose of ethanol in humans and that these manifestations are considered to be symptoms of withdrawal from ethanol (54); the common term for this is "hangover." Redefining our criteria for tolerance and dependence to alcohol and other drugs may be in order (55).

Intervention and Treatment

Importance of Diagnosing Addiction

Although tolerance and dependence are useful in assessing drug effect, the key to a diagnosis of a primary problem with alcohol or drugs is *addictive behavior*. The components of addiction are preoccupation with the acquisition of the drug, compulsive use, and relapse. Once these key behaviors regarding alcohol and drugs are identified as an addiction, then the consequences of an addiction can be more clearly identified. If the essential nature of the addiction is not identified, the misunderstanding that the consequences lead to the "addictive use" of alcohol and drugs may result.

References

1. Jaffe JH (1985). Drug addiction and drug abuse. In *The Pharmacological Basis of Therapeutics*, 7th Ed., Gilman AG, Goodman LS, Rall TW, Murad F, eds., pp. 532-581. New York: Macmillan.
2. Hoffman FG (1983). *A Handbook on Drug and Alcohol Abuse: The Biomedical Aspects*, 2d ed. New York/Oxford: Oxford University Press.
3. Vaillant GE (1983). *The Natural History of Alcoholism*. Cambridge: Harvard University Press.
4. Edwards G, Auf A, Hodgson R (1981). Nomenclature and classification of drug and alcohol-related problems: A WHO memorandum. *Bull WHO* 59:225-242.
5. Jellinek EM (1960). *The Disease Concept of Alcoholism*. New Brunswick: Hillhouse.
6. Tucker JA, Vuchinich RE, Harris CV (1985). Determinants of substance abuse relapse. In *Determinants of Substance Abuse*, Galizio M, Maish SA, eds., pp. 383-424. New York: Plenum.
7. Siegel RK, Albers RW, Agranoff BW, et al. (1981). *Basic Neurochemistry, 3rd Ed.* Boston: Little, Brown.
8. Goldstein DB, Chin JH, Lyon RC (1982). Ethanol disordering of spin-labeled mouse brain membranes. *Proc Nat Acad Sci USA* 79:4321-4323.
9. Lieber CS (1982). *Medical Disorders of Alcoholism Pathogenesis and Treatment*. Philadelphia: W.B. Saunders.
10. Beauge F, Subler H, Borg S (1985). Abnormal fluidity and surface carbohydrate content of the erythrocyte membrane in alcohol patients. *Alcoholism Clin Exp Res* 9:322-326.
11. Chin JH, Goldstein DB (1977). Effects of low concentrations of ethanol on the fluidity of spin-labeled erythrocyte and brain membranes. *J Pharm Pharmacol* 13:435-441.
12. Chin JH, Goldstein DB (1984). Cholesterol blocks the disordering effects of ethanol in biomembranes. *Lipids* 19:929-935.
13. Goldstein DB (1984). The effects of drugs on membrane fluidity. In *Annual Review of Pharmacology and Toxicology*, Vol. 24, Cowan WM, Shooter EM, Stevens CF, Thompson RC, eds., pp. 43-64.
14. Grieve SJ, Littleton JM, Jones P, et al. (1979). Functional tolerance to ethanol in mice: Relationship to lipid metabolism. *J Pharm Pharmacol* 31:737-742.
15. Ingram LO (1976). Adaptation of membrane lipids to alcohols. *J Bacteriol* 125:670-678.
16. LaDroitte P (1984). Sensitivity of individual erythrocyte membrane phospholipids to changes in fatty acid composition in chronic alcoholic patients. *Alcohol Clin Exp Res* 9:135-137.
17. Lee NM, Friedman HJ, Loh HH (1980). Effect of acute and chronic ethanol treatment on rat brain phospholipid turnover. *Biochem Pharmacol* 29:2815-2818.

18. Littleton JM, Geryk JR, Grieve SJ (1979). Alterations in phospholipid composition in ethanol tolerance and dependence. *Alcohol Clin Exp Res* 3:50–56.

19. Feldman RS, Quenzer LF (1984). *Fundamentals of Neuro-psychopharmacology*. Sunderland, MA: Sinauer.

20. Dackis CA, Gold MS (1985a). New concepts in cocaine addiction: The dopamine depletion hypothesis. *Neurosci Biobehav Rev* 9:469–477.

21. Mule SJ (1984). The pharmacodynamics of cocaine abuse. *Psychiatr Ann* 14:724–727.

22. Siegel RK (1984). Cocaine smoking disorders: Diagnosis and treatment. *Psychiatr Ann* 14:728–732.

23. Dackis CA, Gold MS (1985b). Pharmacological approaches to cocaine addiction. *J Subst Abuse Treat* 2:139–145.

24. Schuckit MA (1984). *Drugs and Alcohol Abuse*. New York: Plenum.

25. Green AR, Costain DW (1981). *Pharmacology and Biochemistry of Psychiatric Disorders*. New York: Wiley.

26. Gold MS, Verebey K (1984). The psychopharmacology of cocaine. *Psychiatr Ann* 14:724–727.

27. Goodwin DW, Guze SB (1984). *Psychiatric Diagnosis*. New York/Oxford: Oxford University Press.

28. Melium KL, Morrelli HF (1978). *Clinical Pharmacology*, 2d Ed. New York: Macmillan.

29. Majchrowicz E, Noble EP (1979). *Biochemistry and Pharmacology of Ethanol, Vol. 1.* New York: Plenum.

30. Hill MA, Bangham AD (1975). General depressant drug dependency: A biophysical hypothesis. *Adv Exp Med Biol* 59:1–9.

31. Chin JH, Parsons LM, Goldstein DB (1978). Increased cholesterol content of erythrocyte and brain membranes in ethanol-tolerant mice. *Biochim Biophys Acta* 513:358–363.

32. Vanderkooi JM (1979). Effect of ethanol on membranes: A fluorescent probe study. *Alcohol Clin Exp Res* 3:60–63.

33. Johnson DA, Lee NM, Cooke R, Loh HH (1979). Adaptation to ethanol-induced fluidization of brain lipid bilayers: Cross tolerance and reversibility. *Mol Pharmacol* 17:52–55.

34. Kates M, Manson LA (1984). *Biomembranes: Membrane Fluidity*. New York: Plenum.

35. Beach FA (1974). A review of physiological or psychological studies of sexual behavior in mammals. *Physiol Rev* 27:240–305.

36. Cox AW (1979). Control of "sex centers" in the brain [letter to the editor]. *Medical Aspects of Human Sexuality*, 13:113.

37. Ellison G, Levin E, Potthoff A (1986). Ethanol intake increases during continuous stimulants but not depressants. In *Abstracts*, Third Congress of the International Society for Biomedical Research on Alcoholism, Helsinki, Finland, p. 31.

38. Fadda F, Franch F, Gessa GL (1986). Inhibition of voluntary ethanol consumption in rats by a combination of dihydroergotoxine and thioridazine. In *Abstracts*, Third Congress of the International Society for Biomedical Research on Alcoholism, Helsinki, Finland, p. 32.

39. Gessa GL, Fadda F (1986). Ethanol stimulates mesocortical dopaminergic system in ethanol preferring rats. In *Abstracts*, Third Congress of the International Society for Biomedical Research on Alcoholism, Helsinki, Finland, p. 107.

40. Boismare F, Daoust M, Lhuintre C, et al. (1986). Noradrenaline and GABA brain receptors are co-involved in the voluntary intake of ethanol by rats. In *Abstracts*, Third Congress of the International Society for Biomedical Research on Alcoholism, Helsinki, Finland, p. 30.

41. Lumeng L, Wong DT, Threlkeld, et al. (1986). Neuronal receptors of alcohol-preferring (P) and non-preferring (NP) rats. In *Abstracts*, Third Congress of the International Society for Biomedical Research on Alcoholism, Helsinki, Finland, p. 33.

42. Hunt, WA, Barrett LW, Branch LG (1971). Relapse rates in addiction program. *J Clin Psychol* 90:586–600.

43. Marlatt GA (1980). Craving for alcohol, loss of control, and relapse: A cognitive-behavioral analysis. In *Alcoholism: New Directions in Behavioral Research and Treatment*, Nathan PE, Marlatt GA, Berg TL, eds. New York: Plenum.

44. Schachter S (1982). Recidivism and self-cure of smoking and obesity. *Am Psychol* 37:436–444.

45. Cummings C, Gordon JR, Marlatt GA (1980). Relapse: Prevention and prediction. In *The Addictive Behaviors*, Miller WR, ed. New York: Pergamon.

46. Marlatt GA, Gordon JR (1980). Determinants of relapse: Implications for the maintenance of behavioral change. In *Behavioral Medicine: Changing Health Lifestyles*, Davidson P, Davidson S, eds. New York: Brunner/Mazel.

47. Lichtenstein E (1982). The smoking problem: A behavioral perspective. *J Consult Clin Psychol* 6:804–819.

48. Miller WR, Hester RK (1980). Treating the problem drinker: Modern approaches. In *The Addictive Behaviors*, Miller WR, ed. New York: Pergamon.

49. Ogborne AC (1978). Patient characteristics as predictors of treatment outcomes for alcohol and drug abusers. In *Recent Advances in Alcohol and Drug Problems, Vol. 4*, Israel Y, Glaser RB, Kalant RE, et al., eds. New York: Plenum.

50. Pincus JR, Tucker GJ (1985). *Behavioral Neurology*, 3d Ed. New York/Oxford: Oxford University Press.

51. Heath RG (1972). Pleasure and brain activity in man. *J Nerv Ment Dis* 154:3–18.

52. Tahakoff B, Rothstein JB (1983). *Medical and Social Aspects of Alcohol Abuse*. New York: Plenum.

53. Wilson JR, Erwin G, McClearn GE, et al. (1984). Effects of behavior: II. Behavior sensitivity and acute behavioral tolerance. *Alcoholism* 8:4.

54. Victor M, Adams RP (1953). The effect of alcohol on the nervous system. *Res Pub Assoc Res Nerv Ment Dis* 32:526–573.

55. Millam JR, Ketchum K (1981). *Under the Influence*. Kirkland, WA: Madrona Publishers.

CHAPTER 4

Suicide in Alcoholism and Drug Addiction

History

The word suicide has a Greek derivation, meaning "self-death" (sui, self; cide, kill). Suicide as a consequence of alcoholism and drug addiction has always been found to be common in many sources of inquiry. The association between suicide and alcohol and drugs has been noted by investigators from a variety of disciplines that have assessed suicide. Many past as well as recent studies have confirmed that alcohol and drug addiction are major risk factors for suicide, as causes and precipitants for suicidal behaviors (1-4).

The influence of alcohol and drugs in suicide is both causal and conducive. Chronic use of alcohol and drugs play a primary etiological role in the emergence of suicide thinking and actions. The toxic effects of alcohol and drugs on the brain in part induce suicidal thinking and behaviors by the pharmacological effects that impair judgment and cognition and severely depress mood. Additionally, the crises-oriented life of the alcoholic and drug addict with disruption of interpersonal relationships is conducive to the development of suicidal impulses. Moreover, the alcoholic and drug addict may have comorbid psychiatric disorders that also have suicide as a significant risk factor (5-7).

Prevalence of Suicide in Alcohol and Drug Populations

Importantly, studies have provided substantial agreement that suicidal behavior including completed suicides are highly prevalent among alcoholics and drug addicts (8-13). These findings of a high prevalence of self destructive behaviors are derived from studies of both adult and adolescent populations of alcoholics and drug addicts (14,15). Among the adolescents, suicide ranks as the number two cause of death from all causes behind traumatic accidents. Because alcoholism and drug addiction are youthful disorders, as confirmed by the Epidemiological Catchment Area (ECA) data, it is not surprising that alcohol and drugs are major causes of suicide among adolescents (15,16). The average age of onset of alcoholism is 22 years in males and 25 years in females, according to the findings of the ECA (17).

The most recent and widely cited San Diego studies involving suicides found in a general survey of hospital admissions that 58% of the suicides were associated with drug and alcohol addiction (8,15,18). Moreover, studies in alcoholic and drug addiction populations found that approximately 25% or greater of alcoholics and drug addicts kill themselves by various means according to several studies (6,19,20). The investigations performed by the ECA have confirmed a lifetime prevalence of 18% for suicide among alcoholics and drug addicts in the general population (20). Some investigators have reported that as many as 70% of adolescent suicides are associated with alcohol or drug problems, often of addictive proportions (8,10,15).

The use of alcohol and drugs as poisons represents the most common means of inflicting self-harm by the individual attempting suicide, whether it be by the alcoholic, the drug addict, or the nonaddict. The use of alcohol to induce an intoxicated state or as a drug of overdose, and drugs in inducing similar instances of intoxication and overdoses, are currently the most prevalent methods for suicide attempts and completions from any cause (8,15,18,19).

In terms of relative risk factors, alcohol and drug addiction are the leading factors of all psychiatric disorders, according to studies. Alcoholism and drug addiction are significantly greater contributors to suicide than other psychiatric disorders, such as major depression and schizophrenia. In comparisons of weighted relative risks, depression unrelated to alcoholism was only a moderate predictor of suicidal risks (see Table 4.1) (21). This is an interesting but not a surprising suicidal observation if alcoholism is factored out of depressive disorders. It is possible that many studies reporting higher rates of suicide among affective disorder do not separate alcoholism from the affective disorders. This practice is perpetuated by the propensity for alcoholism to produce a clinical depression indistinguishable from affective disorder as an adverse consequence in conjunction with the denial of abnormal alcohol intake by alcoholics.

Clinical Characteristics of Suicidal Alcoholics and Drug Addicts

Although suicide attempts and completions may occur at any age in alcoholics and drug addicts, there appear to be two peak periods of increased risk, the young and the old. The young in their twenties constituted two-thirds of suicide completions in the recent San Diego study. However, in the same study the rate of suicide by alcohol and drug addicts between the ages of 30 and 40 years is 60% of the remainder of all suicides (8,15). Furthermore, the older male alcoholic is particularly prone to suicide (5,12).

TABLE 4.1. Factors associated with suicide risk.[a]

Variable in rank order	Content of item
1	Age (45 and older)
2	Alcoholism
3	Irritation, rage, violence
4	Prior suicidal behavior
5	Sex (male)
6	Unwilling to accept help
7	Longer duration of current episode of depression
8	Prior inpatient psychiatric treatment
9	Recent loss or separation
10	Depression
11	Loss of physical health
12	Unemployed/retired
13	Single, widowed, divorced

[a]Modified from Litman RE, Faberow NL, Wold CI, Brown TR (1974). Prediction models of suicidal behaviors. In H. Beck, LP Resnik, DJ Jettieri (eds.): *The Prediction of Suicide*, Charles Press, p. 141.

The white male is the most likely race and gender to commit suicide, although the rate for black males is increasing. Being separated, divorced, or widowed provides a greater risk for suicide, as does being unemployed or retired. Poor physical health with an acute or chronic illness also enhances the relative risk (see Table 4.2) (22).

The duration of 9 years for alcohol and drug addiction in suicide cases found in recent studies is shorter than other earlier studies that have shown a later onset of suicide in a more prolonged course of alcoholism (8,15).

Of importance is that suicide risk is most highly correlated with multiple drug use and the diagnosis of the multiple drug and alcohol addiction (8,14); 84% of the addicts who commit suicide are both alcoholics and drug addicts. In the study previously discussed, the mean number of drugs used among the suicide victims was 3.6 for the alcoholics and drug addicts. The drugs used most commonly were alcohol, opiates, sedatives, amphetamines, cocaine, and marijuana. Interestingly, phencyclidine and hallucinogens were less often represented (8,15).

In a review of a large number of reports regarding suicide attempts and completion before 1974, the factors associated with suicide risks were ranked in a relative order of suicide risk (see Table 4.1). The older age is present as the leading risk; however, the relative risk for suicide is increasing for the younger, multiple addicted alcoholic. Common to the young and old, alcoholism was then as now a high risk factor, with drugs enhancing the risk for suicide (21).

The presence of comorbid psychiatric disorders among the alcoholics and

TABLE 4.2. Suicide rate per 1000 population among 3800 attempted suicides by high- and low-risk categories of risk-related factors.

Factor	High-risk category	Suicide rate	Low-risk category	Suicide rate
Age	45 years of age and older	24.0	Under 45 years of age	9.4
Sex	Male	19.9	Female	9.2
Race	White	14.3	Nonwhite	8.7
Marital status	Separated, divorced, widowed	12.5	Single, married	8.6
Living arrangements	Alone	48.4	With others	10.1
Employment status[a]	Unemployed, retired	16.8	Employed[b]	14.3
Physical health	Poor (acute or chronic condition in the 6-month period preceding the attempt)	14.0	Good[b]	12.4
Mental condition	Nervous or mental disorder, mood or behavioral symptoms, including alcoholism	19.1	Presumably normal, including brief situational reactions[b]	7.2
Medical care (within 6 months)	Yes	16.4	No[b]	10.8
Method	Hanging, firearms, jumping, drowning	28.4	Cutting or piercing, gas or carbon monoxide, poison, combination of other methods	12.0
Season	Warm months (April–September)	14.2	Cold months (October–March)	10.9
Time of day	6:00 A.M.–5:59 P.M.	15.1	6:00 P.M.–5:59 A.M.	10.5
Where attempt was made	Own or someone else's home	14.3	Other type of premises, out-of-doors	11.9
Time interval between attempt and discovery	Almost immediately, reported by person making attempt	10.9	Later	7.2
Intent to kill (self-report)	No[b]	14.5	Yes	8.5
Suicide note	Yes	16.7	No[b]	12.3
Previous attempt or threat	Yes	25.2	No[b]	11.0

[a]Does not include housewives and students.
[b]Includes cases for which information on this factor was not given in the police report.
Table by Tuckman J, Youngman WF (1968). A scale for assessing suicide risk of attempted suicides. *J Clin Psychol* 24:17. © 1968, Clinical Psychology Publishing Co., Brandon, VT.

drug addicts is associated with a greater prevalence of suicide in comparison to nonalcoholics and non-drug-addict studies (8,14). The most common comorbid psychiatric syndromes are depression, borderline personality disorder, mania, and schizophrenia. Family histories of depression, suicide, and alcoholism were especially prominent in suicide cases (14).

Prior suicidal behavior is also a significant predictor of subsequent suicide behaviors, as is recent loss or separation. Although depression is a commonly cited risk factor for suicide, it appears that depression associated with alcohol and drug use harbors a greater risk. This may be understandable in light of the dramatic degree of mood and cognitive depression induced by the pharmacological effects of alcohol and drugs. The combination of alcohol and drugs, particularly multiple drugs, may lead to a profound depression, with the hopelessness and helplessness that are central to suicidal thinking and behavior (23).

Mechanisms Underlying Suicide

According to studies, the feeling of hopelessness correlates highly with suicide (23) and is central to the suicidal state whether drug induced or from some other cause. Hopelessness is the imminent feeling that appears to precipitate the self-inflicted destruction. It appears that the mind set requires "hope" not only to sustain sufficient mental inertia for survival but also to avoid self-extinction (23).

As emphasized, many types of drugs are associated with suicidal behavior. Depressants, particularly alcohol, sedatives/hypnotics and opiates, and stimulants such as cocaine and amphetamines are especially prone to produce a sense of hopelessness. The depressant pharmacological actions of these drugs induce a depression that is similar to depressions from other causes, which is characterized by depressed mood, psychomotor retardation, social withdrawal, guilt, and self-reproach (6,24,25). Depressants tend to produce depression during intoxication predominately, whereas the stimulants produce depression during withdrawal most consistently. These drugs of addiction provide a neuropsychopharmacological model for depression and suicide and may provide insights into mechanisms underlying suicidal behavior.

In various studies using different techniques for assessing brain levels in humans and animals by direct and indirect methods, most of the neurotransmitters have been implicated in the neurobiology of depression. Several neurotransmitter hypotheses of suicide and depression may be generated by examining the action of the drugs on the brain. Chronic alcohol use may lead to a deficiency in serotonin in platelets in humans and in brains in animals, whereas chronic cocaine administration produces a marked depletion of many of the neurotransmitters in the brain, including serotonin, norepinephrine, and dopamine, according to human and animal studies.

Antidepressants are purported to work by enhancing the levels of these neurotransmitters in the synapse by a reuptake blockade at the presynaptic neuron after acute and chronic administration as demonstrated in animals. Interesting but yet to be proven, the "neurotransmitter hypothesis" provides a common pathway for the development of the suicidal state for all the drugs of abuse and addiction because so many of the drugs (alcohol) alter the same neurotransmitters (26–28).

Other less convincing theories attempting to explain suicidal behavior are that (i) predisposing personality exists for suicide, and (ii) alcoholics and drug addicts are "self-medicating" an underlying depression or psychosis that is responsible for the suicidal states (29).

According to most studies regarding the first hypothesis, no predisposing personality appears to adequately explain the development of alcohol and drug addiction. Alcoholics and drug addicts are derived from every conceivable personality type and possess all the personality traits that are present in nonalcoholic and drug addicts. Although some personality types are overrepresented among developed drug addicts, such as antisocial and borderline personality disorder, these personality types represent a small proportion of all alcoholics and drug addicts. Furthermore, the evidence supports more clearly that the personality disorder is a consequence of the addiction at this point in investigations (30). Furthermore, if there is a preexisting antisocial or borderline personality, it may only increase the risk of exposure to alcohol and drugs, thereby not conferring a specific vulnerability to the development of alcoholism and drug addiction (19,30). Many personality theorists would defer the diagnosis of personality disorder in the setting of alcoholism and drug addiction until a prolonged period of abstinence had been achieved, allowing time for the pharmacological effects and addictive behaviors pertaining to the alcohol and drugs to subside.

The self-medication concept also is not supported by studies that carefully examine the effects of alcohol and drugs on mood and affect. In one controlled study, three groups of subjects were given alcohol under experimental conditions: (i) depressed alcoholics, (ii) depressed nonalcoholics, and (iii) nondepressed nonalcoholics. By objective measurements, the depressed nonalcoholics experienced the greatest improvement in mood and affect from the ingested alcohol whereas the depressed alcoholics experienced the least benefit. The conclusion of the study was that the alcoholics appear to use alcohol in spite of the depression (often induced by alcohol) and not because of it (31). The depressed nonalcoholics do not appear to use alcohol excessively as the alcoholic or to self-medicate their depression, although they receive a beneficial effect on mood and affect.

Other reports from cocaine addicts find they often experience their greatest euphoria with the initial use of cocaine. With increasing doses and duration of cocaine use, tolerance to the euphoria from cocaine develops while the toxicity from cocaine worsens. Eventually, the cocaine addict is escalating and continuing use in spite of the adverse toxic consequences of severe depression, anxiety, and paranoia in the presence of the significantly diminished euphoria (27).

If self-medication of underlying depression of psychosis were the objective, the use of alcohol and drugs by the alcoholic and drug addict would cease when the depression and psychosis induced by the drugs exceeded the original symptoms. The benefit at that point from self-medication is lost, and to "medicate" psychic distress from the alcohol and drugs is no longer plausible and does not fit the clinical picture. Actual use of drug and alcohol may arise initially from attempts to "feel better," but once the addiction develops the use no longer is dependent on this motivation as addiction appears to be autonomous and has a life of its own (32).

Clinical Care and Treatment

In most instances, the comorbid depression derived from alcohol and drug use, with the concomitant state of hopelessness, will diminish and subside over time with abstinence. In the alcoholic and drug addict, the depression, paranoia, and anxiety are usually induced by alcohol and drugs, and abstinence from alcohol and drugs is essential. However, the tendency to relapse for alcoholics and drug addicts is high, so that specific treatment of the addiction that is generating the alcohol and drug use must be instituted.

Generally, hopefulness reappears with prolonged abstinence especially if specific treatment of the addiction is implemented. Although the suicidal thinking and behavior usually dramatically improve with abstinence and treatment of addiction, they may persist during the early months at chronic, lower levels because of prolonged pharmacological effects of the drugs and the degenerated state of the personality and impaired mental state of the drug addict and the alcoholic (1,3). Because most of these factors respond to treatment, the suicide risk is low for most alcoholics and drug addicts in early recovery despite the recurring suicidal thoughts. Pharmacotherapy with antidepressants and antipsychotics is not indicated in most cases of depression induced by alcohol and drugs, and may actually be harmful in a population that is vulnerable to drug effects such as sedation, reduced cognition, and altered mood, even those from medication. However, for those instances in which imminent and dangerous levels of suicidal thinking and depression may persist, the selective use of antidepressants should be instituted.

In obtaining a history from a known alcoholic or drug addict, a careful inquiry into the suicidal state is necessary, including all the known risk factors associated with suicide. The addict may deny both drug and alcohol use and suicidal ideation and behavior, so that corroborative history from family and friends is highly desirable and sometimes necessary. It can be assumed that suicidal thinking is present in most alcoholics and drug addicts; the clinical necessity is to determine the level of increased risk, especially whether or not suicide is an imminent possibility.

Of critical importance in the setting of a suicide attempt is to obtain a careful screening for the presence of the diagnosis of alcoholism and drug addiction. Unless alcoholism and drug addiction are identified as etiological or precipitating agents in the suicidal attempt and properly treated, the likelihood for another suicide attempt is high. If only specific treatments for the comorbid psychiatric symptoms are initiated, the sense of hopelessness will persist, as well as will the serious risk for suicide.

References

1. Frances RJ, Franklin J, Flavin DK (1986). Suicide and alcoholism. *Ann NY Acad Sci* 487:316–326.
2. Rushing WA (1968). Individual behavior and suicide. In *Suicide*, JP Gibbs, ed., pp. 96–121. New York: Harper and Row.
3. Beck AT, Weissman A, Kovacs M (1976). Alcoholism, hopelessness and suicidal behavior. *J Stud Alcohol* 37:66–76.
4. Marzuk PM, Mann JJ (1988). Suicide and substance abuse. *Psychiatr Ann* 18(11):639–645.
5. Ward NG, Schuckit M (1980). Factors associated with suicidal behavior in poly-drug abusers. *J Clin Psychiatry* 41:379–385.
6. Murphy GE (1988). Suicide and substance abuse. *Arch Gen Psychiatry* 45:593–594.
7. Frances A, Fyer M, Clarkin J (1986). Personality and suicide. *Ann NY Acad Sci* 487:281–293.
8. Fowler RC, Rich CL, Young D (1986). San Diego Suicide Study: II. Substance abuse in young cases. *Arch Gen Psychiatry* 43:962–965.
9. Dorpat TL, Riley HS (1960). A study in the Seattle area. *Compr Psychiatry* 1:349–359.
10. Shaffii M, Carrigan S, Whittinghill JR, et al. (1985). Psychological autopsy of completed suicide in children and adolescents. *Am J Psychiatry* 142:1061–1064.
11. Barraclough B, Bunch J, Nelson B, et al. (1974). A hundred cases of suicide: Clinical Aspects. *Br J Psychiatry* 125:355–373.
12. Kessel N, Grossman G (1961). Suicides in alcoholics. *Br Med J* 2:1671–1672.
13. James IP (1967). Suicide and mortality amongst heroin addicts in Britain. *Br J Addict* 62:391–398.
14. Murphy SL, Rounsaville BJ, Eyre S, et al. (1983). Suicide attempts in treated opiate addicts. *Compr Psychiatry* 24:79–89.
15. Rich CL, Young D, Fowler RC (1986). San Diego Suicide Study: I. Young vs. old subjects. *Arch Gen Psychiatry* 43:577–582.
16. Brent DA, Perper JA, Goldstein CE, et al. (1988). Risk factors for adolescent suicide: A comparison of adolescent suicide victims with suicidal inpatients. *Arch Gen Psychiatry* 45:581–588.
17. Helzer JE, Przybeck TR (1988). The co-occurrence of alcoholism with other psychiatric disorders in the general population and its impact on treatment. *J Stud Alcohol* 49(3):219–221.
18. Rich CL, Fowler RC, Fogarty LA, et al. (1988). San Diego Suicide Study: III. Relationships between diagnoses and stressors. *Arch Gen Psychiatry* 45:589–592.

19. Bouknight RR (1986). Suicide attempt by drug overdose. *Am Fam Physician* 33:137-142.
20. Vaillant GE (1966). A twelve-year follow-up of New York narcotic addicts: I. The relation of treatment to outcome. *Am J Psychiatry* 122:727-737.
21. Litman RE, Feberow NL, Wold CI, Brown TR (1988). Prediction models of suicidal behaviors. In *Prediction of Suicide*, Beck H, Resnik LP, Lettieri DJ, eds., p. 141. Bowier, MD: Charles Press.
22. Tuckman J, Youngman WF (1968). A scale for assessing suicide risk of attempted suicides. *J Clin Psychol* 24:17.
23. Beck AT (1985). Hopelessness and eventual suicide. *Am J Psychiatry* 142:559.
24. Hawton K, Catalan J, eds. (1975). *Attempted Suicide*. New York: Oxford University Press.
25. Mayfield DG, Montgomery D (1972). Alcoholism, alcohol intoxication, and suicide attempts. *Arch Gen Psychiatry* 27:349-355.
26. Brown GL, Goodwin, FK (1986). Cerebrospinal fluid correlates of suicide attempts and aggression. *Ann NY Acad Sci* 487:175-188.
27. Dackis CA, Gold MS (1985). New concepts in cocaine addiction: The dopamine depletion hypothesis. *Neurosci Biobehav Rev* 9:469-477.
28. Post mortem monoamine receptor and enzyme studies on suicide. (1986). In *Psychobiology of Suicidal Behavior. Annals of the New York Academy of Science, Vol. 487,* Mann JJ, Stanley M, eds., pp. 114-121.
29. Khantzian EJ (1985). The self-medicated hypotheses of addictive disorders: Focus on lesion and cocaine dependence. *Am J Psychiatry* 142:1259-1264.
30. Vaillant GE (1983). *The natural history of alcoholism*. Boston: Harvard University Press.
31. Mayfield DG (1979). Alcohol and affect: Experimental studies. In *Alcoholism and Affective Disorders*, Goodwin DW, Erickson, CK, eds., pp. 99-107. New York: SP Medical and Scientific Books.
32. Miller NS, Dackis CA, Gold MS (1987). The relationship of tolerance, dependence and addiction: A neurochemical approach. *J Subst Abuse Treat* 4:197-207.
33. Martin RL, Cloninger CR, Guze SB, Clayton PH (1985). Mortality in a follow-up of 500 psychiatric outpatients. I. Total mortality. *Arch Gen Psychiatry* 42:47-66.

CHAPTER 5

The Genetics of Alcoholism

History

The observation that alcoholism runs in families is relatively certain. Medical experts seem to agree on this point more than any other. Any given alcoholic has a 50% chance of having at least one family member with alcoholism, and a family that has at least one alcoholic is likely to have others; that is, there is a 90% chance of having two or more family members with alcoholism. Furthermore, alcoholics with a family history of alcoholism tend to have a more severe course with greater adverse consequences from alcoholism. Alcoholic parents have alcoholic children about four to five times more often than do parents who are not alcoholics (1,2,3).

The Bible contains references to families with drunkards. Aristotle and Plutarch pondered it, and doctors and preachers of the 19th century were adamant that drunkards beget drunkards. To most of these authorities, alcoholism was a weakness or vice that was inherited as was any other talent or lack of it. The notion that willpower over alcohol is inherited persists today. The moral dilemma of free will for those with alcoholism is thought by many to be coded in genes as is hair color or height or weight. Despite major advancements in alcohol diagnosis and treatment, numerous misconceptions remain popular.

Diagnosis

No other psychiatric illness has so strong a familial dominance. Schizophrenia and affective illness have a family representation of the same illnesses greater than expected in the general population, but not with as high a frequency as alcoholism. Some neurological conditions exceed alcoholism in incidence rates within families; for example, Huntington's chorea is a condition in which a particular offspring has a 50% chance of developing the disease if a parent is affected. The probability of a child developing alcoholism is 25% if one parent is an alcoholic, and the probability increases to greater than 50% if both parents are alcoholics (4,5).

Why the confusion about alcoholism if heredity plays such a large role for so many? Estimates place the rate of alcoholism in the United States between 10 and 20%, meaning that between 20 and 40 million Americans suffer from alcoholism. We all know at least one person, often a family member, who is an alcoholic.

Researchers in recent times have used a variety of techniques to arrive at the same conclusion that alcoholism is inherited rather than determined by environment. By the 1970s, the debate between the nature and nurture approaches diverged. Although many agreed that alcoholism ran in families, it had not been decided if environment or upbringing was more than, less than, or as important as the genes that determined eye and hair color, height, and weight. This natural antagonism is present in many other psychiatric disorders; for example, is schizophrenia produced by schizophrenogic mothers or by faulty genes? If environment is the culprit, then modification of practices and behavioral is indicated. If heredity is the determining cause of alcoholism, then the problem originates in a physical predisposition that initiates alcoholism (6,7).

The research approaches used by medical investigators have been interesting and challenging to understand. Basically, the studies have been designed to try to isolate heredity from environment. The studies have produced good results, but no one type has yielded the entire answer to the question of nature versus nurture. The studies have examined twins, adoptees, families, and offspring of alcoholics (8).

Prevalence

Twin Studies

Researchers in Sweden, Finland, and the United States have found that identical twins were much more concordant or more likely to have a tendency towards alcoholism as a pair than fraternal twins. The assumption is that the inheritance is stronger in identical twins because they have genes or genetic endowments that are identical. In other words, the DNA from one of the identical twins is exactly the same as the DNA from the other twin. DNA is the building block for the genes that are responsible for transmitting inherited information.

Fraternal twins, on the other hand, share only half of their genes. Fraternal twins do not have as strong a tendency to inherit any trait, including alcoholism. A fraternal twin is the same as brothers and sisters in genetic likeness. The only difference is that fraternal twins share a womb at the same time rather than at different times as do brothers and sisters.

Environment still cannot be eliminated, because twins reared in the same environment are treated similarly and thus in effect are subject to the same environment. Even genetically different offspring might have an effect that makes them both alcoholic if environment is responsible for the development of alcoholism.

Adoption Studies

The research on adoptees is interesting because it eliminated environment more than any study to date, although not completely. In Denmark, a study found that the biological parent and not the foster parent determined whether the adopted offspring developed alcoholism. The subjects were adopted away at the age of 6 months from the biological mother; thus, the 9 months in the uterus and the first 6 months of life were still under the influence of the biological mother so that environment was not entirely controlled for. However, the remaining years into adulthood were under the environment of the adopted, foster parents (3). In this milestone study, the adoptees who became alcoholics were much more likely to have biological parents who were alcoholic than foster parents who were alcoholic. Furthermore, even if the foster parents were alcoholic, the adoptees who did not have an alcoholic biological parent did not become alcoholic (9–12).

The biological parents share genes with the adopted-out offspring, so that the hereditary background of the adoptee was seen to be the determining factor in the transmission of alcoholism. The environment of the alcoholic did not play much of a role in the development of alcoholism in the adoptees. Even in homes where alcoholism was active, if the offspring did not share the genes for alcoholism, then no alcoholism in the offspring was present. The probability of becoming an alcoholic is about 25% if the biological father is alcoholic whether the child is a son or daughter. The number of mothers who were alcoholic was too small in this study to make such predictions.

When heredity and environment are both present and operating together, the transmission of alcoholism is still strong and quite common. As might be expected, the probability of having a family history positive for alcoholism is greater if both hereditary and environment are influences on the children. The probability of an alcoholic having a first-degree relative (father, mother, sister, or brother) who is alcoholic is at least 50%. In other words, any given alcoholic has a 50% chance or greater of having at least one close family member who is alcoholic. Also, one can see why alcoholism is a common illness if so many people in the family get it.

Researchers became weary as they tried to unravel the cause of alcoholism by studying alcoholics. The problems are many because of the pharmacological effects of alcohol on people, especially if the alcohol is consumed often and in large amounts. Researchers wanted to know if the greater tolerance for alcohol that alcoholics show was acquired or inherited. Tolerance is defined, in this case, as being able to ingest more alcohol without experiencing as much of alcohol's effect. A person who has increased tolerance for alcohol seems to be able to drink large quantities without showing the effects, that is, without getting as drunk as quickly. Alcoholics appear to have this enhanced tolerance early in their drinking histories, perhaps before the onset of their alcoholism (13).

High Risk Studies

Studies have also examined the children of alcoholics. The children who had not yet started to drink much and who had not yet developed alcoholism were ideal candidates to use. These children are called "high-risk" individuals because their positive family histories of alcoholism put them at higher risk for developing alcoholism than individuals without family histories of alcoholism (14,15).

Tolerance to alcohol was studied in these children before they became alcoholic and was measured objectively and subjectively. Motor coordination and thinking abilities were scored in children with and without a family history of alcoholism. The children who had an alcoholic parent were able to perform better on tests of motor coordination and thinking than children who did not have a parent with alcoholism. Furthermore, as expected if possessing greater tolerance, the high-risk children reported that they did not feel as intoxicated with the same amount of alcohol as did the matched low-risk children (16-18).

What these results tend to show us is that alcoholics may indeed inherit an ability to drink more than others without the genetic predisposition to develop alcoholism. The reason that alcoholics early in their drinking histories drive everyone else home may be that they react differently to alcohol. The brain in alcoholics is probably "wired" in a way that tolerance is greater for alcohol than someone without the genes for alcoholism. The location for tolerance is in the brain, and not in the liver where the metabolism or breakdown and elimination of alcohol occurs. The liver does increase the rate of breakdown of alcohol but not sufficiently to account for the total amount of tolerance.

Tolerance and Dependence

Tolerance is a "physical" sign and symptom that is inherited, and not some personality factor such as low self-esteem or inferiority complex or other deep-rooted psychological problems. The predisposition to alcoholism begins as a physical reaction to alcohol that is called tolerance. Those with a low risk for alcoholism do not adapt well to the presence of alcohol in their brains. The reactions of the lack of tolerance is dysphoria or a disturbed mood, nausea, headache, and perhaps vomiting and a general ill feeling that only gets worse with more alcohol. The nonalcoholic actually feels better as the alcohol leaves the body, so that there appears to be little reinforcement for drinking more alcohol. The alcoholic, on the other hand, feels better as the blood alcohol level rises in the body and brain so that the motivation is to drink more.

This negative reaction or low tolerance to alcohol is also inherited. Orientals and some Occidentals have an intolerance to alcohol that is manifested as a "flushing reaction." The Oriental flushing reaction appears to be inherited. The reaction is characterized by dysphoria, headache, nausea, vomiting, light-headedness, and a red flushing over the face and sometimes body. An Oriental with the flushing reaction usually has several members of the family who also have the reaction to alcohol (19).

The rate of alcoholism among Orientals is low, and this intolerance to alcohol may be a protective mechanism against alcoholism for them. This is an example of a genetic predisposition against alcoholism that is also physical. The families of Orientals who have the flushing reaction have a lower rate of alcoholism than families without this protective reaction.

Tolerance to alcohol or the lack of tolerance appears to be inherited. Whether someone is likely or not to develop alcoholism appears to depend on whether or not he has the genes for alcoholism. Tolerance, in a sense, is a marker for alcoholism. If someone has tolerance for alcohol, they may be at risk for developing alcoholism. The opposite may be true; if someone lacks the tolerance to alcohol, they probably will not develop alcoholism.

There are other markers of alcoholism in addition to tolerance. The electroencephalograph (EEG) and other instruments that also measure brain-wave activity have been used to find some interesting differences between children of alcoholics and other children without alcoholic parents. The high-risk subjects show more slow alpha activity after consuming alcohol than do low-risk children. Alpha activity is normal background in the awake, relaxed state. Also, children of alcoholics show slower onset and progression of other waves, that is, alpha waves when measured in the absence of alcohol. Alpha waves represent the normal background in the awake state with the eyes closed, as recorded on the EEG. These waves may be important in thinking and how fast someone reacts in thinking. The exact interpretation of these findings is unclear at this time. The important conclusion is, as with tolerance, that the brains of alcoholics may be different from the start, even before birth, and may be determined by the genetic makeup (20–22).

The Role of Environment

Caution is urged. There are always exceptions, and other factors than genes are important in the development of alcoholism. Environment with its many and complex interactions with the genetic makeup is also important in the expression of alcoholism. Tolerance to alcohol may be a necessary condition, but not always a sufficient condition, for alcoholism to occur. A particular type of environment may be more conducive to alcoholism for some personalities than others.

A simple and convenient way to view heredity and environment is in an equation in which the predisposition to alcoholism plus the exposure to alcohol equals an addiction to alcohol or alcoholism. Heredity, as discussed, equals the physical predisposition to alcoholism. The exposure is defined by the broad concept of environment. There are many determinants of exposure to alcohol, beginning with the practices, customs, norms, and laws within a given culture. Most cultures, including those in the United States, have a high tolerance for alcohol. Alcohol is relatively cheap, easy to obtain, and a fixed tradition in religious and social practices; its use is even encouraged and enforced by some groups within our society. The powerful media of television, magazines, and roadside billboards inundate and saturate persons of all ages, at all times and in all places. Almost no one can escape the exposure to alcohol, accompanied by varying degrees of overt and tacit approval and disapproval regarding its use.

When the physical predisposition is present, even in varying degrees of vulnerability as may be the case with alcoholism and is with many other genetic disorders such as diabetes mellitus, exposure is required to develop the disease of alcoholism. The intensity of the exposure may vary as may the duration, so that someone will drink much and often if in certain environments as college, or in certain employments as bartending or athletics, or not so much or often in other circumstances. As a rule of thumb, the more the genetic loading — both parents are alcoholic — and the greater and longer the exposure, the more likely it is that alcoholism will develop. Contrariwise, in the absence of a family history with little exposure, a person is least likely to develop alcoholism. Any combination of either hereditary or environment will determine the risk for the development of alcoholism.

We all know of exceptions to this rule, that is, someone with a host of alcoholics in the family who is not alcoholic or someone who is alcoholic but does not have a single relative with alcoholism. The reasons for these exceptions are (i) little opportunity for exposure to alcohol; (ii) denial of alcoholism in the family (e.g., mother or grandfather had a nervous breakdown); (iii) misattribution of alcoholism to another illness, such as, depression (alcoholism causes depression); (iv) nonpenetrance of the alcoholism in a particular generation, as does occur in genetic disorders; or (v) the theory, or some of it, can always be incorrect; it is the evidence in favor of the theory that is convincing.

The Addictive Personality

No one kind of "addictive" personality appears to predict alcoholism. An addictive personality appears to develop in the setting of alcoholism and probably as a consequence of alcoholism. The addictive personality does not seem to be inherited or to be present before the onset of alcoholism (23).

However, some types of personalities seem to be at high risk to develop alcoholism. Antisocial behavior in childhood frequently leads to alcohol drinking and eventual alcoholism. A high proportion of antisocial personalities have alcoholism. It is estimated that between 50% and 90% of those incarcerated in prisons are alcoholic, and many of those are antisocial personalities (23).

Summary

The strongest predictor of future alcoholism is a family history of alcoholism. Every study shows this. About one of every four or five sons and daughters of alcoholics in North America and Western Europe became alcoholic in all studies reviewed. Alcoholism runs in families for the reason of genetic constitution. Environment is important, but plays a different role than the cause; rather, it contributes to the probability of development of alcoholism if the genes for alcoholism are present.

References

1. Goodwin DW (1985). Alcoholism and genetics. *Arch Gen Psychiatry* 42:171–174.
2. Goodwin DW, Schulsinger F, Hermansen L, Guse S, Winokur G (1973). Alcohol problems in adoptees raised apart from alcoholic biological parents. *Arch Gen Psychiatry* 28:238–243.
3. Goodwin DW, Schulinger F, Moller N, Hermansen L, Winokur G, Guze SB (1974). Drinking problems in adopted and nonadopted sons of alcoholics. *Arch Gen Psychiatry* 31:164–169.
4. Goodwin DW, Guze SB (1984). *Psychiatric Diagnosis*. New York: Oxford University Press.
5. Schuckit MA, Haglund RMJ (1982). An overiew of the etiologic theories on alcoholism. In *Alcoholism: Development, Consequences, and Interventions*, Estes N, Heinemann, E, eds., pp. 16–31. St. Louis: Mosby.
6. Cloninger CR, von Knorring AL, Sigvardsson S, Bohman M (1983). *Inheritance of Alcohol Abuse*. Presented at the International Conference on Pharmacological Treatments for Alcoholism Looking to the Future. Alcoholism Education Centre and Institute of Psychiatry, University of London, London, England.
7. Cloninger CR, Reich T, Yokoyama S (1983). Genetic diversity, genome organization, and investigation of the etiology of psychiatric diseases. *Psychiatr Dev* 3:225–246.
8. Miller NS, Gold WS (1988). Research approaches to inheritance of alcoholism and substance abuse. *Substance Abuse* 96:157–168.
9. Schuckit MA, Goodwin DW, Winokur G (1972). A half-sibling study of alcoholism. *Am J Psychiatry* 128:1132–1136.
10. Bohman M (1978). Some genetic aspects of alcoholism and criminality: A population of adoptees. *Arch Gen Psychiatry* 35:269–276.
11. Bohman M, Sivardsson S, Cloninger R (1981). Maternal inheritance of alcohol abuse: Cross-fostering analysis of adopted women. *Arch Gen Psychiatry* 38:965–969.

12. Cadiret RJ, Cain CA, Grove WM (1979). Development of alcoholism in adoptees raised apart from alcoholic biologic relatives. *Arch Gen Psychiatry* 37:561–563.
13. Goodwin DW (1985). Alcoholism and genetics. *Arch Gen Psychiatry* 42:171–174.
14. Schuckit MA, Engstrom D, Alpert R, Duby J (1981). Differences in muscle-tension response to ethanol in young men with and without family histories of alcoholism. *J Stud Alcohol* 42:918–924.
15. Schuckit MA (1985). Studies of populations at high risk for alcoholism. *Psychiatr Dev* 3:31–63.
16. Schuckit MA (1985). Ethanol-induced changes in body sway in men at high alcoholism risk. *Arch Gen Psychiatry* 42:375–379.
17. Schuckit MA (1984). Subjective responses to alcohol in sons of alcoholics and controls. *Arch Gen Psychiatry* 41:879–884.
18. Schuckit MA (1984). Differences in plasma cortisol after ethanol in relatives of alcoholics and controls. *J Clin Psychiatry* 45:374–379.
19. Chan AW (1986). Racial difference in alcohol sensitivity. *Alcohol Alcohol* 21:193–204.
20. Begleiter H, Porjesz B, Bihari B, Kissin B (1984). Event-related brain potentials in boys at risk for alcoholism. *Science* 227:1493–1496.
21. Gabrielli WF, Mednick SA (1983). Intellectual performance in children of alcoholics. *J Nerv Ment Dis* 171:444–447.
22. Gabrielli WF, Mednick SA, Volavka J, et al. (1982). Electroencephalograms in children of alcoholic fathers. *Psychophysiology* 19:404–407.
23. Valliant GE (1983). *The Natural History of Alcoholism.* Cambridge, MA: Harvard University Press.

CHAPTER 6

The Medical Consequences of Alcohol and Drugs of Abuse and Addiction

History

It is important that physicians know in detail the medical complications of alcoholism. However, as important as medical sequelae can be, the majority of alcoholics escape medical consequences. The minority of alcoholics who have medical consequences appear to represent chronic, long-time consumers or have a idiosyncratic reaction to the effects of alcohol (1,2,3).

The medical consequences are related to a host of organ systems in the body. Ethanol is water soluble and reaches virtually every cell that is bathed by water. The toxic effects of ethanol on the body are both direct and indirect. Studies have confirmed that ethanol produces direct toxic damage to organs, for example, brain and muscle, and also influences the development of deficiency states through malnutrition or metabolic derangement (4).

The major systems affected are the cardiovascular, gastrointestinal, hematological, oncological, respiratory, integumentary, traumatic, endocrinological, and neurological. These organ systems are regularly affected by measurable means, although less often to a significant pathological extent. The individual susceptibility appears to vary considerably, and it is difficult to predict who will develop which complications (1–4).

Cardiovascular System

The most common complication from acute and chronic alcohol consumption is an elevation of blood pressure and pulse. After acute administration of alcohol, the physiological response to the elimination of ethanol is a discharge of the sympathetic nervous system with a concomitant rise in blood pressure and pulse. The development of sustained hypertension and tachycardia is a common sequela of regular and chronic alcohol consumption.

An elevation can be detected during the intoxicated state and especially in the early abstinent state while the blood alcohol level is either dropping or has recently reached zero. The absolute values for blood pressure and pulse may or may not be in the abnormal range, depending on the individual reaction to alcohol withdrawal. Those who are young and without existing hypertension are less likely to have an elevation than those who are older and predisposed to some hypertension (5–7).

An elevation in the first 24 to 72 hours of 20–30 mm Hg in systolic blood pressure and 10–20 mm Hg in diastolic blood pressure over that which is baseline for a particular individual is typical following chronic consumption. The values are lower for withdrawal from acute ingestion. The pulse is elevated 10 to 30 beats per minute, in the range of sinus tachycardia, after heavy and more chronic consumption of alcohol.

The blood pressure often returns to normal over a period of a few days without specific therapy. It is important to realize these individuals with an elevated blood pressure and a history of chronic alcohol consumption have acclimated to the sustained increase. The blood pressure and pulse of these individuals should be allowed to gradually subside in the abstinent state with or without specific medical intervention.

Most of those alcoholics with an elevation in blood pressure and pulse will be normotensive. The remainder who continue to have some degree of hypertension will require less medication while in the alcohol-abstinent state. Elevated blood pressures, often in the hypertension range, occur frequently. Any patient with hypertension and tachycardia should be assessed for alcohol intake and alcoholism.

Alcoholic cardiomyopathy is probably more common than is currently believed because of underdiagnosis of alcoholism in general, particularly in medical populations. A significant proportion of the "idiopathic cardiomyopathy" heretofore attributed to a viral etiology almost certainly has an alcohol-induced basis (8,9).

What is generally known about patients with cardiomyopathy (underdiagnosis notwithstanding) is that a chronic drinking history of at least 10 years, especially with heavy intake, is often noted. The signs and symptoms of cardiac insufficiency from cardiomyopathy are generally gradual in onset, although precipitous occurrences have been reported. Patients present most often with heart failure, manifested by breathlessness, fatigability, palpitations, anorexia, and dependent edema as in any syndrome of congestive heart failure. Symptoms of angina pectoris are generally absent, although chest pain of an ischemic type does occur in some patients. The blood pressure may be normal or low, or even elevated (10).

The physical findings are similar to those found in other forms of dilated cardiomyopathy—lateral displacement of the apical pulse, an S-3 and S-4 heart sound, systolic mumurs, elevated venous pressure, hepatomegaly, and edema. The electrocardiogram (EKG) findings are also nonspecific, with atrial and ventricular arrhythmias, intraventicular conduction abnormalities, pathological Q waves, and decreased QRS voltage as common findings.

The chest radiograph generally shows a symmetric cardiomegaly, and cardiac catheterization reveals reduced output, high diastolic pressures, and pulmonary hypertension. The histological features are varied and nonspecific; myocardial fiber hypertrophy and fibrosis as well as lipid or glycogen vacuolization are found (11).

Alcoholic cardiomyopathy is not an inevitably fatal condition, and improvement frequently follows abstinence from alcohol, particularly in those patients in whom cardiac symptoms are of recent onset. It is likely that many of the cases of cardiomyopathy that receive heart transplantations have an alcoholic basis. This is important to note because continued drinking may contribute to a poor outcome post transplantation. All cases of cardiomyopathy should be evaluated for possible alcoholism.

Gastrointestinal System

Disturbances attributable to the gastrointestinal tract commonly occur after alcohol use, particularly in higher and chronic administration. Any complaint arising from the gastrointestinal system deserves an evaluation of alcohol use and possible alcoholism. Alcohol produces irritation and inflammation of the mucosa lining the gastrointestinal tract. Frank ulceration may occur with chronic alcohol use (12).

The well-known condition of "heartburn" is caused by esophageal reflux with esophagitis that commonly occurs with irritation and inflammation of the gastroesophageal junction by alcohol. Severe vomiting may result in mucosal tears at this junction, with hematemesis as in the Mallory–Weiss syndrome. Esophageal varices are an expression of portal hypertension from liver disease, often also induced by alcohol. These varices are engorged, dilated capillaries that represent a collateral circulation. Significant and sometimes fatal hemorrhage may occur from these varices (13).

The stomach and duodenum are vulnerable sites to the corrosive effects of alcohol. Short- and long-term alcohol ingestion is associated with gastritis, erosive gastritis, gastric ulceration, atropic gastritis, and gastric hemorrhage. Furthermore, duodenitis and duodenal ulcerations are a direct result of chronic alcohol irritation and inflammation. Scarring and obstruction may result from chronic ulceration (14).

Chronic administration of alcohol may result in chronic pancreatitis. However, acute ingestion of alcohol is associated with an alteration of the secretion of the pancreatic enzymes, and abnormalities in intestinal absorption with acute and chronic alcohol use. Abdominal pain and vomiting are common during the relapse. The pain is poorly localized to the upper abdomen, radiating to the back. Other signs may be lacking in mild cases, and in more severe cases hypoactive bowel sounds and rebound tenderness suggestive of peritonitis may be present. In cases of high fever, a pancreatic abscess may be suspected; an abdominal mass, a pseudocyst, shifting dullness, and ascites may be encountered. Helpful dianostic features are serum amylase, a KUB (kidney, ureter, bladder), ultrasonography, and computed tomography (CT) or magnetic resonance imaging (MRI) scanning (15,16).

Diabetes mellitus or hyperglycemia is a complication of the eventual destruction of the islet cells in the pancreas from persistent, alcohol-induced, chronic pancreatitis. Often insulin is necessary to compensate for the lost insulin production in the fibrosed and contracted pancreas. At times, replacement therapy for pancreatic enzymes for pancreatic insufficiency may be necessary (17).

Malabsorption and diarrhea are common in alcoholics and result from a number of interactive factors. These include alterations in gastric motility, mucosal erosions, and impaired transport of glucose, amino acids, and vitamins, particularly thiamine and vitamin B_{12}, and minerals such as calcium and magnesium (18).

The liver is a particularly vulnerable organ in alcohol consumption, in part because it is where alcohol is metabolized and broken down for reuse and elimination from the body. The most common manifestation is fatty metamorphosis or fatty liver. For some alcoholics, a fatty liver may precede the onset of alcoholic cirrhosis. However, a large number of those who consume alcohol will develop fat in the liver but not cirrhosis. In fact, evidence from animal studies suggests that fatty metamorphosis occurs regularly with acute ingestion of alcohol. Transient, mild elevations of liver enzymes, particularly alanine aminotransferase (ALT) and aspartate aminotransferase (AST) will occur. These return to normal within a few weeks (19,20).

Alcoholic hepatitis is a severe condition that is characterized by jaundice, fever, anorexia, and right-upper-quadrant pain. The liver histologically shows parenchymal and portal infiltration with polymorphonuclear leukocytes, steatosis, cholestasis, and sometimes hyaline bodies. The serum levels of ALT, AST, and lactate dehydrogenase (LDH) are elevated, at times at high levels. Prolongation of the prothrombin time and ascites may occur (21).

Alcoholic cirrhosis is not a particularly common condition among alcoholics as a total population. However, its prevalence increases in older and more chronic populations of alcoholics. The overall prevalence rate for cirrhosis is 5%–10% of all alcoholics. The most common signs of uncomplicated cirrhosis are weight loss, weakness, and anorexia. The signs may include jaundice, a small or large liver, splenomegaly, ascites, asterixis, testicular atrophy, edema, spontaneous peritonitis, gynecomastia, spider angiomata, palmar erythema, and Dupuytren's contracture. Laboratory findings are hypoalbuminemia and hyperglobinemia, with or without elevation of liver enzymes. Cirrhosis is the scarring of the liver from alcohol; the microscopic picture is that of fibrosis of portal and central zones and an overall distortion of the architecture of the liver, which may be small and shrunken (22,23).

Complications from cirrhosis are ascites, esophageal varices, hepatorenal syndrome (renal failure), and hepatic encephalopathy, coma, and death.

Once cirrhosis has developed, the life expectancy is around 50% if abstinence is maintained and significantly less if the person continues to ingest alcohol. It is not known why which individuals will develop cirrhosis; it tends to occur in chronic, older drinkers, although there are many exceptions to this rule (24,25).

Nutritional Complications

Alcohol consumption and nutritional status are interrelated. Alcohol intake may interfere with the absorption, digestion, metabolism, and utilization of nutrients, particularly vitamins. The use of alcohol as a source of calories to the exclusion of other food sources, including nutrients, may also lead to a nutrient deficiency (25,26).

Alcohol disrupts absorption of nutrients in the various ways outlined in previous sections by acting on the intestinal walls, as in the small intestine, and by damaging organs such as the pancreas, which is responsible for digestion. The effect of alcohol on metabolism is to alter the inactivation and activation of the nutrients. For instance, alcohol decreases the net synthesis of pyridoxal phosphate from pyridoxine. These effects have been linked to the oxidation of ethanol, and may involve the displacement and subsequent degradation of pyridoxal-5-phosphate from its cytosol-binding protein by phosphatase and result in a net decrease in activation. These nutritional effects of alcohol have more than an academic interest. Admissions to hospitals for malnutrition from alcoholism remain a significant cause for admissions for malnutrition. Alcoholism is suggested as the most common cause of vitamin and trace element deficiency in adults in the United States, and malnutrition remains a significant cause of admissions to general hospitals (27,28).

The regular consumption of alcohol itself contributes to the poor intake of other foodstuffs containing proper nutrients. Alcohol contains calories, supplying 7.1 kcal/g. Thus a consumer of 600 ml of 86 proof distilled spirits derives 1500 kcal or more than one-half of his or her daily caloric needs from the alcohol. The calories derived from alcohol are called "empty" calories because of the small amounts of vitamins, minerals, essential amino acids, or essential fatty acids contained in most alcoholic beverages. Primary malnutrition resulting from a decrease in the actual ingestion of nutrients is frequently associated with regular and heavy alcohol use.

1. *Folic acid deficiency.* Megaloblastic anemia is common in malnourished alcoholics and most often results from folate deficiency. Thrombocytopenia and granulocytopenia may accompany the megaloblastic changes, especially if the folate level is severely low. The deficiency results from poor intake and disruption of absorption in the small bowel. The hematological manifestations of the folate deficiency are rapidly reversible despite persistently low serum levels (29,30).
2. *Pyridoxine deficiency.* Pyridoxine deficiency has been implicated in the

development of sideroblastic anemias in the alcoholic. The sideroblastic changes induced by ethanol and a diet low in pyridoxine are reversed by the intake of the vitamin in spite of continued alcohol ingestion (31).

3. *Thiamine deficiency.* Thiamine deficiency in the alcoholic may result from malabsorption and perhaps defective activation of thiamine. Thiamine deficiency is the cause of Wernicke–Korsakoff syndrome. It is certain that latent or subclinical thiamine deficiency is common in the alcoholic, and the administration of parental glucose without thiamine may precipitate Wernicke's encephalopathy in such patients (32).

4. *Iron deficiency.* Iron deficiency usually only occurs when other factors related to iron deficiency are present, such as gastrointestinal bleeding and infection. Iron overload or excess is more likely than deficiency because of increased iron absorption from a pancreatic insufficiency. Because an anemia from another cause may be present, iron may be given incorrectly (33,34).

5. *Zinc deficiency.* Zinc deficiency may be associated with the pathogenesis of night blindness seen in alcoholics because of its role as a cofactor of vitamin A dehydrogenase, the enzymedresponsible for the conversion of retinol to retinal (35).

6. *Fat-soluble vitamin deficiency*
   a. *Vitamin A deficiency.* A deficiency in vitamin A may result from a decreased uptake from malabsorption (steatorrhea), impaired storage, increased degradation, and diminished activation. Chronic consumption of ethanol decreases hepatic vitamin A levels. Clinically, the vitamin A deficiency is related to abnormal dark adaptation and hypogonadism. Repletion of the vitamin A and zinc may reverse these conditions but should be done cautiously because alcohol increases the hepatotoxicity of even moderate doses of vitamin A (36,37).
   b. *Vitamin D deficiency.* Vitamin D deficiency may result from decreased dietary intake, decreased absorption, and altered metabolism. Vitamin D depletion and impairment of calcium transport may lead to a decrease in bone density and increased susceptibility to fractures and asceptic necrosis (38).
   c. *Vitamin K deficiency.* Steatorrhea, decreased intake, and altered colonic microflora may combine to produce vitamin K deficiency. In patients with liver damage, further vitamin K deficiency may result in a depression of an already marginal synthesis of clotting factors and result in bleeding (39).

Endocrinological Effects

Alcohol affects the endocrine system in a variety of ways by interacting at all levels of the endocrine axis. The levels at which alteration from alcohol may occur are the hypothalamus and the pituitary, adrenal, throid, and gonadal glands. Furthermore, liver injury from alcohol disturbs the peripheral metabolism of hormones by changes in hepatic blood flow, protein binding, enzymes, cofactors or receptors.

1. *Adrenocortical function.* Chronic alcohol consumption results in increased plasma cortisol levels. Occasionally the alcohol use is associated with cushingoid changes, which are increased plasma cortisol levels, an abnormal response to dexamethasone, and evidence of pituitary dysfunction. Alcohol activates the hypothalamic–pituitary–adrenal axis to promote adrenocorticotropic hormone (ACTH) release and cortisol secretion (40,41).

2. *Adrenomedullary function.* Alcohol consumption results in stimulation of adrenomedullary secretion of catecholamines. The peripheral metabolism of catecholamines shifts from an oxidative (3-methoxy-4-hydroxymandelic acid) to a reductive pathway (3-methoxy-4-hydroxyphenylglycol), a change that reflects an increase in the NADH/NAD (nicotinamide adenine dinucleotide) ratio or acetaldehyde production. This ratio change may be important in the generation of condensation products in the formation of the tetrahydroisoquinolines (42).

   Chronic alcohol consumption also leads to the stimulation of the secretion of catecholamines from the sympathetic portion of the autonomic nervous system. Alcohol withdrawal is characterized by alterations in vital signs and arousal state that are indicative of a massive release of catecholamines.

3. *Thyroid function.* Alcohol administration increases the liver to plasma ratio of thyroid hormone that may lead to a hepatic "hyperthyroidism." This state is responsible for increased oxygen consumption, local anoxia, and possibly liver injury (43,44).

4. *Gonadal function.* Alcohol consumption decreases plasma testosterone, an effect that results from a decrease in production and increased metabolic clearance of the hormone.

   Alcoholic cirrhosis is known to lead to primary hypogonadism with subsequent feminization. The pathological basis is a multifactorial; destruction of the testosterone-producing cells in the testes, and elevated estradiol and estrone levels and increased conversion of testosterone and androstenediene to estrogen because of decrease breakdown by the liver.

   The clinical manifestations are loss of male secondary sex characteristics and a feminization that include decreased libido, hair, and muscle mass, and the development of gynecomastia, smooth feminine skin. These changes may or may not be reversible, depending on the degree of permanent damage (45,46).

5. *Pituitary function.* The release of the gonadotropin from the hypothalamic–pituitary axis is defective. Also, the release of the antidiuretic hormone in the posterior pituitary gland is inhibited by alcohol. The end

result is a diuretic action of alcohol and subsequent dehydration from a lack of action of the antidiuretic hormone on the reabsorption of free water in the tubules in the kidney (47).

6. *Alcoholic hypoglycemia.* This condition is caused by an inhibition by alcohol of gluconeogenesis in the liver. Gluconeogenesis is the major source of glucose during chronic alcohol consumption, particularly when other dietary sources of glucose are not available to the liver. The symptoms of hypoglycemia may be severe, with fatigue, tremors, seizures, and other manifestations of low blood sugar.

7. *Alcoholic ketosis.* This condition usually follows regular consumption of alcohol, anorexia, and hyperemesis. The level of beta-hydroxybutyrate is higher than that of acetoacetate (48).

Nervous System

Neurological complications from chronic alcohol consumption are numerous and occur in most chronic drinkers. The type and number of neurological complications depend on the severity of the alcohol use, nutritional status, and individual susceptibility to alcohol.

The most common abnormality is a decrease in intellectual functioning or dementia syndrome with a subsequent decrease in recent memory, abstractions, calculations, general knowledge, and other aspects of cognitive functions. Studies show that a reduction in IQ may result from as little as 2 oz of alcohol consumed on a regular basis over a prolonged period of months. Studies of alcoholics show that the depression in IQ may be reversible, improving over a period of months and years from the time of cessation of alcohol use (49,50).

Furthermore, CT scans of the brain have confirmed that cerebral atrophy occurs in alcoholics frequently at any age, but more commonly and more pronounced at later ages. These changes as seen on the CT scans are representative of a decrease in brain mass with a concommitant increase in venticular size. The changes are diffuse and widespread, indicative of a generalized effect of alcohol on the brain. The cerebral atrophy correlates with impairments in the intellect. It is important to note that the atrophy as well as the reduction in IQ is noted to reverse with subsequent CT scanning of the brain and retesting of the IQ.

The underlying mechanism is a direct toxicity by alcohol on the neurons and their processess, the axons and dendrites, as well as on the supporting cells, the astroglia. These neuropathological changes have been noted in animal and human studies when nutritional factors have been controlled for (49).

Interestingly, the most classic neurological syndrome from chronic alcohol consumption may not result from the direct toxic effects of alcohol. The Wernicke–Korsakoff syndrome is the result of a thiamine deficiency that occurs in the setting of alcohol use. Alcohol intake may decrease the absorption and utilization of thiamine but does not play a role in the direct toxicity on nerve cells. The neuropathological changes are caused by alterations in the cerebellum, brainstem, and diencephalon. These changes are often small hemorrhages and infarct in the structures (49).

The clinical manifestations are predictable for Wernicke's syndrome and include a delirium with a clouded sensorium and confusion, ophthalomoplegia, nystagmus, and ataxia. Peripherial neuropathies are commonly associated with the syndrome. All aspects of the syndrome will improve with the administration of thiamine, although not always completely. Many of the patients with Wernicke's syndrome will develop the Korsakoff syndrome, although a few will return to their premorbid state. The Korsakoff syndrome is characterized by a profound loss in recent memory, out of proportion to the other cognitive deficits. In other words, the Korsakoff patient may not remember dates and names but can calculate and abstract reasonably well in an intact personality (49).

Alcoholic peripheral neuropathy is characterized by diminished sensitivity to touch, pinprick, and vibration objectively, and to paraesthesias subjectively. These symptoms appear bilateral and symmetrical, most prominent in the distal portions of the extremities and in greater frequency and severity in the lower extremities. Both sensory and motor nerves are affected (49).

The alcoholic myopathy can be acute, subacute, or chronic in onset. Muscle weakness and atrophy may be present. More often an elevated creatinine phosphokinase (CPK) occurs in association with the symptoms of muscle cramps, weakness, and occasional dark urine (myoglobinuria). In severe cases, the rhabdomyolysis produces significant myoglobinuria with renal failure, which may be fatal. Most likely the etiology of the muscle damage is the direct toxic effect of ethanol on muscle. In most cases, discontinuation of alcohol consumption leads to improvement of the myopathy (1,2,49).

Cancer

Heavy drinking increases the risk of cancer in the tongue, mouth, oropharynx, hypopharynx, esophagus, larynx, and liver. In the United States, these sites represent approximately 10% of all cancers in the white population and 12% in the black population.

1. *Buccal cavity, pharynx, and larynx.* Cancers of the mouth, pharynx, and larynx appear to be related to heavy drinking. Tobacco is the leading risk factor for the development of these cancers, but alcohol carries an additional, increased risk to the development of cancer. Of course, cigarette smoking is common among alcoholics. One study showed that 93% of men and 91% of women in a group of alcoholic outpatients were smokers, proportions far above the prevalence for smoking in the general

population. A study, however, separated out the individual risk for cancer
of the mouth, and concluded that "heavy drinkers" had a 10-fold greater
risk of having cancer of the mouth than minimal drinkers. As the amount
of alcohol consumed is increased, the relative risk of cancer of the
mouth, extrinsic larynx, and esophagus was also increased, much more so
with whiskey than beer and wine.

2. *Esophagus*. Two-thirds of patients with cancer of the esophagus also have
   a history of heavy alcohol use. Investigators have shown a relationship
   between heavy drinking, especially of whiskey or other spirits, and esophageal cancer, after corrections for age and tobacco use were made.
   Smoking has been reported to less important than alcohol in the absence
   of heavy drinking.

3. *Large intestine and rectum*. In studies, a strong association between rectal
   and colonic cancer and alcohol, particularly beer, exists (1).

4. *Liver, primary*. Worldwide, almost 90% of all liver cell cancer arises in
   cirrhotic organs. The typical person with a primary cancer of the liver
   (hepatoma) is an alcoholic with cirrhosis. However, hepatoma may occur
   in alcoholics who do not have cirrhosis. The hepatoma seems to occur 2
   to 8 years after the onset of cirrhosis.

5. *Pancreas*. There may an association between alcohol consumption and
   pancreatic malignancy, particularly if pancreatitis exists before the onset
   of the pancreatic malignancy.

Infectious Diseases

Pneumonia is a frequent cause of illness and death for alcoholics. In some
studies, as many as 50% of all patients admitted with pneumonia were
alcoholics. Also, tuberculosis appears to be prevalent among alcoholics.
Other infectious diseases that are overrepresented among alcoholics are bacterial meningitis, peritonitis, and ascending cholangitis. Less serious infections are chronic sinusitis, pharyngitis and other minor infections (1,2).

The basis for an increased risk for infection among alcoholics is an immune system depressed by alcohol at the various sites of production of the
immune defense in the reticuloenthial system. Studies have demonstrated
decrease white cell production and response in active drinkers, in addition to
impaired antibody production.

References

1. Leiber CS (1982). *Medical Disorders of Alcoholism*. Philadelphia: W. B. Saunders.
2. Peterdorg RG, Adams RD, Braunwald E, et al., eds. (1983). *Harrison's Principles of Internal Medicine, 10th Ed.* New York: McGraw-Hill.
3. Miller NS, Gold MS, Cocores JA, Pottash HC (1988). Alcohol dependence and
   medical consequences. *NY State J Med* 88:476–481.

4. Mendelson JH, Mello NK (1985). *The Diagnosis and Treatment of Alcoholism, 2nd Ed*. New York: McGraw-Hill.
5. Clark LT, Friedman HS (1985). Hypertension associated with alcohol withdrawal: Assessment of mechanisms and complications. *Alcoholism* 9:125-130.
6. Kannel WB, Sorlie P (1974). Hypertension in Framingham. In *Epidemiology and Control of Hypertension*, Paul O, ed. New York: Station Intercontinental Medical Book Corp.
7. Klatsky AL, Friedman GD, Siegelaub AB, et al. (1977). Alcohol consumption and blood pressure. Kaiser-Permanente Multiphasic Health Examination data. *N Engl J Med* 296:1194-1200.
8. Friedman HS, Geller SA, Lieber CS (1982). The effect of alcohol on the heart, skeletal and smooth muscles. In *Medical Disorders of Alcoholism — Pathogenesis and Treatment*, Lieber CS, ed., pp. 436-479. Philadelphia: W.B. Saunders.
9. Fuster V, Gersh BJ, Giulaina ER, Tajik AJ, Brandenberg RO, Frye RL (1981). The natural history of idiopathic dilated cardiomyopathy. *Am J Cardiol* 47:525-531.
10. Demakis JG, Proskey A, Rahimtoola SH, et al. (1974). The natural course of alcoholic cardiomyopathy. *Ann Intern Med* 80:293-297.
11. Evans W (1961). Alcoholic cardiomyopathy. *Am Heart J* 61:556-567.
12. Williams RR, Horn JW (1977). Association of cancer sites with tobacco and alcohol consumption and socioeconomic status of patients: Interview study from the third national cancer survey. *J Natl Cancer Inst* 58:547.
13. Eckardt FF, Grace ND, Kantrowitz PA (1976). Does lower esophageal sphincter incompetency contribute to esophageal variceal bleeding? *Gastroenterology* 71:185-189.
14. Cooke AR (1972). Ethanol and gastric function. *Gastroenterology* 62:501-502.
15. Banks S (1981). Acute and chronic pancreatitis. In *Pancreatic Disease; Diagnosis and Therapy*, Dent TL, ed., pp. 167-188. New York: Grune & Stratton.
16. Sarles H (1974). Chronic calcifying pancreatitis — Chronic alcohol pancreatitis. *Gastroenterology* 66:604-616.
17. Strum WB, Spiro HM (1971). Chronic pancreatitis. *Ann Intern Med* 74:264-277.
18. Arvanitakis C, Greenberger NJ (1976). Diagnosis of pancreatic disease by a synthetic peptide. A new test of exocrine pancreatic function. *Lancet* 1:663-666.
19. Van Waes L, Lieber CS (1977a). Early perivenular sclerosis in alcoholic fatty liver, an index of progressive liver injury. *Gastroenterology* 73:646-650.
20. Van Waes L, Lieber CS (1977b). Glutamate dehydrogenase, a reliable marker of liver cell necrosis in the alcoholic. *Br J Med* 2:1508-1510.
21. DeRitis F, Coltorti M, Giusti G (1972). Serum-transaminase activities in liver disease. *Lancet* 1:685-687.
22. Ratnoff OD, Patek AJ Jr. (1942). Natural history of Laennec's cirrhosis of the liver. An analysis of 386 cases. *Medicine (Baltimore)* 21:207-268.
23. Popper H, Lieber CS (1980). Histogenesis of alcoholic fibrosis and cirrhosis in the baboon. *Am J Pathol* 98:695-716.
24. Powell WJ, Klatskin G (1968). Duration of survival in patients with Laenne's cirrhosis. Influence of alcohol withdrawal and possible effects of recent changes in general management of the disease. *Am J Med* 44:406-420.
25. Rubin E, Lieber CD (1968). Alcohol-induced hepatic injury in nonalcoholic volunteers. *N Engl J Med* 278:869-876.

26. Veitch RL, Lumeg L, Li TK (1974). The effects of ethanol and acetaldehyde on vitamin B_6 metabolism in liver. *Gastroenterology* 66:868.

27. Veitch RL, Lumeg L, Li TK (1975). Vitamin B_6 metabolism in chronic alcohol abuse: The effect of ethanol oxidation on hepatic pyrodosal 5′ phosphate metabolism. *J Clin Invest* 55:1026–1032.

28. Vlahcevic ZR, Buhac I, Ferrar JT, Bell CC, Swell L (1971). Bile acid metabolism of cholic acid metabolism. I. Kinetic aspects of cholic acid metabolism. *Gastroenterology* 60:491–498.

29. Herbert V, Zalusky R, Davidson CS (1963). Correlation of folate deficiency with alcoholism and associated macrocytosis, anemia and liver disease. *Ann Intern Med* 58:977–988.

30. Hermos JA, Adams WH, Liu YK, Sullivan LW, Trier JS (1972). Mucosa of the small intestine in folate-deficient alcoholics. *Ann Intern Med* 76:957–965.

31. Hines JD, Cowan DH (1970). Studies on the pathogenesis of alcohol-induced sideroblastic bone marrow abnormalities. *N Engl J Med* 283:441–446.

32. Tomasulo PA, Kater RMH, Iber FL (1968). Impairment of thiamine absorption in alcoholism. *Am J Clin Nutr* 21:1340–1344.

33. Eichner ER, Buchanan B, Smith JW, Hillman RS (1972). Variations in the hematologic and medical status of alcoholics. *Am J Med* 263:35–42.

34. Charlton RW, Jacobs P, Seftel H, Bothwell TH (1964). Effect of alcohol on iron absorption. *Br Med J* 2:1427–1429.

35. Russell RM, Morrison SA, Smith FR, Oaks EV, Carney E (1978). Vitamin A reversal of abnormal dark adaptation in cirrhosis. *Ann Intern Med* 88:622–626.

36. Sato M, Lieber CS (1981). Hepatic vitamin A depletion after chronic ethanol consumption in baboons and rats. *J Nutr* 111:2015–2023.

37. Leo MA, Lieber CS (1982). Hepatic vitamin A depletion in alcoholic liver injury. *N Engl J Med* 307:597–601.

38. Baran DT, Teitelbaum SL, Berfield MA, Parker G, Cruvant EM, Avoli LV (1980). Effect of alcohol ingestion on bone and mineral metabolism in rats. *Am J Physiol* 238:507–510.

39. Cederbaum AI, Lieber CS, Toth A, Beatty DS, Rubin E (1973). Effects of ethanol and fat on the transport of reducing equivalents into rat liver mitochondria. *J Biol Chem* 248:4977–4986.

40. Mendelson JH, Stein S (1966). Serum cortisol levels in alcoholic and nonalcoholic subject during experimentally induced alcohol intoxication. *Psychosom Med* 28:616–626.

41. Mendelson JH, Ogata M, Mello NK (1971). Adrenal function and alcoholism. I. Serum cortisol. *Psychosom Med* 33:145–157.

42. Davis VE, Brown H, Huff JA, Cashaw JL (1967). Ethanol-induced alterations of norepinephrine metabolism in man *J Lab Clin Med* 69:787–799.

43. Bleecker M, Ford DH, Rhines RK (1969). A comparison of 131-itriiodothyronine accumulation and degradation in ethanol-treated and control rats. *Life Sci* 8:267–275.

44. Bernstein J, Videla L, Israel Y (1975). Hormonal influences in the development of the hypermetabolic state of the liver produced by chronic administration of ethanol. *J Pharmacol Exp Ther* 192:583–591.

45. Medelson JH, Ellingboe J, Mello NK, Kuehnle J (1978). Effects of alcohol on plasma testosterone and luteinizing hormone levels. *Alcohol Clin Exp Res* 2:255–258.

46. Bhalla VK, Chen CJ, Gnanprakasam MS (1979). Effect of in vivo administration of human chorionic gonadotropin and ethanol on the process of testicular receptor depletion and replenishment. *Life Sci* 24:1315–1324.
47. Linkola J, Ylikhari R, Fyhrquist F, Wallenius M (1978). Plasma vasopressin in ethanol intoxication and hangover. *Acta Physiol Scand* 104:180–187.
48. Feinkel N, Singer DL, Arky RA, et al. (1963). Alcohol hypoglycemia. I. Carbohydrate metabolism in patients with clinical alcohol hypoglycemia and the experimental reproduction of the syndrome with pure ethanol. *J Clin Invest* 42:1112–1133.
49. Adams RP, Victor M (1985). *Principles of Neurology, 3d Ed.* New York: McGraw-Hill.
50. Parsons OA, Leber WR (1981). The relationship between cognitive dysfunction and brain damage in alcoholics: Casual, interactive, or epiphenomenal. *Alcoholism* 5:326–343.

CHAPTER 7

The Psychiatric Consequences of Alcohol and Drugs of Abuse and Addiction

History

Psychiatric symptoms are commonly associated with alcohol and drug use, particularly in chronic addictive use. The relationship between alcohol and drug addiction and idiopathic psychiatric disorders is complex and requires a thorough understanding of both categories of disorders. Not only are the etiology and prognosis of each disorder different, but each requires a unique and sophisticated approach to treatment (1–4).

It is important to bear in mind that there are no specific symptoms, including alcohol and drug addiction, that are peculiar to only a single psychiatric disorder. Typically, psychiatric symptoms cluster to form psychiatric syndromes in particular patterns that distinguish one syndrome from another. Furthermore, the relationship between psychiatric symptoms and alcohol and drug addiction provides significant overlap, with virtually all the psychiatric symptoms occurring between them (5,6). Furthermore, alcohol and drug addiction is an autonomous and primary disorder with a clinical course of its own.

The fundamental criteria of each disorder must be considered before the important aspects of the relationship between the addiction and psychiatric disorders are appreciated. Understanding and utilizing only one approach, such as "psychiatric" or "addictive," will yield less success and lead to errors in diagnosis and treatment. The basic definitions of the alcohol and drug addiction and psychiatric disorders must be comprehended before contemplating diagnosis and treatment. The definition for addiction is behavioral and includes three major and two minor criteria. The major criteria are essential to make the diagnosis, and the minor criteria are frequent accompaniments of the addictive process to alcohol and drugs but are not essential to the diagnosis of alcohol and drug addiction (7).

Diagnosis

Addiction

The major criteria are preoccupation with acquiring alcohol and drugs, the compulsive use of alcohol and drugs in spite of adverse consequences, and

77

the relapse to alcohol and drugs in spite of adverse consequences from their continued use. The minor criteria are tolerance and dependence to alcohol and drugs. Tolerance is the diminishing effect of alcohol and drugs at a constant dose or the need to increase the dose to maintain the same effect from the alcohol and drugs. Dependence is the onset of stereotypic and predictable signs and symptoms on the cessation of the use of a drug (7,8,9).

The development of tolerance and dependence is an expected occurrence in response to regular use of alcohol and drugs as an adaptation; however, neither is specific for addiction. Tolerance and dependence occur in the absence of addiction, although because of frequent use addiction usually involves the development of tolerance and dependence. Furthermore, addiction implies a loss of control over the use of alcohol and drugs because it is pervasive in the three major criteria of preoccupation, compulsivity, and relapse.

The acute and chronic use of alcohol and drugs produces signs and symptoms that occur predictably in susceptible individuals, particularly those who have developed an addiction to alcohol and drugs. A review of these signs and symptoms are necessary to appreciate the permutations of syndromes that are induced by alcohol and drugs. Acute use of alcohol and drugs does not ordinarily produce definable psychiatric syndromes beyond intoxication states that persist and require diagnosis and treatment, except in exceptional cases of intoxication overdose by the naive user. However, the chronic use of alcohol and drugs is particularly prone to the development of the signs and symptoms that constitute identifiable psychiatric syndromes. Characteristically, these signs and symptoms tend to cluster in aggregates to form a particular pattern as a syndrome for a particular drug or, more commonly, a combination of drugs and alcohol (7,10).

Other drugs produce the same symptoms that are produced by alcohol. Cocaine, marijuana, and phencyclidine (PCP) induce, during intoxication and withdrawal, intense anxiety and profound depression as well as hallucinations and delusions. The additive effect with alcohol is expected and does occur regularly. The concurrent use of alcohol and other drugs makes it difficult to distinguish between the separate effects of these respective drugs, although a clear predominance may emerge with careful inquiry (11).

Intoxication (Acute and Chronic)

Depression is a common syndrome that is induced by the state of chronic alcohol and drug intoxication. The depression may be mild and intermittent or severe and persistent, and is characterized by a lowered mood or decreased spirits and a depressed or constricted affect. Typically, boredom and lack of enthusiasm, energy, and interest in daily living accompany the depressed mood. In more severe cases, frank psychomotor retardation with dulled thought processes, impaired concentration and memory, slowed motor movements, and anhedonia with a lack of motivation for self-care may be manifested (12–14).

The depression is frequently associated with suicidal ideation, with a high rate of suicide attempts and completion. Twenty-five to 50% of all suicides involve the use of alcohol, often in alcoholics. One of the single most important risk factors for suicide is alcohol and drug addiction. A significant proportion, as many as 25% of alcoholics, die of suicide as a consequence of their alcoholism. The exact percentage of alcoholics that die of suicide because of associated drug use is unknown but is considered to be high (15,16).

Anxiety

Anxiety is also a common disorder that occurs almost inevitably in chronic alcohol and drug consumption. The acute and chronic use of alcohol and many drugs is always accompanied by some discharge of the sympathetic nervous system during the withdrawal state. The sympathetic nervous system when firing releases catecholamines, which produce the signs and symptoms of anxiety. The spectrum of the anxiety disorders induced by alcohol and drugs is wide, varying from mild anxiety to severe generalized anxiety and phobic states. Virtually all the states of the anxiety disorders can be produced by alcohol and drugs, including generalized anxiety, panic attacks, simple phobias, and agoraphobia. The alcoholic frequently has anxiety and irrational fears that are phobic and range from being afraid to leave the house to a diffuse fear of people, places, and things, such as driving an automobile, appearing in public, and socializing in outside drinking situations (17–24).

These symptoms of anxiety and depression may be particularly troublesome and may prompt the alcoholic and drug addict to seek treatment for the anxiety – but unfortunately, not for the alcoholism and drug addiction. The clinician must be vigilant and attentive to the possibility and likelihood that these symptoms are being produced by alcoholism and drug addiction and their effects. A persistent history with corroborative sources such as the family and employer is often necessary to establish alcoholism and drug addiction as the source of the anxiety.

Hallucinations and Delusions

Classical hallucinations and delusions are less frequent occurrences in chronic alcoholics and drug addicts; however, the denial regarding the consequences of alcoholism that is always present in alcoholics and drug addicts is of delusional nature and proportions, although not considered a classical delusion. With alcohol, the hallucinations typically occur as part of the abstinence syndrome in the form of auditory or visual hallucinations. The alcoholic hallucinosis, as it is termed, occurs in a clear sensorium that is to be distinguished from the hallucinations that occur in a clouded sensorium as a part of delirium tremens. The auditory hallucinations are usually of a derogatory nature, condemning and accusatory, and resolve eventually with continued abstinence; however, months may pass before they do. The visual hallucinations are less frequent and are typically, as in delirium tremens, zooscopic in type with animals being visualized, often insects or rodents or snakes. These also may take months to subside with abstinence from alcohol (25).

The predominant delusions are paranoid in nature, and originate in part from the toxic disturbance of the brain from the alcohol and drugs, as do the hallucinations. The delusions take the form of irrational fear that someone or something is out to get the alcoholic and drug addict. They are a part of the delirium tremens, but often occur on their own in a clear sensorium (25). The cocaine-induced delusional syndrome is characterized by paranoia that can persist for days, weeks, or months.

Personality

The effect on personality of alcohol and drugs is clear and dramatic. Because of the cumulative toxic effects of alcohol and drugs, insight and judgment become impaired and are exercised in improper and self-destructive ways. The typical syndromes of personality disturbances that arise are antisocial, narcissistic, borderline, histrionic, schizoid, dependent, immature, and passive-dependent. The deterioration in personality that occurs as a result of the toxic and addictive process of alcohol and drugs is often devastating. However, the changes in the personality occur insidiously over time and almost imperceptibly at any moment in the progression, but become obvious when a sufficient interval of time has passed for a comparison to be made. These personality changes are frequently reversible with abstinence and specific treatment for the addiction. For some changes, only a relatively brief time is required for reversibility whereas other changes in personality may require a prolonged period; months and years may be required after specific treatment of the alcoholism (26–28).

Denial

The denial of the alcoholism and drug addiction and its consequences is delusional, and can taken the form of a fixed, false belief that is irrational and contrary to the evidence. The denial is accompanied by minimization, rationalization, and projection, which are utilized to deflect the focus of the alcoholism and drug addiction away from the alcoholic to some other reason or person. Typically, the focus is shifted from the responsibility of the alcoholic to those close to the alcoholic such as a family member, an employer, or "society." When the denial is confronted, it is often resistant to rational evidence of the consequences of the alcoholism and drug addiction.

The denial is a mixture of diffuse disruption of the brain from the chemical effect of alcohol and drugs and the intrapsychic, intradynamic defense mechanisms of repression, rationalization, and projection (29).

Other Causes

The nonspecific nature of the psychiatric symptoms are also seen in other conditions that produce a diffuse disruption of brain function. Primary systemic illnesses occurring throughout the body affecting the brain secondarily are common causes of anxiety, depression, hallucinations, and delusions. These symptoms of underlying illnesses are abundant in medical and surgical practices. Primary diseases of the brain such as meningoencephalitis, tumors, and degenerative processes are also common etiologies of anxiety, depressions, hallucinations, and delusions (30).

Psychiatric Syndromes

Idiopathic psychiatric syndromes are typically of unknown origin and consist of signs and symptoms that tend to cluster in a pattern sufficiently common to produce a definable syndrome that serves as a diagnostic category. Anxiety disorders are separated into generalized anxiety, panic attacks, phobic states, and posttraumatic stress disorders. Depression is either termed a major depression as a diagnosis or part of the spectrum of bipolar illness that includes unipolar depression or manic-depressive illness. Schizophrenia is a syndrome of psychotic symptoms such as hallucinations, delusions, and personality deterioration, which may have multiple etiologies with schizophrenia as a final common pathway. Personality disorders are many and include antisocial, borderline, histrionic, schizotypal, passive, aggressive, and other disorders. A personality disorder is defined as a collection of personality traits that are maladaptive and develop during early childhood before the age of 15 years. These traits are constant and enduring, and do not vary over time or depend on circumstances for expression. Personality disorders define the individual in a predominant pattern of behavior that is characteristic for that type of personality disorder. Considerable overlap may occur in the personality traits so that multiple personality disorders may occur in the same individual.

Differentiating Induced from Idiopathic Psychiatric Illness

Some guidelines can be employed to distinguish between the psychiatric syndromes that are caused by alcohol and drugs and those that exist as idiopathic syndromes by themselves. The first important step is to recognize that alcohol and drugs produce psychiatric syndromes, and that the reverse concept, that idiopathic psychiatric disorders cause "addictive" alcohol and drug use, is not a clinically relevant approach. Once an addictive pattern has established itself, the preoccupation with acquiring alcohol, compulsive use of alcohol, and recurrent relapse to alcohol take precedence over other aspects of the clinical picture and tend to determine the course of both the addiction and the additional idiopathic psychiatric disorder. The behaviors of addiction are autonomous, having a life of their own, and do not depend on another psychiatric condition to sustain them. The addiction supplants the symptoms of the other disorder to produce a clinical course that will not be altered significantly by treating only the "underlying," "other," idiopathic psychiatric disorder.

It is clinically useful to separate the two conditions according to their diagnostic criteria, prognosis, and response to treatment. Although the addiction and the idiopathic psychiatric disorder are interrelated, and each affects the course of the other, it is essential to diagnosis and treatment to keep in mind the individual characteristics of each. The idiopathic psychiatric disorder may or may not predispose to the use of alcohol. The self-medication concept of "addictive" use of alcohol and drugs is used to explain addictive use but it fails to account for salient features of addiction. Both the psychiatrically disordered and the relatively normal individual begin using alcohol and drugs for similar reasons. The reasons for alcohol use are numerous and include happiness, sadness, celebration, mourning, victory, and defeat. The use of alcohol and drugs is often predicated on normal and abnormal states that in themselves are not specific and distinguishing. At some point either early or late in the course of alcohol and drug use, the addictive process is initiated, with ensuing consequences that are often psychiatric in nature. The resultant adverse consequences from the addictive process are often worse than the original symptoms that are ascribing as initiating the addictive use. The addiction supersedes the other psychiatric conditions, and the addictive use continues in spite of the accruing psychiatric consequences and not because of them (29,31,32).

An illustrative example is provided by a study conducted to examine the effect of alcohol on mood. Three groups of subjects were given alcohol to record the response in the mood to the effects of alcohol. The groups of depressed alcoholics, depressed nonalcoholics, and nondepressed nonalcoholics responded differently than expected to the ingestion of a small amount of alcohol. The depressed alcoholic experienced the least benefit with a lowered mood in response to alcohol, whereas the depressed nonalcoholic experienced the greatest improvement in mood followed by the nondepressed nonalcoholic, whose mood improvement was between the other two groups (33).

Furthermore, when the drinking histories of nonalcoholic, manic-depressive individuals are studied, some interesting findings are available. The alcohol consumption of the manic-depressives shows no consistent pattern during a depressive episode; it will either decrease, remain the same, or increase. The drinking will increase during a manic phase, most likely consistent with the increased activity of behaviors of many types that are associated with the excesses, indiscretions, and manifestations of poor judgment of the manic state (33,34).

The conclusions from these studies are that alcoholics continue to drink alcohol in spite of adverse reactions of mood from alcohol or the alcohol-induced depression, and not because of it. The other important conclusion is that it is erroneous to view addictive alcohol use on the basis of a nonalcoholic experience with alcohol. The nonalcoholic may drink for pleasure or mood elevation but stops short of the adverse consequences because addictive use is not occurring. Ironically, the alcoholic does not appear to "feel good," because drinking makes them "feel bad" (33,34).

Studies have characterized the course of depression in alcoholics, particularly, in the active phase of drinking and the acute withdrawal period. These studies have also been performed on chronic users of other drugs such as cocaine, PCP, marijuana, and sedative/hypnotic drugs. The alcohol and drug-induced depression becomes increasingly severe with larger doses and longer duration of use, particularly heavy chronic use. The depression often diminishes with decreasing doses and intermittent periods of abstinence and disappears with prolonged abstinence from the alcohol and drugs (35–38).

In the majority of cases, the depression will remit within days of the cessation of use of alcohol and drugs, although perhaps as many as 10% to 20% of those who are depressed will have a more lasting depression that may take weeks, perhaps months, to subside. Specific treatment of the addiction and additional psychotherapy as needed will usually suffice to treat most casesdof lingering depression (39,40). In a few cases, 1% to 2%, the depression will persist and be attributable to another form of intervention in addition to the treatment of addiction. Antidepressants may be employed in those 1% to 2% of the cases of a persistent depression but are not indicated in the instances of the transient depressions that eventually subside. Additionally, a large number of alcoholics and drug addicts will have suicidal thinking during the course of the addictive use; some will actually attempt suicide, and of those, some will succeed.

Anxiety is another symptom that is commonly associated with alcohol and drug use and is similar to depression; the larger the doses and the longer the duration of use, the more frequent and severe the anxiety. The anxiety takes many forms as previously discussed and generally will subside with less alcohol and drug use, particularly with some periods of abstinence intermixed. The anxiety tends to remit with time with prolonged abstinence from alcohol and drugs. The acute withdrawal from alcohol and drugs is characterized by intense anxiety, followed by lower intensity over sometimes a protracted course of weeks and months, and perhaps years (18). Persistent, incapacitating anxiety may be treated with low-dose antidepressants with the plan of attempting to discontinue them at some point to determine the continued need.

Intervention and Treatment

Laboratory drug testing is a particularly valuable diagnostic tool in evaluating new and old patients and distinguishing between a drug-induced syndrome from an idiopathic psychiatric syndrome. At times the history of drug use is not available or denied during the interview, and a properly obtained blood and urine screen for drugs is very useful.

The laboratory can aid in making a differential diagnosis and identifying drugs as an active consideration as a cause of psychosis, depression, mania, and personality changes as well as other psychiatric symptoms. Treatment planning and prevention of serious medical consequences often rest on the use of drug screening. Moreover, testing is widely used to monitor progress or relapse in the treatment of alcohol and drug addiction in inpatient and outpatient settings.

The appropriate use of analytical technology in drug testing requires an understanding of available test methodologies. These include drug screening by thin-layer chromatography, comprehensive testing using enzyme immunoassay, and confirmation by gas chromatography-mass spectrometry (GC-MS).

Pharmacological Interventions

Pharmacological intervention is relatively contraindicated in this population, as most drugs that are used in the treatment of anxiety such as benzodiazepines are highly addicting in the alcoholic and drug addict. The benzodiazepines and other sedatives-hypnotics share pharmacological cross-tolerance and dependence with alcohol. The specific treatment of addiction and other behavioral techniques are most often indicated for the treatment of anxiety in this population (19,35).

Significant anxiety is usually induced by the alcohol and drugs, although recovery from alcoholism and drug addiction is marked by anxiety and depression from other nonpharmacological causes. The anxiety and depression result from a number of nonpharmacological reasons, derived from the psychological changes that must occur in the recovering alcoholic to abstain from alcohol and drugs and from the external factors that may have reached crisis proportions because of neglect and poor judgment by the alcohol and drug addict. These external factors are often difficulties in the areas of major life concerns such as marriage, employment, and legal matters.

Occasionally, the delusions and hallucinations from alcohol and drugs may persist beyond the period of intoxication and acute detoxification. These symptoms persist uncommonly in alcoholics, although they do occur as in alcoholic hallucinosis. Persisting delusions are more common from heavy, high-dose use of cocaine, PCP, and other hallucinogens. These aberrations in thinking are often paranoid in nature and may range from ideas of reference to frank delusions of persecution. A protracted period of weeks to months may be required for these effects from the drugs to subside. If these symptoms are troublesome and of a magnitude that interfere with adequate psychological functioning, short-term use of neuroleptics may be employed to treat the delusions and hallucinations as they occur in the drug-induced states (41).

The use of medications in the alcoholic and drug addict as a rule should be conservative because their basic problem is loss of control over alcohol and drugs. They have difficulties in controlling medications similar to those they have in controlling alcohol and drugs of addiction. A common attitude among alcoholics and drug addicts is that if one pill works, then two or three must be better. The judgment regarding self-medication in the alcoholic is sometimes as distorted toward medications as it is toward the alcohol and drugs of addiction.

Further, most psychotropic medications have adverse sedative and other mood-altering effects on the mentation and emotions of the alcoholic. Antidepressants produce alterations in mood and thinking, and thus they may have an adverse pharmacological effect on the alcoholic. Some antihypertensives are sedating and produce aberrations in thinking. There are many other medications that should be used with special consideration and caution in the alcoholic and drug addict. The clinical rule of thumb is that any condition that is not a result of the alcoholism and drug addiction should be treated, if required, by weighing the risks and benefits of the use of medications in a population with a relative contraindication for pharmacological effects.

Finally, the signs and symptoms of alcoholism and drug addiction do not respond to pharmacological intervention because there is no specific pharmacological treatment for addiction. The exceptional medication in the treatment of alcoholism may be antabuse, used as an adjunct to the mainstay treatment of the addiction to reduce the likelihood of impulsive drinking.

The idiopathic psychiatric and medical disorders should be treated as they would be ordinarily with important considerations. The need for medications may be less frequent and in smaller doses when the alcohol and drug use has been eliminated because of diminishing cross-tolerance and dependence. Also the practice of empirical, trial-and-error medicating for atypical symptoms should be avoided in the high-risk populations of alcoholics and drug addicts. Importantly, the proper treatment of the additional idiopathic psychiatric disorder has a greater likelihood of success by treating the alcohol and drug addiction. The persistence of a schizophrenic syndrome in an alcoholic will significantly reduce the probability of resisting alcohol use originating from the addictive process. The adequate treatment of a depression will allow the alcoholic to continue to treat the addiction to alcohol. Incapacitating anxiety will also interfere with an acceptable level of functioning to abstain from alcohol and drugs. Finally, behavioral programs and intensive psychotherapy may be needed to treat significant personality problems that may be obstructing proper treatment of the alcohol and drug addiction.

References

1. Helzer JE, Prysbeck TR (1988). The co-occurrence of alcoholism with other psychiatric disorders in the general population and its impact on treatment. *J Stud Alcohol* 49(3):219–224.
2. Schuckit MA (1982). The history of psychotic symptoms in alcoholics. *J Clin Psychiatry* 43(2):53–57.
3. Powell BJ, Penick EC, Othmer E, Bingham SF, Rice A (1982). Prevalence of additional psychiatric syndromes among male alcoholics. *J Clin Psychiatry* 43(10):404–407.
4. Wolf AW, Schubert DSP, Patterson MB, Grande TP, Brocco KJ, Pendleton L (1988). Association among major psychiatric diagnoses. *J Consult Clin Psychol* 56(2):292–294.
5. Schuckit MA (1983). Alcoholism and other psychiatric disorders. *Hosp Community Psychiatry* 34(11):1022–1027.
6. Schuckit M (1983). Alcoholic patients with secondary depression. *Am J Psychiatry* 140:6.
7. Miller NS, Gold MS (1989). Suggestions for changes in DSM-III-R criteria for substance use disorders. *Am J Drug Alcohol Abuse* 15(2):223–230.
8. Jaffe JH (1985). Drug addiction and drug abuse. In *The Pharmacological Bases of Therapeutics*, 6th Ed., Gilman GS, Goodman LS, Rall TW, Murad F, eds., pp. 532–540. New York: Macmillan.
9. APA (1987). *Psychoactive Substance Use Disorders Diagnostic and Statistical Manual of Mental Disorders*, 3d Ed (revised). Washington, DC: American Psychiatric Association.
10. Woodruff RA, Guze SB, Clayton PJ, Carr D (1979). Alcoholism and depression. In *Alcoholism and Affective Disorders*, Goodwin RA, Erickson CK, eds., pp. 39–47. New York: SP Medical and Scientific Books.
11. Miller NS, Mirin SM (1982). Multiple drug use in alcoholics: Practical and theoretical implications. *Psychiatr Ann* 19(5):248–253.
12. Schuckit MA (1982). Prevalence of affective disorder in a sample of young men. *Am J Psychiatry* 139(11):1431–1436.
13. Peace K, Mellsop G (1987). Alcoholism and psychiatric disorder. *Aust NZ J Psychiatry* 21:94–101.
14. Martin RL, Cloninger CR, Guze SB (1985). Alcohol misuse and depression in women criminals. *J Stud Alcohol* 46(1):65–71.
15. Martin RL, Cloninger CR, Guze SB, Clayton PJ (1985). Mortality in a follow-up of 500 psychiatric outpatients. I. Total mortality. *Arch Gen Psychiatry* 42:47–66.
16. Litman RF, Feberow NL, Wold CI, Brown TR (1974). Prediction models of suicidal behaviors. In *The Prediction of Suicide*, Beck H, Resick LP, Letteri DJ, eds., p. 141. Bowie, MD: Charles Press.
17. Small P, Stockwell T, Cantar S, Hodgson R (1984). Alcohol dependence and phobic anxiety states. I. A prevalence study. *Br J Psychiatry* 144:53–57.
18. Stockwell T, Small P, Hodgson R, Cantar S (1984). Alcohol dependence and phobic anxiety stated. II. A retrospective study. *Br J Psychiatry* 144:58–63.
19. Schuckit MA (1987). Dual diagnosis: Substance abuse and anxiety. *Psychiatr Times* 20–21.

20. Rounsaville BJ, Dolinsky ZS, Babor TF, Meyer RE (1987). Psychopathology as a predictor of treatment outcome in alcoholics. *Arch Gen Psychiatry* 44:505–513.
21. Stavynski A, Lamontagne Y, Lavallee YJ (1986). Clinical phobias and avoidant personality disorder among alcoholics admitted to an alcoholism rehabilitation setting. *Can J Psychiatry* 31:714–719.
22. Bibb JL, Chambless DL (1986). Alcohol use and abuse among diagnosed agoraphobics. *Behav Res Ther* 24(1):49–58.
23. Bowen RC, Cipywnyk CMD, D'Arcy C, Keegan D (1984). Alcoholism, anxiety disorders and agoraphobia. *Alcohol Clin Exp Res* 8(1):48–50.
24. Weiss KJ, Rosenberg DJ (1985). Prevalence of anxiety disorder among alcoholics. *J Clin Psychiatry* 46:3–5.
25. Adams RP, Victor M (1985). *Principles of Neurology*, 3d Ed. New York: McGraw-Hill.
26. Mirin SM, Weiss RD (1986). Psychopathology in chronic cocaine abusers. *Am J Drug Alcohol Abuse* 12(1/2):17–29.
27. Reich J, Chaudry D (1987). Personality of panic disorder of alcoholics. *J Nerv Ment Dis* 175:224–228.
28. Gawin FH, Kleber HD (1986). Abstinence symptomatology and psychiatric diagnosis in cocaine abusers: Clinical observations. *Arch Gen Psychiatry* 43:107–113.
29. Miller NS (1987). A primer of the treatment process for alcoholism and drug addiction. *Psychiatry Lett* 5(7):30–37.
30. Peterdorg RG, Adams RD, Braunwald F, eds. (1983). *Harrison's Principles of Internal Medicine*, 10th Ed. New York: McGraw-Hill.
31. Goodwin DW, Guze SB (1980). *Psychiatric Diagnosis*. New York: Oxford University Press.
32. Milam JR, Ketcham K (1981). *Under the Influence*. Kirkland, WA: Madrona.
33. Mayfield DG (1979). Alcohol and affect: Experimental studies. In *Alcoholism and Affective Disorders*, Goodwin DW, Erickson CK, eds., pp. 99–107. New York: SP Medical and Scientific Books.
34. Schuckit MA (1979). Alcoholism and affective disorder: Diagnostic confusion. In *Alcoholism and Affective Disorders*, Goodwin DW, Erickson CK, eds., pp. 9–19. New York: SP Medical and Scientific Books.
35. Lader M, Petursson H (1983). Long-term effects of benzodiazepines. *Neuropharmacology* 22:527–533.
36. Liskow B, Mayfield D, Thiele J (1982). Alcohol and affective disorder: Assessment and treatment. *J Clin Psychiatry* 43(4):144–147.
37. Post RM, Kotin J, Goodwin FK (1974). The effects of cocaine on depressed patients. *Am J Psychiatry* 131(5):511–517.
38. Blankfield A (1986). Psychiatric symptoms in alcohol dependence: Diagnostic and treatment implications. *J Subst Abuse Treat* 3:275–278.
39. Schuckit MA (1985). The clinical implications of primary diagnostic groups among alcoholics. *Arch Gen Psychiatry* 42:1043–1049.
40. Miller NS (1988). PCP: A dangerous drug. *Am Fam Physician* 38(3):215–218.
41. Miller NS, Gold MS, Millman RB (1989). Cocaine. *Am Fam Physician* 39(2):115–120.

CHAPTER 8

The Pharmacology of Alcohol and Drugs and Sexual Responsivity

History

The human sexual response has been divided into four phases by Masters and Johnson on the basis of identifiable and measurable responses during sexual activity. The first phase is excitement, followed sequentially by the plateau, orgasmic, and resolution phases. The derivation of these phases has been based on interviewing and measuring the behavioral and physiological accompaniments of the human sexual response in hundreds of subjects (1).

The excitement phase is the arousal produced by stimulation, either physical or psychological, for the achievement of adequate sexual excitement (Figure 8.1). In the male, adequate arousal results in penile erection, which occurs within 3 to 8 seconds. As the phase is prolonged, thickening and

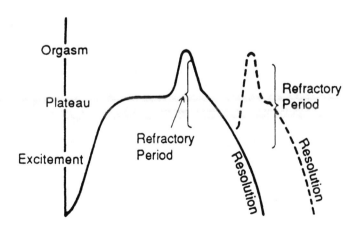

FIGURE 8.1. The male sexual response cycle. From: Masters WH, Johnson VE (1966). *Human Sexual Response*, p. 5. Boston: Little, Brown.

elevation of the scrotal sac is followed by partial testicular elevation and size increase. In the female, vaginal lubrication occurs within 10 to 30 seconds, with thickening of vaginal walls and labia, followed by expansion of the inner two-thirds of the vagina and elevation of the cervix and corpus with eventual tumescence of the clitoris (1) (Figure 8.2).

The plateau is characterized by an increase in the penile coronal circumference and testicular tumescence (50%–100% enlarged) (see Figure 8.1). Full testicular elevation and rotation occur with a purple hue of the corona of the penis, and mucoid secretion flow from the Cowper's gland. In the female, the orgasmic platform in the outer third of the vagina expands with full expansion of the inner two-thirds of the vagina, and uterine and cervical elevation further inward. The body skin acquires a reddish or rosy hue. Enlargement of the clitoris and mucoid secretions from Bartholin's glands subsequently occur. The plateau phase is characterized by an intensification of sexual tension, which can be brief or prolonged depending on the intensity of the stimuli and drive for orgasm (1).

The orgasmic phase is also called an involuntary climax. The duration is only a few seconds in which the vasocongestion and myotonia, which have developed from sexual stimulation in the excitement and plateau phases, are released during orgasm (see Figure 8.1). The orgasmic phase on an average lasts less than a minute. The subjective awareness of the orgasm is pelvic in focus, specifically concentrated in the clitoral body of the vagina and uterus in the female (Fig. 8.2) and in the penis in the male, particularly the prostate and seminal vesicles. There is a great variation in both intensity and duration in the female orgasmic experience, while the male tends to follow standard patterns of ejaculatory reaction with less individual variation. In the male, there are contractions of accessory organs of reproduction, including the vas deferens, seminal vesicles, ejaculatory duct, and prostate, with

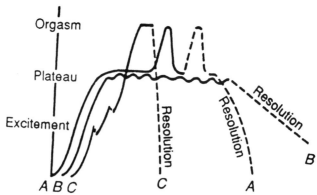

FIGURE 8.2. The female sexual response. From: Masters WH, Johnson VE (1966). *Human Sexual Response,* p. 5. Boston: Little, Brown.

relaxation of the external bladder sphincter. The contraction of the penile urethra occurs at 0.8-sec intervals for 3 or 4 contractions, slowing thereafter for 2 to 4 or more contractions. The anal sphincter may contract 2 to 4 times at 0.8-sec intervals. The female experiences a pelvic response but no ejaculation. The uterus in the female contracts from the fundus toward the lower uterine segment with minimal relaxation of the external cervical opening. Contractions of the orgasmic platform occurs at 0.8-sec intervals for 5 to 12 contractions, slowing thereafter for 3 to 6 contractions. The 2 to 4 external rectal sphincter contractions occur at 0.8-sec intervals. The external urethral sphincter contractions occur 2 or 3 times at irregular intervals in a small number of subjects (1).

The resolution phase is also involuntary (see Figure 8.1). During this phase, a reversal of the reaction pattern to the previously developed tension returns the individual through the plateau and excitement levels to the un- stimulated state. The females have less potential for returning to another orgasmic experience from any point beyond an initial part of the resolution phase if they submit to reapplication of effective stimuli (see Figure 8.2). However, the females do have facility for multiple orgasms if the reversal is instituted at the plateau tension level before resolution has begun. The males on the other hand have an obligatory refractory period after orgasm during which the physiological ability to respond to restimulation is much slower than that of the female. The physiological residuals of sexual myotonic tension usually are dissipated slowly in both male and female. Total involu- tion is completed only after all manner of sexual stimuli have been with- drawn. In the male, the refractory period occurs with a rapid loss of pelvic vasocongestion and loss of penile erection in a rapid and in a slower stage. In the female, during the period of the potential for ready return to orgasm, there is a retarded loss of pelvic vasocongestion. The loss of the sex skin color change and of the orgasmic platform occurs with the loss of the remainder of pelvic vasocongestion, which resolves more slowly in the fe- male. The clitoral tumescence subsides and returns to the normal position in the female (1).

General Reactions

General body reactions during the human sexual response as measured by Masters and Johnson are the following: in the male, 30% experienced nipple erection, 25% sexual flush, and most experienced carpopedal spasms, gener- alized skeletal muscle tension, hyperventilation, and tachycardia between 100 and 160 beats per minute. During the orgasmic phase, specific "convul- sive," skeletal, muscle contraction occurs with hyperventilation and continu- ing tachycardia. During the resolution phase the sweating, hyperventilation, and tachycardia resolve. In the female the events are essentially the same except the sex tension flush occurred in 75% (1).

Orgasm has a steeper onset for younger individuals and a more gradual

onset for older persons. The physiological evidence is that women can respond in all phases of the human sexual response almost as quickly as
males. The average female takes 4 minutes to reach orgasm during mastur-
bation whereas the average male takes 2 to 4 minutes. Some women can
achieve orgasm in 15 to 30 seconds, however. According to the Greeks,
orgasm was one of the most intense feelings, as an explosive discharge
ensues from the accumulated vascular and neuromuscular tension. Men and
women are similar physiologically in the human sexual response. Orgasm
may be very subdued, but most commonly a combination of genital and
total body responses is visible. The face is distorted, the extremities are
extended, the abdomen is hard, the neck stiff, and the eyes huge, as the
whole body convulses in synchrony with genital throbs or twitches. Moans
or screams and carpopedal spasms usually occur. The male has a sensation
that ejaculation is imminent with urethral contractions and fluids moving
out under pressure. The female experience is momentary suspension, followed by a peak, intense sensation in the clitoris that spreads through the
pelvis with a suffusion of warmth in the pelvis and body and with a throb-
bing of the pelvis (1).

According to psychoanalytic theory, the more mature the orgasm, the
more vaginal it is in nature. Physiologically there is only one type of orgasm;
the clitoris and vagina respond identically whether directly involved or not.
Subjectively they may differ, as a clitoral orgasm may be more intense and
vaginal more satisfying (the vaginal wall is less sensitive). The aftereffects of
orgasm are muscle relaxation, decreased vasocongestion, mind reawakening,
return of the senses, peace, gratification, and feeling sleepy or exhilarated,
and thirsty or hungry (1).

The Autonomic Nervous System and Sexual Performance

The mechanism of arousal involves memory and imagination through con-
nections from cerebral centers to the autonomic innervations. The sensory
nerves are the same as for other nonsexual functions, including touch perception which is transmitted from receptors in the periphery to the spinal
cord and brain. The mechanism of erection for both men and women includes impulses to the spinal cord through the autonomic spinal nerves in
the sacrum. The parasympathetic nervous system causes arterial dilatation,
and the sympathetic nervous system causes arterial constriction. Sexual
stimulation involves activation of the parasympathetic nerves so that there is
a rush of blood into the cavernous and spongy tissue of the penis. A loss of
erection consists of inhibition of the parasympathetic nerves and constriction of the blood vessels by activation of the sympathetic nerves. The mechanism of ejaculation involves sympathetic nervous stimulation with vasoconstriction and contractions of the penis. The homologous equivalence of
erection in females is vasoengorgement in the labia, clitoris, and vagina, and
ejaculation equals orgasmic contractions that occur in the orgasmic platform of the outer one-third of the vagina and other pelvic organs (2).

Sexual Dysfunction

The three basic categories of sexual function include desire, performance, and satisfaction. Disorders of sexual function are termed disinterest, dysfunction, and dissatisfaction.

Prevalence

Because various forms of sexual dysfunction are so commonly associated with alcohol and drug use, complaints in the area of sexual performance should suggest obtaining a history of alcohol and drug use. Decreased desire (libido) regularly occurs in men and women who frequently consume alcohol or use drugs and medications. Paradoxically, alcohol and drugs may induce uninhibited, aggressive sexual behavior that is offensive and violent.

Acute or chronic use of alcohol and drugs produce sexual dysfunction in both men and women that can be measured by the physiological responses. More subtly, these agents may dull the emotional responses and impair the ability to experience the intimacy required for mutual satisfaction and adequacy in sexual performance (3–5).

Intoxication

Disinterest is a lack of desire for sexual activity. The reasons for disinterest are frequently mental or emotional, although specific definition is complex. Drugs that affect the cerebral cortex and the limbic system interfere with motivation, judgment, and emotionality. Many drugs can enhance sexual desire and performance in small or low doses. These "aphrodisiacs" include nitrates, bromocriptine, L-dopa, alcohol, cocaine, marijuana, heroin, and phenylcyclidine (PCP). However, beyond a low threshold dose, and in chronic use, the higher cortical functions and limbic systems are diffusely impaired to result in a reduction in the desire for sexual activity. Other drugs that decrease desire include central-acting sympatholytic antihypertensives such as reserpine, alpha methyldopa, clonidine, and propranolol. Tranquilizers such as benzodiazepines, barbiturates, tricyclic antidepressants, and phenothiazines diffusely impair higher cortical functioning and the limbic system and therefore interfere with desire and motivation. Moreover, any drug that acts diffusely on the neurons in the brain, as many do, can frequently decrease the interest or desire (6–9) (Table 8.1).

Performance

Requisite for sexual performance are vasocongestion and myotonia. Impotence is defined as dysfunction with either or both erection and orgasm (ejaculation). Any process that interferes with the congestion or myotonia produces dysfunction by interfering with erection and orgasm in males and

TABLE 8.1. Summary of alcohol and drug effects.[a]

	Cerebral cortex and limbic system			Autonomic nervous system			Endocrine gland		
	Cell membranes	Neuro-transmitters	Pre- and postsynaptic receptors	Cell membranes	Neuro-transmitters	Pre- and postsynaptic receptors	Testosterone	Estrogen	Prolactin
Alcohol	+	+[b]	+	+	−	+	+	+	+
Barbiturates	+	GABA	+	+	−	+	−	−	−
Benzodiazepines	+	GABA	+	+	−	+	−	−	−
Cannabis	+	−	+	+	−	−	−	−	−
Cocaine	−	+[c]	+	−	+[c]	+	−	−	+
Heroin	−	−	+[d]	−	−	+	−	−	−
Antidepressants	−	+[c]	+	−	+[c]	−	−	−	−
Antipsychotics	−	+[c]	+	−	+[c]	−	−	−	+
Antihypertensives	−	+[c]	+	−	+[c]	−	−	−	+
Bromocriptine	−	−	+	−	−	−	−	−	+
L-Dopa	−	−	+	−	−	−	−	−	+

[a]From Gilman AG, Goodman LS, Rall TW, Murad F (1985). *The Pharmacological Basis of Therapeutics*, 7th Ed. New York: Macmillan.
[b]May affect many neurotransmitters.
[c]Catecholamines.
[d]Opiate receptors.

females. Specifically, drugs can act in the cerebral cortex, the limbic system, the spinal cord, spinal nerves, and receptor endings to interfere with autonomic nervous system function and therefore with erection and orgasm. This dysfunction applies to both males and females because the neurophysiology for both sexes is similar. Drugs that enhance sexual activity in low doses actually interfere at higher doses and (at low doses) with chronic use. Nitrates, which promote vasodilation, enhance vasocongestion in low doses, but in higher doses decrease peripheral resistance to a level too low to allow for perfusion and accumulation of blood in the penis, resulting in dysfunction. Alcohol in chronic administration results in decreased erections and premature orgasm (6,7,10).

Adrenergic blocking agents can inhibit the innervation to the vas deferens and epididymis so that less semen is presented to the posterior urethra, resulting in less stimulation for ejaculation. Adrenergic blockade also results in decreased erection, secondary to lowered blood flow because of decreased peripheral resistance in the vasculature. Retrograde ejaculation may occur from sympathetic blockade of the internal urethra sphincter, which does not close as it ordinarily does during ejaculation. Alcohol, barbiturates, benzodiazepines, and other general depressants decrease erection and orgasm by decreasing spinal reflexes and transmission in peripheral nerves. Also, decreased vaginal secretions and responses occur secondary to these depressant drugs. Other drugs that have anticholinergic activity, such as antidepressants, antihistamines, and anticholinergic agents, decrease blood flow by blockade of the parasympathetic nervous system and result in decreased erection and ejaculation of the penis in the male and decreased engorgement and enlargement of the vagina, clitoris, vulva, and uterus and decreased orgasm in the female (6,7,10).

Amphetamines and cocaine in small doses may cause a sustained erection and delay in orgasm (ejaculation), although in moderate to high doses these drugs result in impotence and inorgasmia secondary to poor erection, ejaculation, engorgement, and orgasm. Heroin also produces decreased erection and orgasm in moderate to high doses, especially with chronic use (6,7,10).

Alcohol in low doses may aid in erection and orgasm by decreasing cortical excitement and enhancing inhibition of the sympathetic nervous system. However, in moderate to high doses, and especially in chronic use, spinal reflexes are inhibited, serum testosterone level is decreased, and estrogen is increased secondary to alcohol-induced testicular and liver damage. The dysfunction is often reversible but may be permanent if significant testicular and liver damage occur. In women, subjective perceptions of sexual arousal and vaginal vasocongestion are less with increasing intoxication with alcohol. Also, premature ejaculation commonly occurs during withdrawal from alcohol and other drugs, particularly depressants; withdrawal from alcohol and drugs stimulates and activates the sympathetic nervous system, which promotes ejaculation (6,7,10).

Antipsychotic medications that block dopamine transmission result in decreased motor activity, and many have increased adrenergic blockade action, resulting in decreased erections secondary to reduced peripheral resistance and blood flow (6,7,10).

Satisfaction

In low doses, as discussed, certain drugs such as alcohol benzodiazepines, and cocaine enhance sexual pleasure directly through stimulation of the limbic system and indirectly by inhibiting anxiety and promoting a relaxed emotional state. In higher doses and with chronic use, however, many drugs blunt affect, produce depression and anxiety, alter values and attitudes, distort sensory and subjective sensations, and impair intimacy, erotic pleasure, aesthetic enjoyment, sensitivity to self and others, increase guilt, release instinctive behaviors, and promote selfish, misdirected gratifications. The dissatisfaction can be severe and long lasting, resulting in decreased or nonexistent pursuits of sexual activity.

The primary purpose of the human sexual response is to derive pleasurable satisfaction, and not to reproduce or procreate, as is commonly believed. The sex drive itself is reduced when satisfaction is impaired (11). Dissatisfaction affects sexual performance in all phases of the human sexual response.

Diagnosis

1. *Desire*. Alteration occurs in the psychological appreciation in the phases of excitement, plateau, orgasm, and resolution. Desire and other subjective experiences are primarily affected.
2. *Performance*. Alteration occurs in the physiological performance in the phases of excitement, plateau, orgasm, and resolution. Arousal, erection, and orgasm are primarily affected.
3. *Satisfaction*. Alteration occurs in the emotional appreciation in the excitement phase: erotic versus intimate feelings, self-gratification versus sensitivity, instinct versus aesthetic enjoyment, pure sexual pursuit versus romance, guilt versus satisfaction.

Neurochemistry

Sexual dysfunction can be arbitrarily divided into three categories for purposes of illustrating the ways in which alcohol/drugs/medications affect the human sexual response. Desire, performance, and satisfaction are three major functions in the human sexual response that are altered by alcohol and drugs.

The desire is defined in psychological terms as libido (12). Libido has an underlying neurochemical substrate in the limbic system of the brain. Major structures located in the limbic system are arranged in a ring located deep on the medical surface of the brain and include the cingulate gyrus, hippocampal gyrus, fornix, mammillary bodies, hypothalamus, amygdala, and septal area. These structures constitute an integrated network with communications between each other and with other parts of the central nervous system, such as the cerebral hemispheres and the autonomic nervous system (13).

Stimulation of different locations within the limbic system elicits visceral, aggressive (fight), defensive (flight), and sexual responses. Stimulation of the septal region elicits penile erection, mounting, and grooming in the male animal. Stimulation of a reward center located in combined areas of the hypothalamus, thalamus, and midbrain induced an experimental rat to press a lever 5000 times per hour to the extent of exhaustion and exclusion of food and water (14). In humans, stimulation of the septal region produced pleasure clearly of a sexual nature. Various provocations of erotic stimuli (pictures), self-fantasy, drugs delivered directly to the septal region or given systemically, and electrical stimulation all produced subjective sensations of sexual pleasure and brain-wave changes emanating from the septal area (15). The patients pressed a lever for self-stimulation in the septal area as many as 1500 times during a 3-hour span, as did the rat (16). These pleasure or reward centers are located close to the regions where stimulation leads to an erection of the penis in males and, presumably, the clitoris and vaginal platform in females.

Sexual responsiveness and performance are served by a complex set of neural subsystems that include components from the cerebral cortex down to the spinal cord and peripheral nervous system (17). These areas in the central and peripheral nervous systems are rich in the neurotransmitters dopamine, norepinephrine, and serotonin (18–21). The autonomic nervous system is subserved by these neurotransmitters as well as others such as epinephrine and acetylcholine. The cerebral cortex and spinal cord are ubiquitously supplied by gamma-amino butyric acid (GABA) (22). Alcohol and drugs affect and interact with the neural structures of the limbic system in addition to the other major contributors to the human sexual response: the cerebral cortex, autonomic nervous system, spinal cord, and nerves.

The hormones involved in the maintenance and stimulation of the human sexual response are produced by the endocrine glands. These hormones exert a profound physiological effect on the target organs to which they are transported by the bloodstream. Major endocrine structures affected by alcohol and drugs are the hypothalamus and pituitary gland.

The important hypothalamic hormones in the sexual response are short-chained polypeptides, the follicle-stimulating hormone releasing factor (FSH-RF), the luteinizing hormone-releasing factor (LH-RF), and the pro-lactin-inhibiting factor (PIF). These neurohormones stimulate the release of the follicle-stimulating hormone (FSH) and the luteinizing hormone (LH), and inhibit prolactin secretion from the pituitary gland. These gonadotro-pins, FSH and LH and prolactin (P), in turn stimulate the sex glands. FSH and LH stimulate the ovaries to manufacture and secrete the female sex hormones estrogens and progesterone. LH stimulates the interstitial (Leydig's) cells of the testes to manufacture and secrete the male sex hormone testosterone. Prolactin stimulates milk production and secretion in the breasts (23).

Desire, performance, and satisfaction are determined by the production of these sex hormones. Ovulation, spermatogenesis, and the female and male secondary sex characteristics are dependent on the effect of these sex hormones as well. A negative feedback mechanism involving the sex hormones and the hypothalamus, pituitary, ovaries, and testes exists to regulate the human sexual response.

Chronic alcohol and drug use may lead to severe disorders of reproductive function. Menstrual abnormalities including anovulatory cycles and luteal-phase deficits are common. Risk is high for spontaneous abortions and fetal abnormalities during pregnancy. The hypothalamic–pituitary–gonadal axis may be affected adversely by alcohol and drug use (24,25).

Other Drug Use

The neurochemical mechanisms by which the cerebral cortex, the limbic system, and the autonomic nervous system are altered may include perturbation of cell membranes, manipulation of neurotransmitters, and alteration in presynaptic and postsynaptic neurons. Alcohol, benzodiazepines, barbiturates, and marijuana change the membrane fluidity of the cell membranes that affect the function of the neurons (26–28). The effect of alcohol is mediated by direct perturbation in cell membranes and by manipulations of neurotransmitter release, uptake, and action on presynaptic and postsynaptic receptor sites and alterations in postsynaptic receptor structure and function (29).

Reserpine and methyldopa deplete the presynaptic supply of the catecholamines, whereas clonidine acts on alpha$_2$ receptors to inhibit the release of catecholamines from the presynaptic neuron. Bromocriptine and l-dopa are dopamine agonists that acts directly on postsynaptic dopamine neurons. Propranolol inhibits beta receptors on postsynaptic adrenergic neurons. Cocaine and tricyclic antidepressants inhibit reuptake of catecholamines by the presynaptic neurons to enhance catecholamine effect with acute use and cause dopamine depletion with chronic use. Nitrates produce vasodilation by relaxing the muscle walls of the arterioles and arteries. Heroin acts at opiate receptors on presynaptic and postsynaptic neurons. Alcohol, barbiturates, and benzodiazepines may enhance GABA transmission in postsynaptic neurons (6,30,31).

Intervention and Treatment

The specific treatment of sexual dysfunction that is caused by alcohol and drugs is to remove the etiological agents. The diagnosis of sexual dysfunction is difficult in itself because of the personal nature and reluctance to offer complaints in a clinical interview. Once the diagnosis of sexual dysfunction has been made, then a screen for alcohol and drug use should be performed.

Further difficulty is often encountered at this point because of the denial surrounding alcohol and drug use. The denial is in the form of minimization of the amount and frequency of use and rationalizations for the use. The physician is oriented toward encouraging compliant use of the medication, that is, the physician is biased against discontinuing an effective antihypertensive agent unless the patient is vigorously opposed. A patient may, in fact, think that sexual dysfunction is something he or she must accept, or the patient may not make the connection between the medication and sexual dysfunction.

Usually sexual dysfunction remits with abstinence from alcohol and drugs and discontinuation of the offending medications, even after chronic use. Long-standing sexual dysfunction from alcohol and/or cocaine will gradually subside with the institution of normal physiological functioning.

Furthermore, psychotherapy, marital therapy, or other treatments such as 12-Step programs for alcohol and drug addiction may be required. Specific behavioral techniques are available through sex therapists for sexual dysfunctions such as premature ejaculation in males and inorgasmia in females if impairment in sexual function persists after the alcohol, drugs, or medication have been discontinued.

References

1. Masters WH, Johnson VE (1966). *Human Sexual Response*. Boston: Little, Brown.
2. Adams RP, Victor M (1985). *Principles of Neurology*, 3d Ed. New York: McGraw-Hill.
3. Masters DW, Johnson VE (1970). Secondary impotence. In *Human Sexual Inadequacy*, pp. 161–185. Boston: Little, Brown.
4. Schuckit MA (1984). *Drug and Alcohol Abuse*, pp. 53–54. New York: Plenum Press.
5. Mendelson JH, Mello NK (1979). Biologic concomitants of alcoholism. *New Engl J Med* 301:912–921.
6. Gilman AG, Goodman LS, Rall TW, et al. (1985). *The Pharmacological Bases of Therapeutics*, 7th Ed. New York: Macmillan.
7. Smith CM (1977). Morphine, sedative/hypnotics and alcohol dependence. In *Drug Addiction I: Morphine, Sedative-Hypnotics and Alcohol Dependence*, Marten WR, ed. New York: Springer-Verlag.
8. Gold MS, Dackis CA, Pottash ALC, et al. (1982). Naltrexone, opiate addiction and endorphins. *Med Res Rev*. 2:211–246.
9. Miller NS (1987). A primer of the treatment process for alcoholism and drug addiction. *Psychiatry Lett* 5:30–37.
10. Melium KL, Morrelli HF (1978). *Clinical Pharmacology*, 2d Ed. New York: Macmillan.
11. Katchadourian HA, Lunde DT (1983). *Fundamentals of Human Sexuality*, 3d Ed. New York: Holt, Rinehart & Winston.

12. Freud S (1951). Letter to an American mother. *Am J Psychiatry* 107:787.
13. Isaacson RL (1982). *The Limbic System*, pp. 1–60. New York: Plenum Press.
14. Olds J (1956). Pleasure centers in the brain. *Sci Am* 193:1005–1006.
15. Cox AW (1979). Control of "sex centers" in the brain [Letter to the editor]. *Medical Aspects of Human Sexuality* 13:113.
16. Heath RG (1972). Pleasure and brain activity in man. *J Nerv Ment Dis* 154:3–18.
17. Beach FA (1947). Reviews of physiological and psychological studies of sexual behavior in mammals. *Physiol Rev* 27:240–305.
18. Baxter BL, Gluckman MI, Scerni RA (1976). Apomorphine self-injection is not affected by alpha-methylparatyrosine treatment: Support for dopaminergic reward. *Physiol Behav* 4:611–612.
19. Davis WM, Smith SG (1973). Blocking effect of alpha-methyltyrosine in amphetamine-based reinforcement. *J Pharm Pharmacol* 25:174–177.
20. DeWit H, Wise RA (1977). A blockade of cocaine reinforcement in rats with the dopamine receptor blockade pimozide but not with the adrenergic blockers phentolamine or phenoxybenzamine. *Can J Psychol* 31:195–203.
21. Wise, RA (1978). Catecholamine theories of reward: A critical review. *Brain Res* 152:215–247.
22. Siegel GJ, Albers RW, Agranoff AW, et al. (1981). *Basic Neurochemistry*. Boston: Little, Brown.
23. Wilson JD, Foster DW (1985). *William's Textbook of Endocrinology*, 7th Ed. Philadelphia: Saunders.
24. Mendelson, JH (1986). Alcohol effects on reproductive function in women. *Psychiatry Lett* 4:35–38.
25. Vanthiel DH, Gavaler JS (1982). The adverse effects of ethanol upon hypothalamic–pituitary–gonadal function in males and females compared and contrasted. *Alcohol Clin Exp Res* 6:179–185.
26. Goldstein DB (1984). The effects of drugs on membrane fluidity. *Annu Rev Pharmacol* 24:43–64.
27. Johnson DA, Lee NM, Cooke R, et al. (1979). Adaptation to ethanol-induced fluidization of brain lipid bilayers: Cross tolerance and reversibility. *Mol Pharmacol* 17:52–55.
28. Kates M, Manson LA (1984). *Biomembranes: Membrane Fluidity*. New York: Plenum Press.
29. Miller NS, Dackis CA, Gold MS (1987). The relationship of addiction, tolerance and dependence to alcohol and drugs: A neurochemical approach. *J Subst Abuse Treat* 4:197–207.
30. Dackis CA, Gold MS (1985a). New concepts in cocaine addiction: The dopamine-depleting hypothesis. *Neurosci Biobehav Rev* 9:469–467.
31. Dackis CA, Gold MS (1985b). Pharmacological approaches to cocaine addiction. *J Subst Abuse Treat* 2:139–145.

CHAPTER 9

The Pharmacology of Alcohol

History

Alcoholism is an illness or disease that requires medical diagnosis and treatment. Alcoholism is not a moral problem; rather, moral problems result from the alcoholism. Much of what appears to be alcoholism are the consequences of alcoholism. Alcoholism begins simply as an addiction to alcohol that is physical in origin. From the pursuit, compulsivity, and relapse to alcohol ensue the mental, medical, psychiatric, and spiritual consequences. The essential core of the alcoholism needs to be identified because the consequences will abate. Treating only the consequences will serve to distract the attention from the primary disease of alcoholism and enable the consequences to continue (1–3).

Mental illness has reached the correct status of inclusion in the domain of medicine. Alcoholism is not yet a medical disease as medicine is practiced. Although the American Medical Association has officially called alcoholism a disease, its members still struggle with that decision. Approximately 25% to 50% of a general medical practice is composed of alcoholics, according to surveys. The problem is not likely to go away.

Prevalence

The prevalence rates for alcoholism by age, sex, and race and the age of onset of alcoholism as determined at the time of interview in the Epidemiologic Catchment Area Study (ECA). The ECA show clearly that alcoholism and drug addiction are common youthful disorders. The lifetime prevalence for alcohol dependence in the general population is 28.8% – 23.8% in men and 46% in women – but alcoholism and drug dependence are rising rapidly among women. The prevalence is greater among those under 45 years old than those over 45. The age of risk for alcoholism is young: almost 40% began drinking between ages 15 and 19, and the proportion of cases that began by 30 years old is 80%. At all ages, women have a later onset than men (1).

Finally, self-recognition of excessive drinking by the alcoholics was high in this study, as the majority of alcoholics thought they were consuming more than they should even when reluctant to admit it in a treatment setting. Only 12% of the alcoholics had talked to their doctors about a drinking problem. The rate of medical contact because of drinking was greater for those with severe alcoholism (27%) as compared to 11% with less severe forms, although the rate was low overall. Obviously, denial of alcoholism and its associated psychiatric syndromes was great (1).

A common association with drug dependence was alcoholism, as among those with drug dependence the prevalence of alcoholism ranged from 36% to 84% depending on the type of drug used. The prevalence of alcoholism was highest among cocaine addicts, 84%, and lowest among tetrahydrocannabinol (THC) addicts, 36% (1).

The cooccurrence of alcoholism with drug addiction is particularly common in younger populations. As many as 90% of alcoholics under the age of 30 are addicted to another drug, most often marijuana, followed in frequency by cocaine, sedatives/hypnotics (benzodiazepines/barbiturates), and opiates. Studies of inpatient and outpatient populations have found that 80% of cocaine addicts, 50% of marijuana addicts, and 50%–75% of opiate addicts are alcoholics; 25%–50% of alcoholics are benzodiazepine addicts (4,5). The young age of the multiple addicted (20–35 predominately) is clearly predominant in medical practice.

Several studies have found a prevalence rate of alcoholism/drug addiction between 25% and 50% for general medical populations, more for inpatients than outpatients, and between 50% and 75% for general psychiatric populations; also, the rate is higher for inpatients (2,6,7). In actual clinical practice, the diagnosis of alcohol and drug addiction is underestimated and underdiagnosed in these populations. The reverse, the presence of psychiatric disorders in alcohol and drug treatment populations is less although significant according to some studies (3, 4,8–11). The most common psychiatric syndrome is depression, followed by anxiety and personality disorders.

Patterns of Use

The duration of alcoholism is also a relatively predictable aspect. Alcoholism tends to be a progressive illness overall with a steady deterioration in personality and health over time. According to the studies, the mean duration of alcoholism is 9 years for those who eventually experience a remission of 1 year or more. Because the mean age of alcoholism is in the early and middle twenties, the typical duration of alcoholism is between 1 and 5 years, followed by 6 to 10 years in duration. This is in contradistinction to the popular conception that the typical alcoholic is old and a long-standing drinker. What is very interesting is that alcoholism can and does develop within 1 year, as 17% of those in remission from alcoholism for more than 1 year were alcoholic within 1 year from the onset of the drinking histories (5).

These findings are enlightening for understanding the diagnosis and treatment for alcoholism. The importance of early diagnosis and treatment is clearly suggested by the data. The majority of the alcoholics are diagnosable and treatable by 5 years after the onset of drinking. This is so because the distribution of the duration of alcoholism is skewed toward its shorter duration. A small but significant number report a duration of greater than 10 years, with a large range between 10 and more than 50 years. The mode, or most frequent duration, is 1 to 5 years for alcoholism, and almost 50% of those who report a remission of alcoholism for more than 1 year experienced a duration of alcoholism of 5 years or less (3,6).

The diagnosis of alcoholism can be made earlier in the natural history of alcoholism than most have suspected. Effective treatment for alcoholism does exist, so earlier intervention is desirable. Many of the medical complications that are usually relied on for the diagnosis occur later in onset; although they are reliable indicators of adverse consequences of alcoholism, medical complications are not particularly useful earlier in its course. The behavioral criteria describe the loss of control over alcohol that leads to the adverse consequences in disruption in interpersonal relationships, manifested in marital, legal, employment, and other arenas of the alcoholic's life.

Any discussion of the younger alcoholic of today is remiss without attention to the prevalence of other drug use in addition to alcohol. The alcoholic under the age of 30 years old, which constitutes the majority of the alcoholics today, is addicted to at least one other drug in addition to alcohol. The most common drug is marijuana, followed by cocaine, sedative/hypnotics, hallucinogens, and others. Reversing the index drug—of those who are addicted to marijuana, 36% are alcoholics; of those who are addicted to barbiturates, 71% are alcoholics; of those who are addicted to cocaine, 84% are alcoholics; of those who are addicted to opioids, 67% are alcoholics (5).

The contemporary alcoholic is a polydrug addict who combines and substitutes one drug for another. In a history session during a medical evaluation this observation must be used so that an accurate diagnosis can be made and correct treatment can be instituted. Carefully planned detoxification schedules are based on accurate histories and diagnoses. Also, prescribing practices must be modified to take into account the vulnerability that alcoholics have for other drugs, particularly sedatives/hypnotics and tranquilizers. Alcoholics become easily addicted to a wide variety of drugs, presumably because of generalized vulnerability to drug and alcohol addiction (9,10).

The locations where alcoholics can be found are well known. To summarize: Households average an alcoholism rate of 14%, meaning that 1 of 6 people living in a household will suffer from alcoholism at some point, most likely early in their lives. Among men, 1 of 4 will suffer from alcoholism, and among women, 1 of 12 (11,12).

The prevalence of alcoholic patients seen in clinical practice is common. Approximately 25% to 50% of patients in a general medical practice are composed of alcoholics (a general medical practice is defined as being composed of the typical household, in a middle-class population, with no predominance of a particular illness). The consequences of alcoholism are commonly hypertension, gastrointestinal problems, upper respiratory illness, cardiac complaints, trauma, and other abnormalities.

Because a general medical practice is devoted to a large number of chronic care patients, it is not surprising that the proportion of alcoholics in a general medical practice is so high. The prevalence of alcoholism is 14.4% among chronic care patients, defined as chronic illnesses. Some of these chronic illnesses are a consequence of alcoholism and some are not. Certainly, the alcoholism aggravates or contributes to the severity, course, and prognosis of the chronic illness (5).

A not too surprising figure is that the prevalence of alcoholism among the psychiatric population is 37%. Alcoholism itself produces psychiatric symptoms, so that many of these patients have alcoholism as the primary problem. The diagnosis and treatment of the alcoholism in many instances will resolve the psychiatric symptoms. However, the correct diagnosis of alcoholism must be made before proper treatment can be instituted (13).

The prevalence of alcoholism among the incarcerated is alarmingly high. Of those incarcerated, 57% qualify for the diagnosis of alcoholism in their lifetime, and approximately half of them have had active alcoholism in the past year. Other well-known statistics: more than 80% of murders involve someone who was intoxicated with alcohol at the time of the murder, 80% of domestic violence involves someone who was intoxicated at the time of the violence, and more than 50% of automobile deaths involve someone who was drinking.

If these statistics seem alarming to some, it might be because the previous epidemiological studies did not ascertain diagnoses. The most recent, comprehensive epidemiological study from which the data in this chapter were derived is the first to use diagnostic criteria, the DSM-III. The ECA data actually diagnosed alcoholism and did not estimate it. The criteria from the DSM-III were derived from other operationally defined criteria that have been used extensively in research protocols. The DSM-III criteria have a universal application and have been verified in clinical trials; they describe addictive use, tolerance, and dependence. The most critical addition are the criteria for addictive use. These criteria reflect the loss of control over alcohol that is central to the diagnosis of alcoholism as recommended by the World Health Organization. Tolerance and dependence are not specific for alcoholism, as they occur in normal drinkers who do not demonstrate alcoholism or the loss of control over alcohol. Also, younger healthier alcoholics do not show significant tolerance and dependence as do older, more chronic alcoholics.

Tolerance

Tolerance is defined as the need to increase the dose or the amount of alcohol or "thing" to maintain the same effect from alcohol or that "thing." Another way of stating tolerance is that the effect is diminished or lost at a particular dose or amount of drug or "thing." Tolerance represents an adaptation of the brain or body to the continuous presence of a foreign substance, such as alcohol. The adaptation occurs at the pharmacodynamic site where the receptor is located on the target organ. In the instance of alcohol, the brain is the site where the addiction to alcohol most logically would appear to occur (1,14).

The brain and body must function as normally as possible, and homeostatic mechanisms operate to ensure that the brain and body are within psychological and physiological boundaries of normal functioning. When alcohol is present in the brain, the cells are changed by the alcohol to produce observable behaviors and subjective experiences that are characteristic of intoxication. The brain "resists" this alcohol-induced change by adapting in various ways at different levels. The brain is operating at a new and adjusted set point in the presence of alcohol to offset the effects, that is, the brain opposes the alcohol effect. The net result of the combination of alcohol and the brain is to remain as near normal as the limits of tolerance by the brain allows and the amount of alcohol that needs to be neutralized (2,5,14).

Dependence is defined as the onset of signs and symptoms of withdrawal on the cessation of the use of alcohol or "thing." Withdrawal is a set or spectrum of predictable and stereotypic signs and symptoms that represent a deadaptation to the presence of alcohol or "thing." Frequently, the best anecdote for the signs and symptoms of withdrawal is the cause or alcohol. "The hair of the dog that bit you" is another way of stating that the drug, in this case alcohol, that induced the dependence syndrome will suppress the withdrawal (3,6,7).

The brain adjusts itself to a different level of functioning in the presence of alcohol but when the alcohol is withdrawn, the brain is "out on the limb" in the adapted state. In this state, the functioning is not in the normal range without the inducement of alcohol, and the observable signs and symptoms are characteristic of the brain's and body's attempts to return themselves to the previous set point for normal functioning. Dependence is a deadaptation of the body to the absence of alcohol, and the deadaptation is expressed in the typical signs and symptoms of withdrawal (1,4).

Tolerance and dependence are on a continuum. As the tolerance is increased, the severity of the dependence is also increased. If the tolerance to alcohol in someone is particularly striking and great, then the dependence syndrome will be severe and significant. This direct relationship is seen with other drugs. The short-acting barbiturates show a rapid onset of tolerance and also have a more severe withdrawal syndrome than the longer acting barbiturates. Alcohol is a relatively short-acting drug, so that the withdrawal syndromes tend to be noticeable and severe (14).

There are many types of tolerance to alcohol. Tolerance is separated into two major categories for convenience – pharmacokinetic and pharmacodynamic tolerance. Pharmacokinetic tolerance is the dispositional capacity of an individual to dispose of alcohol. The dispositional tolerance is determined by a variety of physiological parameters that include absorption, distribution, and elimination of alcohol.

The absorption of alcohol is through the small intestine, mainly the duodenum. After alcohol is ingested, it passes down the esophagus to enter the stomach, which acts as a reservoir. The emptying time of the stomach determines how long the alcohol is retained before it passes down to the duodenum for absorption. Contrary to popular belief, only a small amount of alcohol is absorbed from the stomach. Anything that delays the time that alcohol remains in the stomach will prolong the absorption. Food, particularly fatty foods, certain drugs, and the volume of liquid will slow the passage of alcohol out of the stomach. Also, the concentration of alcohol is important as too high and low percentages of alcohol will not be absorbed as just the right dilution. Absolute alcohol (100%) irritates and inflames the lining of the stomach to impede its own absorption, whereas a dilute concentration (less than 20%) will also not be absorbed as quickly. The optimum dilution is about 40%, which happens to be the percent concentrations of most liquors distilled for distribution. The proof of alcohol is equal to twice its percent so that 80 proof vodka is equal to 40% alcohol.

The buzz or euphoria that some drinkers seek is dependent on how fast and how high the blood level of alcohol is reached. The faster and higher the blood alcohol peak, the greater the euphoria or high. Anything that slows the absorption or dilutes the concentration of alcohol will lower both the time it takes to reach the blood and the height of the peak blood level of alcohol. Food and dilute mixed drinks will not get some persons as drunk as fast as a moderately concentrated alcoholic beverage on an empty stomach.

Alcohol is distributed everywhere. Alcohol is a polar molecule that is soluble in water so it goes wherever water goes, and water is a constituent of all living cells in the body. One can readily see that alcohol in the form of ethanol gets around inside the body, thus enabling it to produce a wide variety of effects. Although alcohol does not mix well with fats, it is such a small molecule in comparison to the barriers to it that it enters sanctuaries that are closed to other larger molecules.

Alcohol is eliminated chiefly by a metabolic breakdown in the liver. A series of enzymes are responsible for the alteration of ethanol into various forms that are excreted, or used elsewhere in the body for energy, or as building blocks for protein and storage. The enzyme alcohol dehydrogenase converts alcohol to acetaldehyde. Acetaldehyde is a noxious chemical that, when injected into humans, produces a violent, nauseating reaction that resembles a severe hangover. In fact, acetaldehyde is the best single explanation we have for the hangover. Acetaldehyde is further converted by the enzyme acetaldehyde dehydrogenase to acetic acid. Acetic acid has many fates that include carbohydrates, fats, proteins, and carbon dioxide and water.

A small amount of alcohol is excreted unchanged in the lungs, urine, and sweat; this accounts for about 2%, as 98% of the alcohol is metabolized by the liver. This form of tolerance does not account for the tolerance that develops to alcohol because the blood level remains the same as tolerance appears. If breakdown by the liver were responsible for tolerance, then the blood alcohol level would decrease as the alcohol was metabolized.

The tolerance with which an individual is born is called innate tolerance. Innate or inborn tolerance varies widely from individual to individual and according to ethnicity. Larger individuals as a rule have a larger capacity for alcohol, as shown by an ability to drink larger amounts of alcohol with less effect of intoxication. The reason is that the blood volume is greater for larger individuals so that the concentration of a given dose of alcohol is less. In other words, larger people have more body water to dilute the peak of the blood alcohol level during absorption.

Other examples of innate tolerance are orientals and alcoholics, at least, those who are at high risk for the development of alcoholism. As many as 80% of Orientals have an aversive response to small amounts of alcohol. This aversive reaction runs in families and appears to be a genetically transferable condition. The reaction consists of signs and symptoms of a severe hangover that include nausea, vomiting, lightheadedness, a red facial and truncal flush, palpitations, and sleepiness. As little as an ounce or less of wine will trigger this reaction. Because the reaction is genetically determined, it represents an innate intolerance to alcohol.

Alcoholics and high-risk individuals have an increased, innate tolerance to alcohol. Innate tolerance to alcohol is tolerance that is present before alcohol has been consumed and is an inherited trait. Innate tolerance is to be differentiated from acquired tolerance, which develops in the presence of and as a result of alcohol use. Alcoholics appear to have this enhanced tolerance early in their drinking history, often at the start of alcohol drinking. High-risk individuals before becoming alcoholic also have this increased capacity to drink alcohol without as great an effect that low-risk individuals have. The innate tolerance or an inborn capacity to drink alcohol may be a marker for alcoholism before its onset (12,13).

Acquired tolerance begins with the use of alcohol. Acquired tolerance is sometimes divided into acute and chronic tolerance to distinguish between what happens after a single dose of alcohol and after continuous use of alcohol. Studies have shown that tolerance develops after one dose of alcohol. When tolerance is measured objectively and subjectively in nonalcoholics and plotted along the blood alcohol curve, tolerance to alcohol is noted at a higher blood level on the descending limb of the curve as compared to the ascending limb. The tolerance that develops so rapidly is nonetheless the same as that expressed after chronic or regular use of alcohol (2).

Chronic tolerance, although probably qualitatively not different from acute tolerance, takes more time to develop and has a greater capacity. How much greater may not be that significant, especially when compared to the degree of tolerance that develops in opiate use. The minimum lethal dose of morphine is about 10 times higher in opiate addicts with tolerance than in users without tolerance to opiates. The lethal dose of ethanol (alcohol) is essentially the same for alcoholics with tolerance to alcohol as those without tolerance to alcohol.

The reason for increased tolerance in alcoholics may be for more than the obvious one, that one can drink more with a greater capacity without suffering the toxic effects of overdose. Tolerance appears to correlate with the euphoric effects of alcohol; the greater the tolerance to alcohol, the greater the euphoria. Euphoria is that elusive sensation of feeling "high," or a sense of well-being, that all is right with oneself and the world. Drugs of abuse and addiction have both these effects, but differ in the proportion of either feeling high or a sense of well-being. Alcohol gives the user more of the latter effect of well-being whereas cocaine provides an intense euphoria. Actually, the amount of euphoria from alcohol is milder than that provided by many drugs of abuse and addiction, such as cocaine and heroin.

Alcohol may be a drug of the higher intellect. Animal studies suggest that alcohol has low reinforcing properties. Most animals do not prefer alcohol over water and do not use alcohol to excess or at all, unless no other liquid is available. The animal's aversion to alcohol suggests that feeling good is not a critical reason for using alcohol. Furthermore, alcoholics tend to lose this tolerance over time after chronic consumption and with aging. The loss of tolerance to alcohol probably is what is responsible for the decrease in euphoria and the sense of well-being that occurs with an alcoholic-level consumption of alcohol. The mystery of addiction to alcohol or alcoholism is why the alcoholic continues to drink after the loss of tolerance and euphoria or well-being. The advanced alcoholic usually drinks to the stage of sedation, bypassing any high. Feeling good is not a reason for drinking in abnormal drinkers. Feeling bad is a reason to avoid drinking by the alcoholic. The time course for the loss in tolerance may be months, more often, a few years.

Pharmacodynamic Tolerance

The mechanism that explains tolerance most economically and logically is found at the receptor site where alcohol acts. Pharmacodynamic tolerance to alcohol is tolerance that develops at the receptor site, which is the cell membrane in the case of alcohol. Alcohol acts to disrupt cell membranes. Cell membranes are the outer covering of mammalian cells, analogous to the skin in the human body. The cell membrane is composed of "phospholipids," which contain long-chain fatty acids. These fatty acids point toward the center of the cell in an alignment with each other that provides for order in the membrane. The order of the membrane is important for normal functioning of the cell. Alcohol causes these fatty acids to move about in a more fluid or disorderly way (15,16).

The cell resists the action of alcohol to cause disordering so that it can maintain as normal an order as possible under the influence of alcohol. What the cell membrane does is to increase its intrinsic order so as to reset the set point of the membrane closer to the prealcohol order. In the presence of alcohol, the membrane order is near normal, and in the absence of alcohol, the membrane is more ordered. A more ordered membrane is more rigid because the fatty acids are more resistant to the motion that is caused by alcohol. The tolerance to alcohol is correlated with these rigid membranes. The development of more rigid membranes is an example of pharmacodynamic tolerance (17,18).

The red blood cells of alcoholics are actually more rigid than those of nonalcoholics, when membranes are tested for their degree of fluidity or order. It cannot be determined by these studies if the more rigid red blood cells in the alcoholics represent innate or acquired pharmacodynamic tolerance. The hope is to develop a blood test that will measure the amount of tolerance to alcohol if tolerance turns out to be a marker for alcoholism (19).

Cross-tolerance between alcohol and other drugs is an interesting but predictable occurrence. What this means is that someone who is tolerant to alcohol will also be tolerant to those drugs that share cross-tolerance with alcohol. Barbiturates and benzodiazepines are two classes of sedatives/hypnotics that have cross-tolerance with alcohol. A well-known example is that alcoholics frequently require higher doses of these drugs to obtain the desired effect. Also, benzodiazepines such as librium, valium, and ativan are used to detoxify alcoholics during withdrawal. Because of the cross-tolerance, the signs and symptoms of alcohol withdrawal are suppressed by librium. Librium can also be used to suppress the signs and symptoms of withdrawal from barbiturates such as secobarbital and pentobarbital (15).

Dependence

Dependence is a term that has undergone a lot of change in meaning as applied to alcohol and drugs. The term dependence has many meanings and derivations to professionals and nonprofessionals. The pharmacological definition of dependence is "the onset of withdrawal on the cessation of the drug or alcohol." The pharmacological definition is the same as "physical dependence." Withdrawal is characterized by a predictable and stereotypic set of signs and symptoms that are typical for alcohol or a given drug. Withdrawal is a deadaptation of the brain and body to the absence of alcohol after a period of adaptation during the development of tolerance.

The signs and symptoms of the withdrawal of various drugs have some commonality and some uniqueness. The withdrawal is a hyperexcitable state in response to the depressant action of alcohol. The sympathetic nervous system is discharging in withdrawal from many drugs, particularly alcohol. The sympathetic nervous system is responsible for the anxiety, apprehension, tremor, palpitations, sweating, irritability, high blood pressure, and other manifestations of an excited state. Anxiety and depression are common to the withdrawal of many drugs, including alcohol. As is evident, withdrawal is an unpleasant state that has negative feelings and significant medical consequences.

Alcohol withdrawal should be considered as a spectrum of signs and symptoms of the abstinence state. At one end of the spectrum is anxiety, tremor, palpitations, and hypertension, while the more severe part of the spectrum consists of seizures, delusions, hallucinations, delirium tremens, and death. Delirium tremens (DTs), when untreated, has a mortality rate of 50%. DTs constitute a confused and cloudy sensorium with disorientation as to time and place, a hypervigilant and agitated state, marked tremors of extremities and body, significant elevations of blood pressure and pulse, terrifying visual hallucinations, usually of animals such as snakes, severe dehydration from the hypermetabolic state, and prostration. The causes of death in DTs are self-inflicted injury as a result of the confusion and hallucinations, heart failure from arrhythmias, and pneumonias. With proper treatment the mortality and morbidity can be reduced to less than 25% (3,4).

Other features of the abstinence syndrome or spectrum are auditory hallucinations or hearing voices in the absence of a source, visual hallucinations (again, animals such as bugs or worms), and paranoid delusions that someone is out to harm them despite the absence of harm toward them. The abstinence syndrome can mimic other known psychiatric conditions such as anxiety disorders, manic-depression, schizophrenia, phobias, and obsessive-compulsive disorders.

The dependence syndrome in its milder forms develops after a small dose of alcohol in a nondrinker. Fluctuations in mood, blood pressure and pulse, and disturbances in sleep and appetite can occur after only a few ounces of alcohol. It is a myth that high doses of alcohol over prolonged periods of time are necessary to develop "physical dependence." The hangover is an example of alcohol withdrawal or a dependence syndrome. The hangover occursdin response to the cessation of the use of alcohol and is characterized by anxiety, depression, headache, malaise, and elevated blood pressure and pulse. Furthermore, the more severe signs of withdrawal that include seizures and DTs can develop only after a few weeks of regular alcohol use in susceptible individuals.

References

1. Victor M, Adams RP (1953). The effect of alcohol on the nervous system. *Res Pub Assoc Res Nerv Ment Dis* 32:526–573.
2. Wilson JR, Erwin G, McClearn GE, et al. (1984). Effects of behavior: II. Behavioral sensitivity and acute behavioral tolerance. *Alcoholism* 8:4.
3. Edwards G, Auf A, Hodgson R (1981). Nomenclature and classification of drug and alcohol-related problems: A WHO memorandum. *Bull Who* 59:225–242.
4. Jaffe JH (1985). Drug addiction and drug abuse. In *The Pharmacological Basis of Therapeutics*, 7th Ed., Gilman AG, Goodman LS, Rall TW, Murad F, eds., pp. 532–581. New York: Macmillan.
5. Majchrowicz E, Nobel EP (1979). *Biochemistry and Pharmacology of Ethanol, Vol. 1.* New York: Plenum.
6. Jellinek EM (1960). The disease concept of alcoholism. New Brunswick, NJ: Hillhouse Press.
7. Goldstein DB (1984). The effect of drugs on membrane fluidity, Cowan WM, Shooter EM, Stevens CF, Thompson RC, eds. *Ann Rev Pharmacol* 24:43–64.
8. Miller NS, Dackis CA, Gold MS (1987). The relationship of addiction, tolerance and dependence to alcohol and drugs. A neurochemical approach. *J Subst Abuse Treat* 4:197–207.
9. Lieber CA (1982). *Medical Disorders of Alcoholism: Pathogenesis and Treatment.* Philadelphia: W.B. Saunders.
10. Melium KL, Morrelli HF (1978). *Clinical Pharmacology,* 2d Ed. New York: Macmillan.
11. Miller NS, Goodwin DW, Jones FC, et al. Antihistamine blockade of alcohol-induced flushing in Orientals. *J Nerv Ment Dis* 175(11):661–667.
12. Goodwin DW (1979). Alcoholism and heredity. *Arch Gen Psychiatry* 36:57–61.
13. Goodwin DW (1985). Alcoholism and genetics. *Arch Gen Psychiatry* 42:171–174.
14. Hill MA, Bangham AD (1975). General depressant drug dependency: A biophysical hypothesis. *Adv Exp Med Biol* 59:1–9.
15. Goldstein DB (1984). The effects of drugs on membrane fluidity. *Ann Rev Pharmacol Toxicol* 24:43–64.
16. Chin JH, Goldstein DB (1977). Drug tolerance in biomembranes: A spin label study on the effects of ethanol. *Science* 196:684–685.
17. Chin JH, Parsons LM, Goldstein DB (1978). Increased cholesterol content of erythrocyte and brain membranes in ethanol tolerant mice. *Biochim Biophys Acta* 13:358–363.
18. Chin JH, Goldstein DB (1981). Membrane disordering action of ethanol: Variation with membrane cholesterol content and depth of the spin label probe. *Mol Pharmacol* 19:425–531.
19. Miller NS (1987). A blood marker for pharmacodynamic tolerance to alcohol. *J Subst Abuse Treat* 4:93–102.

CHAPTER 10

The Pharmacology of Amphetamines

History

The amphetamine molecule is chemically simple with a number of intriguing actions. Attempts to refine and emphasize desired effects and minimize the less useful effects have led to the development of derivatives of amphetamines that are of clinical, experimental, and illicit interest (1).

The similarity in chemical structures between amphetamines and the catecholamines is significant for understanding the sympathomimetic properties of amphetamines. The mechanism of action of amphetamines can be inferred from the actions of the catecholamines, which are structural analogues (2).

The various sympathomimetic molecules that are chemically related to amphetamine by substitutions in the amphetamine molecule are drugs that include diethylproprion, phentermine, chlorphentermine, fenfluramine, furfenorex, benzphetamine, methyl phenidate, and phenmetrazine (2).

Psychostimulants such as mescaline are produced by substitution of the aromatic ring of the amphetamine molecule with one or more methoxy groups. These methoxylated amphetamines appear to act directly on receptors rather than indirectly by release of neurotransmitter. STP (2,5-dimethoxy-r-methylamphetamine) is the most potent methoxylated derivative of amphetamine (2).

The presence of a methyl group in the side chain alpha to the nitrogen results in a molecule that confers inhibitory action on the enzyme monoamine oxidase. This particular chemical modification of the amphetamine molecule has resulted in two clinically useful monoamine oxidase inhibitors, tranylcypromine and pheniprazene.

Prevalence

Estimation of Prevalence

Patterns of use are difficult to determine for a variety of reasons. Estimates of amphetamine use are always significantly low and probably represent only the "tip of the iceberg." The indifference of society, the practices of the medical profession, and the denial of the user/addict contribute heavily to the resistance to assess drug use in the United States. The enormous professional pressures to prescribe medicines and the profitability of the manufacture and sales of drugs make surveillance and estimation impractical and even undesirable. Another source of resistance is the reluctance of legislative and medical bodies to pass effective laws regarding drug use. Only a modest amount of literature regarding amphetamine abuse and addiction exists as a result of these factors.

The addictive potential and nature of amphetamines were established in the late 1950s. By the early 1970s, the medical and psychiatric literature contained significant evidence and admonishments of a worldwide epidemic of amphetamine use from Peru and Mexico to Switzerland and France, from Great Britain and Sweden to the United States and Canada. Only recently studies in Great Britain have found that the availability and the use of amphetamines were second only to marijuana as the drug of choice of adolescents.

Amphetamine abuse and addiction gradually increased in prevalence in this country from the 1930s to the early 1960s, and accelerated in the mid-1960s until amphetamines were classified as Schedule II drugs by the U.S. government. Even then, various state governments needed to pass "amphetamine acts" to further restrict the prescribing of the drug by physicians for medical and psychiatric disorders.

Patterns of Use

Racemic beta-phenylisopropylamine or amphetamine (Benzedrine) contains two isomers. The dextrorotatory isomer has the greater pharmacological activity. Dextroamphetamine (Dexedrine) was marketed as a more potent form (on a weight basis) of amphetamine. Except for the matter of dosage, no therapeutic distinction can be made between the levoisomer and the dextroisomer, as their pharmacological effects are identical.

Methamphetamine (speed, "crystal," Methedrine) is one of the many amphetamine derivatives that were synthesized by the pharmaceutical industry following the enthusiastic acceptance of amphetamine as a pressor drug, although clearly more potent as a central nervous system (CNS) stimulant. It has been marketed by many drug houses for pressor and CNS stimulatory purposes. The popularity of amphetamine and methamphetamine relative to the other CNS stimulants does not reflect any great pharmacological difference between these two groups of drugs, but rather the highly important factors of their potency, ready availability, low cost, and wide publicity.

Ephedrine occurs naturally in various plants. It was used in China for at least 2000 years before it was introduced into Western medicine in 1924. Its central actions are less pronounced than those of the amphetamines.

Phenylephrine differs chemically from epinephrine in lacking an OH in the 4 position on the benzene ring.

Phenylpropanolamine is available in a wide variety of "over-the-counter" anorexants in tablets or capsules or in combination with other drugs such as caffeine. Continuation of this CNS stimulant as an over-the-counter drug is controversial (3).

Sympathomimetic agents appearing in Schedule IV of the Controlled Substance Act are diethylproprion, mazindol, and phentermine. Diethylproprion possesses pharmacological actions that are similar to amphetamine, although the CNS stimulation is less and the cardiovascular side effects are minimal. Mazindol, an imidazoline derivative, resembles tricyclic antidepressants. Mazindol is a weaker CNS stimulant than amphetamine, with modest effects on the cardiovascular system. Phentermene is a sympathomimetic agent that is similar to amphetamine, only with weaker actions (3).

Drugs introduced in Schedule III of the Controlled Substance Act are benzphetamine and phendimetrazine. These drugs are similar to amphetamines, but have less CNS stimulation and cardiovascular effects. Phenmetrazine and methamphetamine are included with dextroamphetamine in Schedule II of the Controlled Substance Act (3).

Intoxication

Acute Intoxication

The subjective effects were first systematically quantified in 1938 (4). When amphetamines are taken by mouth, or inhaled as snuff, the user typically experiences sensations of euphoria, anxiety, enhanced self-awareness and self-confidence, heightened alertness, greater energy, and an increased capacity for concentration. Sensations of hunger and fatigue are reduced. The behavior of the user becomes hyperactive, talkative, irritable, and restless. The user moves around frequently with adventitious movements of the body. Judgment is compromised, with decisions and actions that reflect poor discretion. The user may say things or attempt actions that are foolish and hasty. Overt sexual behavior that is out of character may occur. Distortion in thinking and perceptions arise. Suspiciousness, guarded, and hypervigilant scanning of the environment characterizes some users. Illusions of movement in space add to the elevated arousal. The emotional affect may appear more or less spontaneously (5–8).

Physiological responses are sympathomimetic. The physiological effects that accompany the psychological effects are those predicted from adrenergic drugs such as amphetamines acting positively on the sympathetic nervous system to mimic effects of norepinephrine and epinephrine. A rise in blood pressure, increase in pulse rate, pupillary dilation, and anorexia are regular concomitants of almost any acute dose. Blood glucose may increase as does blood coagulability. Skeletal muscle tension increases while the smooth muscle contraction in the bronchial tubes and gastrointestinal tract decreases. The cardiovascular effects may manifest themselves not only by an increase in heart rate, but by ectopic atrial and ventricular beats such as paroxysmal arterial tachycardias and premature ventricular contractions. An initial increase in cardiac output results from positive chronotropic and inotropic effects, and a later reflexive drop in cardiac output occurs from increased peripheral resistance of the vasoconstrictive effects of the amphetamines.

Dry mouth and dysphagia for solid foods may develop. The skin is cool from peripheral vasoconstriction. The pupils are dilated with a gaze that may be fixed or glassy or normal. The deep tendon reflexes are increased, and fine tremors may be observable in the hands — especially when held in a position. Urinary retention and constipation result from the inhibitory effect of the sympathetic nerve supply to the bladder and bowel. The physiological effects are dose related, but tolerance develops over time to some degree to most of the cardiovascular, neurological, and gastrointestinal effects (3,9).

In increasing doses, the mood may be predominantly anxious and the speech rapid, slurred, and incoherent. Stereotypic movements may intermix with fidgety, jerky, random motions. Grinding of the teeth may occur. An ataxic gait may be present. The thoughts may be loosely connected, illogical, and tangential. Affect may appear silly and irrelevant. Headache, nausea, vomiting, and malaise may predominate. Frank delusions, especially paranoia, may develop (3,9).

An abstinence withdrawal syndrome from amphetamines that indicates physical dependence follows even small, acute doses. The effects are generally opposite to those of the intoxicating state; the mood may be depressed, thinking and behavior are slowed, movements are deliberate and methodical; fatigue, somnolence, increased appetite, ennui, and perhaps a "craving" or "drive" to use further stimulants may be present (10,11).

These symptoms are more intense and appear sooner with intravenous administration, but otherwise are the same qualitatively for oral and intravenous routes. The oral and intravenous experiences are different because of a faster and greater rise in peak blood levels of amphetamines with the latter.

Chronic Administration

Increasingly, with continued use and the passage of time, the pace of the thoughts quickens and concentration is impaired. Abrupt mood changes replace the initial euphoria, to which tolerance develops. Misperceptions and illusions appear and are often disturbing and frightening to the user. Movements, lights, and actions by people in the surroundings are distorted and exaggerated. Frank visual, tactile, olfactory, and auditory hallucinations may follow further amphetamine use. These occur less often with prolonged consecutive oral administrations than with intravenous use. Shadows become people, and the user may see his body as covered with sores and vermin (12,13).

The auditory hallucinations are usually voices that make derogatory statements about the person. The voices may be singular or in groups. The individual may or may not recognize the voices. These voices are frightening and sometimes prompt aggressive and violent actions toward the self or others (14,15).

The suspicious and guarded thinking may progress to the frank paranoia of a delusional degree. The delusions may be well formed or vague and are often paranoid in content and affect. The individual may act accordingly toward a delusion in a frightened or violent manner. Violent behaviors have been in response to the paranoid state toward self and others (16).

The primary characteristics of amphetamine psychosis are ideas of reference, paranoid delusions (delusions of persecution and grandiosity), and auditory and visual hallucinations in the setting of a clear consciousness. Many of these patients with a drug-induced psychosis are diagnosed as acute or chronic paranoid schizophrenics. The similarities between the idiopathic and drug-induced schizophrenia have led to the formulation of a biochemical model of schizophrenia (17-19).

The psychosis is associated with a large individual variation of response, both qualitatively and quantitatively. The psychosis may ensue after administration of a few small doses — or larger doses of amphetamines are required over a longer period of time to induce the psychoses (20,21).

The amphetamine-induced psychosis is antagonized in humans by haloperidol. Haloperidol is a dopamine blocker that neutralizes the effect of dopamine at the postsynaptic site. Haloperidol also is effective in idiopathic schizophrenia in reducing the delusions and hallucinations. Other dopamine blockers such as phenothiazines are also effective in both idiopathic schizophrenia and the amphetamine-induced psychoses.

Amphetamine-derivative psychosis does occur. Phenmetrazine by oral, but particularly by intravenous, administration produces a psychosis identical to that produced by amphetamines. Paranoid ideation, stereotyped behavior, hallucinations, and thought disorders all occur from phenmetrazine use. Similarly, other sympathomimetic agents such as diethylpropiron and methylphenidate have also been documented as etiological agents in the "amphetamine psychosis."

Diagnosis

A simplistic formulation that is useful for conceptualization is "exposure plus vulnerability" equals use, abuse, and addiction. The supply of amphetamines through legal and illegal production and the prescribing practices of physicians determine the exposure. The vulnerability of individuals and groups to seek out, use, abuse, and become addicted to the amphetamines is derived from psychological and physical predisposition. A complete discussion is complex and outside the range of this chapter. Characterization of the etiology of drug use is at best descriptive at this juncture in our objective understanding, although some sound theoretical formulations have significant support (22–25).

Exposure contributes significantly to abuse and addiction in that an estimated 85% of the population has used some form of an illicit drug by the age of 25. Controversy exists over whether drug use per se is causally related to drug abuse and addiction. The position that addicts have a narrow range of vulnerability is naive. Certainly, high-risk populations do exist. These populations may abuse and become addicted to drugs in low levels of exposure. However, higher level exposures may select out less vulnerable populations (22,26,27).

The American pharmaceutical industry has probably been making 8 to 10 billion doses of stimulant drugs annually. The FDA estimated in 1968 that approximately 4 to 5 billion conventional doses of amphetamines were sold illegally and diverted into channels of illegal usage. The ease with which distributors of illicit drugs could obtain substantial properties of stimulants in bulk or individual dosage forms made possible the rapid spread of amphetamine abuse in the 1960s. Some diversion of legally manufactured amphetamines to illicit markets may still occur.

Regulation of drug manufacture and sale is not stringent. As a result, some of the "speed" offered for sale, and particularly that in a form suitable for intravenous injection, is now derived from the "basement" chemist (28).

The addictive potential is high with amphetamines. Classification of amphetamines as a Schedule II drug emphasizes that characteristic. The addictive potential, although well established, has not been appreciated by everyone. In a controlled study under double-blind conditions, normal subjects preferred amphetamine's effects over those of all other drugs, including morphine. Some studies have even demonstrated that amphetamines are preferred over morphine by heroin addicts. These findings suggest the reasons why amphetamines remain prevalent and popular out of proportion to the extent of their chemical utility (29).

Many people find the effects of "uppers" useful and gratifying. Individuals who use "downers" such as alcohol, sedatives, tranquilizers, and hypnotics may use an "upper" to "get going" in the morning. This downer-and-upper cycle has been increasingly common with the cocaine and alcohol combination, but is seen with a variety of other stimulants including amphetamines and amphetamine derivatives prescribed over the counter and obtained illicitly. A plethora of possible combinations include "speed-balling" in which heroin or a barbiturate is mixed with amphetamines or cocaine. A businessman may use alcohol in the evening and a nasal decongestant in the morning. A housewife may take benzodiazepines or barbiturates during the day and evening and use an amphetamine derivative in the morning.

Frequent entries to amphetamine use are for weight reduction in obesity, as an aphrodisiac to stimulate and prolong sexual pleasure, the emotional "blues," depression, a desire "to get a kick out of life," and psychiatric diagnoses such as attention deficit disorder in children and narcolepsy in adults. The mode of introduction to these drugs may serve only as an explanation for exposure but not as a sufficient cause for continued use once the adverse consequences have begun to appear. At that point, an addiction may be operative that signals a preoccupation, compulsive use and recurrent use in spite of costly physical, mental, and emotional consequences.

The treatment of depression with amphetamines is transient and ineffective for the reason similar to the loss of an anorectic effect with the development of tolerance. Dependence develops as well, to result in symptoms that worsen the depression because depression is a withdrawal effect of amphetamines. The depression can be profound and worse than the original depression for which amphetamines were prescribed.

The least controversial indications for the use of amphetamines seem to be in the treatment of narcolepsy and attention deficit disorders in children and adults. These conditions are rare and uncommon, respectively, so that the number of legal prescriptions should be minuscule. Amphetamines have been classified as a Schedule II drug in the United States, and since 1969 most of the use of amphetamines has been restricted by voluntary bases on prescribing and by official prohibitions in the United Kingdom.

Tolerance and Dependence

Tolerance develops to many of the actions of amphetamines and related drugs, to the euphoria, anorexia, hyperthermia, hypertension, and the increased excretion of noradrenalin. Tolerance implies a relative loss of an effect at a particular dose so that only a transient and less intense euphoria or anorexia may occur in response to amphetamines after chronic administration. Continued use and an increase in dose only produce a short-lived enhancement of an effect that eventually diminishes for that dose (30).

Tolerance to the cardiovascular effects of the amphetamines, and more specifically to their vasoconstrictor actions, is strongly suggested by the fact that speed addicts can survive single intravenous doses of 1000 mg or more with only an occasional untoward physiological effect. The risk of a cardiovascular disturbance would be high if a nontolerant user were similarly exposed to amphetamines (25,31).

Little tolerance seems to develop to the "awakening" or "antisleep" actions of these drugs. The undiminished effectiveness of amphetamine in the treatment of narcolepsy, and the state of persistent wakefulness during chronic use, lend support to this view.

Chronic administration may lead to a depletion of neurotransmitters at the presynaptic site. Less neurotransmitter is available for release into the synaptic cleft to act on the postsynaptic site. A deficiency in the neurotransmitter leads to the development of tolerance to the particular effect produced by the neurotransmitter. Less dopamine for release by the presynaptic neuron is manifested as less euphoria and locomotion (32,33).

Withdrawal states or the expression of physical dependence may be attributable to compensatory postsynaptic changes that occur in response to a depletion in neurotransmitters. Postsynaptic supersensitivity develops from an increased proliferation of receptor sites to compensate for a lack of stimulation from the neurotransmitter. The supersensitivity may underlie the various mood changes and stereotypic behaviors that are seen in the chronic withdrawal states from amphetamine (32–34).

A denervation supersensitivity of postsynaptic sites may develop such as in the caudate nucleus. The increased sensitivity of the caudate nucleus may underlie some of the stereotypic movements. Postsynaptic supersensitivity is similarly an explanation for neuroleptic-induced tardive dyskinesia that may result from a chronic postsynaptic dopamine receptor blockade (32–34).

Often, a significant improvement in mood, energy, and paranoid thinking occurs within days. However, a slow recovery over weeks, months, and perhaps years may be required for complete resolution of the signs and symptoms of withdrawal from chronic amphetamine use. Mood lability, memory loss, confusion, and paranoid thinking and perceptual abnormalities may persist for over a year or perhaps indefinitely.

Neurochemistry

Neurons containing dopamine originate in the substantia nigra and the ventral tegmentum in the interpeduncular nucleus. The neurons of the substantia nigra project to the corpus striatum. A feedback pathway from the caudate nucleus to the substantia nigra is mediated by the neurotransmitters acetylcholine (ACh) and gamma-aminobutyric acid (GABA), which inhibit neuronal firing. In addition, presynaptic autoreceptors regulate the release of dopamine by inhibition. Dopamine neurons also project from the ventral tegmentum to the mesolimbic and mesocortical areas of the brain. The reward center where reinforcement occurs originates in neurons in the lateral hypothalamus that project in the median forebrain bundle through the septal area to the ventral tegmentum. The presynaptic neurons from the lateral hypothalamus may release opioid peptides because the neurons of the ventral tegmentum contain opiate receptors (34,35). Amphetamines and related drugs may act on the postsynaptic dopamine neurons of the reward center to enhance drug-seeking behavior.

Norepinephrine-containing neurons originate in the brainstem. The major sites are the locus ceruleus in the pons and the midbrain. The presynaptic neurons from these areas project diffusely to hypothalamic, mesolimbic, and cortical regions. Norepinephrine neurons are involved both in the ascending and descending reticular activating system and in mediating food reinforcement and promoting satiety effects (36,37).

The action of amphetamines on the dopamine neurons in the mesolimbic area may be responsible for changes in mood such as euphoria, anxiety, and depression. Similar action on the mesocortical DA neurons may mediate effects on judgment and insight by amphetamines (34,35). Increased arousal seen with amphetamines may result from amphetamine-enhanced activity of norepinephrine neurons in the reticular activating system in the midbrain.

Amphetamine and related drugs appear to affect the neurotransmitter systems to enhance their activity by two major mechanisms. The first and probably the most significant is promoting release of dopamine and norepinephrine from the presynaptic neurons, and the second is blocking of the reuptake of catecholamines by the presynaptic neuron. Reuptake is the major route of elimination of catecholamines that are released into the synaptic cleft. More catecholamines are present at the postsynaptic site because of their increased release, and their termination of action by reuptake by the presynaptic neuron is blocked by amphetamine. A greater sustained action of the catecholamines at the postsynaptic site may be responsible for the behavioral effects of the amphetamines (38,39).

Evidence suggests that amphetamines act on the presynaptic neurons that provide the adrenergic supply to the hunger center in the lateral hypothalamus. Amphetamines may act to block hunger by enhancing catecholaminergic effects at that site. The dopamine innervation to the caudate nucleus is involved in mediating the amphetamine-induced motor stereotypic behavior, perhaps with a contribution from the amygdala. The mesolimbic system and the olfactory tubercle appear to be involved in locomotor activity associated with amphetamine-induced locomotor behavior through effects on dopamine (40–42).

References

1. Weiner, N (1985). Norepinephrine, epinephrine and the sympathomimetic amines. In *Pharmacological Basis of Therapeutics*, 7th Ed., Gilman A, Goodman L, Rall TW, Murad F, eds., 145–180. New York: MacMillan.
2. Biel JH (1970). Structure-activity relationships of amphetamine and derivatives. In *Amphetamines and Related Compounds*, Costa E, Garattini S, eds., p. 3. New York: Raven Press.
3. Gilman A, Goodman L, Rall TW, Murad F, eds. (1985). *Pharmacological Basis of Therapeutics*, 7th Ed. New York: Macmillan.
4. Bahnsen P, Jacobsen E, Thesleff H (1938). The subjective effect of beta-phenylisopropylamin-sulfate on normal adults. *Acta Med Scand* 97:89–92.
5. Jacobsen E, Wollstein A (1939). Studies on the subjective effects of the cephalotropic amines in men. *Acta Med Scand* 100:159–162.
6. Schroeder DJ, Collins WE (1974). Effects of secobarbital and D-amphetamine on tracking performance during angular acceleration. *Ergonomics* 17(5):813–821.
7. Smith GM, Beecher HK (1959). Amphetamine sulfate and athletic performance: Objective effects. *JAMA* 170:542–557.
8. Cameron JS, Specht PG, Wendt GR (1965). Effects of amphetamines on moods, emotions and motivation. *J Psychol* 61:93–121.

9. Martin WR, Sloan JW, Sapira JD, et al. (1971). Physiologic, subjective and behavioral effects of amphetamine, methamphetamine, ephedrine, phenmetrazine and methylphenidate in man. *Clin Pharmacol Ther* 12:245–258.

10. Lasagna L, Von Felsinger JM, Beecher HK (1955). Drug-induced mood changes in man. I. Observations on healthy subjects, chronically ill patients, and post addicts. *JAMA* 157:1066–1120.

11. Kilbey MM, Ellinwood EH, eds. (1977). Chronic administration of stimulant drugs: Response modification. In *Cocaine and Other Stimulants*, pp. 410–429. New York: Plenum Press.

12. Griffith JD, Cavanaugh JH, Oates JA (1968). Paranoid episodes induced by drug. *JAMA* 205:39–40.

13. Ellinwood EH, Jr. (1967). Amphetamine psychosis. I. Description of the individuals and process. *J Nerv Ment Dis* 144:273–283.

14. Angrist B, Sathananthan G, Wilk S (1974). Amphetamine psychosis: Behavioral and biochemical aspects. *J Psychiatr Res* 11:13–23.

15. Davis JM (1975). Catecholamines and psychosis. In *Catecholamines and Behavior, Vol. 2*, Freidhoff AJ, ed. New York: Plenum Press.

16. Kalant OJ (1966). Abuse of amphetamine-like drugs. In *The Amphetamines: Toxicity and Addiction*. Springfield, IL: C. C. Thomas.

17. Prinzmetal M, Bloomberg W (1935). The use of benzedrine for the treatment of narcolepsy. *JAMA* 105:2051–2055.

18. Bell DS (1965). Comparison of amphetamine psychosis and schizophrenia. *Br J Psychiatry* 3:701–707.

19. Segal DS, Janowsky DS (1978). Psychostimulant-induced behavioral effects: Possible models of schizophrenia. In *Psychopharmacology: A Generation of Progress*, Lipton MA, DiMasco A, Killam KF, eds., p. 461. New York: Raven Press.

20. Connell PH (1958). Amphetamine psychosis. *Maudsley Monograph No. 5*. London: Oxford University Press.

21. Bell DS (1973). The experimental reproduction of amphetamine psychosis. *Arch Gen Psychiatry* 29:35–40.

22. National Commission on Marijuana and Drug Abuse (1973). Drug use in America: Problems in perspective. In *Second Report of the National Commission on Marijuana and Drug Abuse*. Washington, DC: National Institute on Drug Abuse.

23. Mayfield DG (1979). Alcohol and affect: Experimental studies. In *Alcoholism and Affective Disorders*, Goodwin DW, Erickson CK, eds., pp. 99–107. New York: SP Medical and Scientific Books.

24. Schuckit MA (1983). Alcoholic patients with secondary depression. *Am J Psychiatry* 140(6):711–714.

25. Kramer JC, Fischman VS, Littlefield DC (1967). Amphetamine abuse. *J Am Med Ass* 201:305–309.

26. Grinspoon L, Bakalar JB (1980). Drug dependence: Nonnarcotic agents. In *Comprehensive Textbook of Psychiatry*, 3d Ed., Kaplan HI, Freedman AM, Sadock BJ, eds. Baltimore: Williams & Wilkins.

27. Strategy Council on Drug Abuse (1973). *Federal Strategy for Drug Abuse and Drug Traffic Prevention, 1973*. Washington, DC: U.S. Govt. Printing Office.

28. Canadian Medical Association (1969). Nonmedical use of drugs, with particular reference to youth. Report of the special committee on drug misuse, council on community health care, Canadian Medical Association. *Can Med Assoc J* 101.

29. Knapp P (1952). Amphetamine and addiction. *J Nerv Ment Dis* 115:406–410.
30. Rylander G (1971). Stereotype behavior in man following amphetamine abuse. *Proc Eur Soc Study Drug Tox* 12:28–34.
31. Cox C, Smart RG (1970). The nature and extent of speed use in North America. *Can Med Assoc J* 102:724–729.
32. Dominic JA, Moore KE (1969). Supersensitivity to the central stimulant actions of adrenergic drugs following discontinuation of a chronic diet of α-methyltyrosine. *Psychopharmacologia* (Berlin) 15:96–101.
33. Creese I, Burt DR, Snyder SH (1977). Dopamine receptor binding enhancement accompanies lesions-induced behavioral supersensitivity. *Science* 197:596–598.
34. Dackis CA, Gold MS (1985). Pharmacological approaches to cocaine addiction. *J Subst Abuse Treat* 2:139–145.
35. Miller NS, Dackis CA, Gold MS (1987). The relationship of addiction, tolerance and dependence: A neurochemical approach. *J Subst Abuse Treat* 4(3–4):197–207.
36. Ungerstedt U (1971). Stereotaxic mapping of the monoamine pathway in the rat brain. *Acta Physiol Scand (Suppl)* 83:1–48.
37. Von Voigtlander PF, Moore KE (1970). Behavioral and brain catecholamine depleting actions of U-14.624, an inhibitor of dopamine-β-hydroxylase. *Proc Soc Exp Biol Med* 133:817.
38. Chiueh CC, Moore KE (1975). D-amphetamine-induced release of "newly-synthesized" and "stored" dopamine from the caudate nucleus in vitro. *J Pharmacol Exp Ther* 192:642–653.
39. Azzaro AJ, Ziance RJ, Rutledge CO (1974). The importance of neuronal intake of amines for amphetamine-induced release of ³H-norepinephrine from isolated brain tissue. *J Pharmacol Exp Ther* 189:110–118.
40. Thornburg JE, Moore KE (1973). The relative importance of dopaminergic and noradrenergic neuronal systems for the stimulation of locomotor activity induced by amphetamine and other drugs. *Neuropharmacology* 12:853–866.
41. Russek M, Rodrigues-Zendejas AM, Teitelbaum P (1973). The action of adrenergic anorexigenic substances on rats recovered from lateral hypothalamus lesions. *Physiol Behav* 10:329–333.
42. Hoebel BG (1975). Satiety: Hypothalamic stimulation, anorectic drugs, neurochemical substrates. In *Hunger: Basic Mechanisms and Clinical Implications*, Novin D, Wyrujicka W, Bray G, eds. New York: Raven Press.

CHAPTER 11

The Pharmacology of Anabolic-Androgen Steroids

History

The anabolic-androgen steroids (AAS) are chemicals that have both properties contained in the same molecule. Therefore, it is impossible to discuss one type of action without including the other because the effects of intoxication from these compounds are both anabolic and androgenic. Anabolic action is the performance-enhancing and muscle-mass-proliferation property, whereas the androgenic action is characteristic of male sex hormones. The pharmacological objective in use by athletes is to promote the anabolic or performance-enhancing effect while attempting to minimize the androgenic effect (1,2).

These chemicals were first studied for their capacity to increase muscle mass in 1935. The researchers demonstrated a increase in the catabolism (breakdown) of protein following administration of androgens, resulting in a positive nitrogen balance in castrated dogs. During World War II, anabolic steroids were used to enhance the aggressive behavior of troops as well as to build up the weight of those who survived severe starvation (3,4).

In the early 1950s, anabolic steroids began to be used by athletes to improve their athletic abilities, particularly by weightlifters to improve their strength. The contemporary competitive athlete in many fields of sport is currently using these anabolic-androgenic compounds to become bigger, faster, and more aggressive. In fact, reports are emerging that coaches have come to expect that athletes use steroids to maintain and gain a competitive edge at the high-school, college, and professional levels of sports (5,6).

These chemicals, however, are not without toxicities. The medical and psychiatric complications, aside from the illegality of their use, are becoming increasingly apparent. Of importance is that the anabolic-androgen steroids are being used addictively with the characteristic loss of control that accompanies addiction to other drugs. This is a particularly disturbing feature of steroid use because no apparent benefit results from addictive use, and the adverse consequences are especially severe (7,8).

Prevalence

In surveys in the United States, more than 90% of body builders are found to use anabolic steroids. Many athletes believe that anabolic steroids increase their performance, strength, muscle mass, and aggressiveness. Of critical importance is the finding that as many as 700,000 high-school students in the United States have tried these steroids. The prevalence rates for high-school boys range from 4% to 11% and for girls from 0.5% to 2.5%. Estimates place the total number of steroid users at 1 million or more. Among college athletes in the United States, a rate of 20% has been reported, although actual estimates of prevalence are hard to obtain (9–11).

Most users purchase AAS illicitly through illegal sources, although some are able to find physicians who are willing to prescribe these chemicals. Only recently have the prevalence and toxicities of AAS been apparent to the practicing physicians so that the demand from the illicit sources may increase (12,13).

Patterns of Use

The user typically uses 10 to 100 times the therapeutic doses, and often does not know the exact composition of the AAS because of the illicit source. The steroids are often mixed from more than one source to achieve the high doses desired, and when used in combination is referred to as "stacking." The combination may be given entirely intramuscularly or with oral preparations. For performance enhancing, the user typically uses the drugs in cycles for weeks with intervening periods of time of abstinence or reduced dose to attempt to avoid toxicity or to prevent detection by drug testing (14,15).

The steroid user frequently consumes other drugs to control side effects from the steroids. Diuretics are taken to reduce the fluid retention from the mineralocorticoid effect of steroids. Estrogen blockers such as clomiphene or tamoxifen are used to prevent the steroid-induced gynecomastia. Human chorionic gonadotropin is used to reduce the testicular atrophy that is induced by the androgenic effect on the pituitary secretions of the male gonadotropin, follicle-stimulating hormone (FSH) (16,17).

A significant number of AAS users are addicted to the steroids, and as in most contemporary drug addicts, are additionally addicted to multiple drugs, including alcohol, marijuana, cocaine, and benzodiazepines. It is not always clear if the users of these steroids were attracted to their use for the performance-enhancing ability or the addictive quality of the drugs as with other drugs of addiction (15,16).

Neurochemistry

The AAS differ in their chemical structure, route of administration, duration of action, and relative androgenic and anabolic effects and toxicities. All anabolic steroids can be classified into two major chemical groups: 17-α-alkylated and 17-esterified steroids. The esters are given mainly intramuscularly, and thus are slowly released from the depot following parental injection, producing a longer duration of action than the oral administration. Because there is substantial breakdown of the testosterone molecule after oral administration by the first pass through the liver via the portal system, alkylation with methyl or ethyl group protects hepatic oxidation of the 17-β-hydroxyl moiety following an oral dose. However, the alkylated derivatives are not as safe as testosterone itself because of the higher risk of hepatic toxicity (17,18).

The androgens are four-ring structures with 19 carbon-containing steroids. Testosterone, the major androgen in humans, is secreted mainly by the Leydig's cells of the interstitial tissues of the testes. Androgens are responsible for the male phenotype in utero, and stimulate the development of the testes, scrotum, penis, seminal vesicles, prostate, vas deferens, and epididymis. Overproduction of androgens in adults is responsible for the aggressive sexual behavior in males. Androgens promote the deepening of the voice, sebaceous gland secretion and acne, and body hair on the axilla, trunk, limbs, and face (19).

The anabolic effect is to stimulate the growth of the muscle mass during its normal development. Because no anabolic steroid is free from androgenic effects, the unavoidable consequence of high-dose AAS use is the unwanted masculinization. It may not be possible to separate the androgenic from the anabolic properties because they do not result from different actions of the same hormone, but represent the same actions in different tissues. The actions of these steroids are less specific because the androgen-responsive muscles contain the same androgen-receptor system as the other androgen-target tissues. Therefore all anabolic agents have androgenic activity, and in sufficient doses can produce androgen effects and be used as replacement therapy for androgens (20).

In the body, testosterone is converted to more active metabolites such as dihydrotestosterone (DHT) and estradiol. About 98% of testosterone is bound to plasma proteins, testosterone-estradiol-binding globulin (TeBG) or SHBG and albumin, and only 1% to 2% of the hormone remains unbound or free. The free hormone enters the target cell by passive diffusion and is converted to DHT by 5-α-reductase enzyme. DHT binds to specific receptors on the nucleus, which generates a new mRNA so that new proteins are synthesized by the ribosomes (21).

The administration of high doses of anabolic steroids to athletes causes a significant decrease in serum luteinizing hormone (LH), FSH, and adrenocorticotropin hormone (ACTH), because of the hypothalamic negative feed-back effects of administering exogenous steroids. The synthesis of proteins causes a positive nitrogen balance, increases lean body mass, and enhances muscle growth in hypogonadial males. In normal adult males, these effects occur at about half of the levels seen in the hypogonadial male (22).

Pharmacokinetics

Testosterone is readily absorbed orally, but has poor bioavailability because of the rapid first-pass effect so that only 50% reaches the circulation. Methyltestosterone, a synthetic androgen, is less extensively metabolized by the liver and has a longer half-life, which improves the bioavailability after oral administration. The half-life of testosterone is highly variable, ranging from 10 to 100 minutes. Nandrolone decanoate given intramuscularly has a mean half-life of 6 days. Nandrolone exhibits a linear pharmacokinetics behavior (dose-independent) similar to other types of steroids, including prednisolone and methylprednisolone (18,23).

In the presence of liver disease, there is a decrease in both the rate of metabolism of the anabolic steroids and the synthesis of the plasma proteins responsible for their binding. Because anabolic steroids can cause liver dam-age, repetitive use of large doses of these steroids by athletes will increase their plasma-free concentration, with saturation of receptor sites and conse-quent toxicity. Alcohol ingestion also interferes with the metabolism of certain androgens by promoting increased levels of conjugated estradiol that tends to produce feminization in males (23).

Testosterone metabolism results in four main metabolites: dihydrotestos-terone (DHT), estradiol (E), androsterone (A), and etiocholanolone (ET). Testosterone and its metabolites are excreted in the urine mainly as glu-curonic and sulfuric acid conjugates. The plasma levels of androsterone glucuronide and estradiol glucuronide are good markers of androgen metab-olism (23).

Most injectable steroids are released slowly so that they can be adminis-tered every 2 to 4 weeks, and thus are considered long-acting agents. Testos-terone esters, testosterone propionate, testosterone enanthate, and testos-terone cypionate are intramuscular forms. The oral steroids need to be given daily because of their short half-life (18).

Intoxication

The effects of intoxication have medical and psychiatric consequences. The AAS have been associated with heart attacks, strokes, liver disease, tumors and cancer, high blood pressure, fluid retention, altered immunity, and skin abnormalities. Men may develop sterility, testicular atrophy, painful gyneco-mastia, prostatic hypertrophy, and hair loss. Women may develop sterility, menstrual irregularities, masculinization with deepening of voice, increase in body hair, and clitoral hypertrophy (24–28).

Psychological effects include depression, suicidal thinking, insomnia, marked aggression and violent behavior, mood swings and frank psychosis. Many steroid users suffer from psychotic and depressive disorders that are similar to DSM-III-R criteria for these diagnostic categories (29).

Adolescents and preadolescents may experience premature epiphyseal closure of their bones and an exaggerated response to the mood and mental changes induced by steroids. Children may also develop virilization and gynecomastia, and male children have a higher rate of feminizing effects than adult males (24).

Tolerance and Dependence

The development of tolerance and dependence to AAS has been documented in studies. The occurrence of clinically evident withdrawal symptoms occurs at a high rate in steroid users. Studies show that tolerance was detectable in 20%, and withdrawal in 84% of a group of users, many of whom were also addicted to steroids. The withdrawal syndrome is characterized by fatigue, depression, restlessness, anorexia, insomnia, and decreased libido as well as a craving or desire to use more of the drug (30).

Diagnosis

The preoccupation with acquiring, compulsive use, and relapse to these steroids has been documented in clinical practice and in research studies. Some steroid users maintain that they would not stop taking AAS even if it was proven beyond a doubt that these steroids caused permanent sterility, liver cancer, or heart attacks. Further evidence for addictive use appears to be mounting as the toxicity from the use of these drugs become more apparent with the compulsive use (30).

Obviously, weight lifters and athletes are at high risk to develop an addiction to steroids, and the addiction should be suspected in any athlete having medical and psychiatric problems. Careful and thorough evaluations may yield rewarding results if a sufficiently high index of suspicion is maintained (30).

Other Drug Use

The use of other drugs in conjunction with or before the onset of steroid use by steroid users and addicts is significant. Many steroid users are addicted to alcohol, cocaine, marijuana, and other drugs in a manner similar to the multiple addicted. Many steroid addicts were addicted to other drugs before becoming addicted to AAS (15).

Intervention and Treatment

High-risk groups for using and being addicted to these drugs are weight lifters, other athletes, adolescents, and young adults. Also, anyone who is addicted to drugs and alcohol should be screened for steroid use as a matter of routine and complete evaluation. During a medical evaluation, any liver, cardiac, or endocrine abnormality should be investigated for AAS use. Psychiatric manifestations such as depression, fatigue, and psychosis should be evaluated for AAS use, particularly in the high-risk groups. A diagnostic interview, as with any other suspected drug problem, is to be used.

Drug testing for detection of steroid use involves identification of the steroid and the metabolite. Because some of the exogenously administered AAS such as testosterone esters are metabolized to testosterone, it is necessary to calculate ratios to distinguish quantitative differences from endogenous sources of testosterone. Normally, the ratio of testosterone to epitestosterone in the urine of males is 1–2.5 to 1. When the ratio exceeds 6 to 1, the administration of exogenous testosterone compounds is likely. The steroids that are not metabolized in the urine can be detected by their presence in the urine as foreign (31).

It is important to employ a high-quality laboratory that can competently perform testing for these drugs. As discussed in chapter   , false-negative results are far more common than false-positive results; thus, a well-regulated laboratory can be expected to minimize the likelihood of either. Drug testing for steroids is intricate and involves testing for 40 different steroid compounds, using expensive GC-MS methodology that is expensive and difficult for many laboratories to do.

Just as with any other drug addiction, denial and rationalization must be confronted. A peculiar justification in this regard is that the user may emphasize the performance and masculinization of these drugs in spite of the lack of objective verification of this claim in the scientific literature, as well as their illicit nature and medical and psychiatric complications. This is addictive use.

Detoxification for withdrawal does not ordinarily require specific pharmacological interventions. Supportive medical and psychiatric care for the sequelae of the use of these drugs may be needed, that is, hepatic toxicity or suicidal intent. Administration of hormonal replacement may be indicated in severe cases of hypothalamic suppression of the gonadotropins.

Because the addiction to AAS is essentially the same as to any drugs, the use of specific principles in the treatment of addiction is indicated. Because many of the AAS addicts are also addicted to alcohol and other drugs, standard treatment for these addictions will work for the AAS. The addicts may be referred to 12-step-based treatment programs, and the recovery programs such as Alcoholics Anonymous and Narcotics Anonymous.

References

1. Redda KK, Walker CA, Barnett G (1989). *Cocaine, Marijuana, Designer Drugs: Chemistry, Pharmacology and Behavior*. Boca Raton, FL: CRC Press.
2. Haupt HA, Rovere GD (1984). Anabolic steroids: A review of the literature. *Am J Sports Med* 12:469–484.
3. Kochakian CD, Murlin JR (1935). The effect of male hormone on problem and energy metabolism of castrated dogs. *J Nutr* 10:437.
4. Kopera H (1985). The history of anabolic steroids and a review of clinical experience with anabolic steroids. *Acta Endocrinol (Suppl)* 271:11–18.
5. Wilson JD (1988). Androgen abuse by athletes. *Endocrinol Rev* 9:181–199.
6. Lamb DR (1984). Anabolic steroids in athletics: How well do they work and how dangerous are they? *Am J Sports Med* 12:31–38 .
7. Murad F, Haynes RC (1985). Androgens. In *The Pharmacological Basis of Therapeutics*, 7th Ed., Gilman AG, Goodman LS, Rall TW, Murad F, eds. New York: Macmillan.
8. Rogers HJ, Spector RG, Trounce JR (1981). *A Textbook of Clinical Pharmacology*. London: Hodder and Stoughton.
9. Council on Scientific Affairs (1988). Drug abuse in athletes: Anabolic steroids and human growth hormone. *JAMA* 259:1703–1705.
10. Buckley WE, Yesalis CE, Friedl K, et al. (1988). Estimated prevalence of anabolic steroid use among male high school seniors. *JAMA* 260:3441–3445.
11. Dezelsky TL, Toohey JV, Shaw RS (1985). Non-medical drug use behavior at five United States universities: 1 15-year study. *Bull Narc* 37(2–3):49–53.
12. Coward V (1987). Steroids in sports: After four decades, time to return these genies to bottle? *JAMA* 257:421–427.
13. Bergman R, Leach RE (1985). The use and abuse of anabolic steroids in Olympic-caliber athletes. *Clin Orthop Relat Res* 198:169–172.
14. Frankle MA, Cicero GJ, Payne J (1984). Use of androgenic anabolic steroids by athletes. *JAMA* 252:482 .
15. Pope HG Jr, Katz DL, Champoux R (1988). Anabolic-androgenic steroid use among 1,010 college men. *Physician Sportsmed* 16:75–81.
16. Pope HG Jr, Katz DL (1988). Affective and psychotic symptoms associated with anabolic steroid use. *Am J Psychiatry* 145:487–490.
17. Gower DB (1979). *Steroid Hormones*. London: Croom Helm.
18. Van Wayjen RGA, Buyze G (1962). Clinical pharmacological evaluation of certain anabolic steroids. *Acta Endocrinol (Suppl)* 63:18.
19. Griffin JE, Wilson JD (1985). Disorders of the testes and male reproductive tract. In *Textbook of Endocrinology*, 7th Ed., Wilson JD, Foster DW, eds., pp. 259–311. Philadelphia: Saunders.
20. Desauller PA, Krahenbhl C (1962). Evaluation and mode of action of anabolic steroids: Differentiation of action of various anabolic steroids. In *Protein Metabolism*, p. 185. Berlin: Springer-Verlag.
21. Smith RG, Nag A, Syms AL, Norris JSH (1986). Steroid receptor, gene structure and molecular biology. *J Steroid Biochem* 214:51.
22. Tepperman J (1973). *Metabolic and Endocrine Physiology*, p. 70. Chicago: Yearbook Medical Publisher.
23. Nowakowski H (1962). Metabolic studies with anabolic steroids. *Acta Endocrinol (Suppl)* 63:37.

24. Kibble MW, Ross MB (1987). Adverse effects of anabolic steroids in athletes. *Clin Pharm* 6:686–692.
25. McNutt RA, Ferenchick GS, Kirlin PC, et al. (1988). Acute myocardial infarction in a 22-year-old world-class weight lifter using anabolic steroids. *Am J Cardiol* 62:164.
26. Mochizuki RH, Richter KJ (1988). Cardiomyopathy and cerebrovascular accident associated with anabolic-androgenic steroid use. *Physician Sportsmed* 16: 109–114.
27. Ishak KG, Zimmerman HJ (1987). Hepatotoxic effects of the anabolic/androgenic steroids. *Semin Liver Dis* 7:230–236.
28. Creagh TM, Rubin A, Evans DJ (1988). Hepatic tumours induced by anabolic steroids in an athlete. *J Clin Pathol* 41:441–443.
29. APA (1987). *DSM-III-R: Diagnostic and Statistical Manual of Mental Disorders*, 3d Ed. Washington, DC: American Psychiatric Association.
30. Brower KJ, Blow FC, Beresford TP, Fuelling C (1989). Anabolic-androgenic steroid dependence. *J Clin Psychiatry* 50:31–33.
31. Hatton CK, Catlin DH (1987). Detection of androgenic anabolic steroids in urine. *Clin Lab Med* 7:655–668.

CHAPTER 12

The Pharmacology of Benzodiazepines

History

The benzodiazepines have been and remain among the most prescribed drugs in the United States and the world since their introduction in 1961. Of interest is that four of the 10 most commonly written prescriptions in 1987 were for drugs used for the relief of pain and anxiety; currently, 1 of these is the benzodiazepine Xanax (1).

Physicians continue to prescribe substantial numbers of benzodiazepines. The seven best-selling psychiatric drugs sold in community drug stores in 1988 were all benzodiazepines: alprazolam (Xanax), triazolam (Halcion), diazepam (Valium), lorazepam (Ativan), clorazepate (Tranxene), temazepam (Restoril), and flurazepam (Dalmane) (1). These prescribing practices have continued in spite of a large number of studies providing considerable evidence that pharmacological tolerance, dependence, abuse, and addiction occur frequently with these agents in both medical and nonmedical settings (2,3). Because of the documented adverse consequences from extended benzodiazepine administration and the availability of alternative methods of effective treatment for the disorders treated with benzodiazepines, the justifications for their use beyond the short term are few (4–10).

The confusion that exists in medical practice regarding the pharmacology, risks, and benefits of benzodiazepines arises in part from the significant misunderstanding and misuse of definitions concerning diagnosis, drug treatment, drug effects, abuse and addiction, and tolerance and dependence (3,11,12). The seeming orientation of the medical profession toward prescribing medications for physical and psychological disorders in the general population, and particularly in high-risk groups such as persons with alcoholism, drug addiction, and chronic illness, may account for the substantial overprescribing of the benzodiazepines. The nature of the complaints for which benzodiazepines are prescribed are extraordinarily common and include anxiety, depression, insomnia, and pain. The pervasiveness and persistence of these symptoms in medical and nonmedical populations make benzodiazepines particularly attractive to both patients and physicians.

Prevalence

Three principal methods of study are used to assess the prevalence of benzo-diazepine use. The first is by enumerating the number of prescriptions writ-ten, as performed by the National Prescription Audit; the second and third methods are surveys periodically sponsored by the National Institute on Drug Abuse (NIDA), such as the National Household Survey and the Drug Abuse Warning Network (DAWN), respectively (2,13).

The past and current findings are that the benzodiazepines are the most frequently prescribed class of psychotropic medications in the United States and Europe. Diazepam had been the single most commonly prescribed ben-zodiazepine until 1987 when it dropped in rank below alprazolam, which has been experiencing a sharp increase in sales in recent years to reach the number four position among all medications prescribed in 1987. Although the overall use of benzodiazepines has been declining since the peak level of 100 million prescriptions per year in 1975, their use continues at an extraor-dinarily high rate as 81 million prescriptions were filled in 1985 (2,14).

The most widely cited study for prevalence of benzodiazepine use was based on self-reports from those who were interviewed in the 1979 National Household Survey. The study found that long-term use, defined as regular daily use for a year or longer, occurred in 15% of those for whom benzo-diazepines were prescribed (13). This 15% constituted 1.6% of all adults between the ages of 18 and 79 years in the general population (15,16).

The 1985 National Household Survey found significant increases oc-curred with the nonmedical use of tranquilizers among adults who were 26 years or older. The percent of these respondents reporting ever having used a tranquilizer, nonmedically, increased from 3.6% in 1982 to 7.1% in 1985. Among persons of all ages in 1985 having used tranquilizers during the preceding year, 17% were 12 to 17 years of age, 25% were 18 to 25, 31% were 26 to 34, and 26% were 35 and older. The group was composed of 61% males; 89% were whites, 7% blacks, and 4% hispanics. The reported fre-quency of use in the past year for 10 times or fewer was 55%; 11 to 99 times, 32%; and more than 100 times, 13% (14).

Patterns of Use

Although many studies and reviews are available that examine the potential for developing dependence on benzodiazepines, most suffer from problems in definitions, interpretations, and conclusions regarding the diagnosis of benzodiazepine "dependence" (2,3,11,17,18). Essentially none of the studies use clear definitions of abuse, addiction, tolerance, and dependence. Most studies on the medical use of benzodiazepines concentrate on the pharmaco-logical tolerance and dependence. Few studies address the addictive use and potential in medical populations.

Nonetheless, these studies clearly establish the following: (i) pharmacological dependence on benzodiazepines occurs often with a rapid onset measured in weeks; (ii) the development of pharmacological dependence adheres to known pharmacokinetic and pharmacodynamic models; (iii) the dependence syndrome consists of withdrawal symptoms of anxiety, panic, depression, seizures and delirium, and other expressions of excessive autonomic nervous system discharge; (iv) the signs and symptoms are indistinguishable from those present in anxiety disorders and other drug withdrawals except in time course; and (v) the long-term efficacy of benzodiazepines has not been established (19–26). Furthermore, other studies strongly suggest that (i) the benzodiazepines are not as effective in the treatment of anxiety as once surmised; (ii) the drugs are not as safe as once proposed; (iii) the indications for benzodiazepines are narrower than previously defined; (iv) other acceptable methods for treating anxiety are available; (v) abuse and addiction occur in greater prevalence than previously realized; and (vi) the distinction between medical and nonmedical use is not sharp, and significant overlap is present (27–32).

The intent of the following discussion is to review critically the problems in the definitions and concepts of abuse, addiction, tolerance, and dependence that lead to difficulties in interpreting and applying the findings of these reports and reviews. The relevance and purpose of clarifying them is to provide guidelines for the clinician in considering the safety and efficacy of the benzodiazepines in clinical practice.

It is interesting and important to note that the nonmedical users of benzodiazepines reported in the National Household Survey in 1985 consisted essentially of polydrug-addicted abusers. The prevalence of use of other substances among these benzodiazepine users in 1985 included alcohol, 95%; marijuana, 72%; cigarettes, 63%; cocaine, 49%; and heroin, 2%. As expected, the rate of nonmedical use of tranquilizers was higher among young adults, ages 18 to 25 years, than in any other group in the general population. In contrast, the highest rate of medical use of benzodiazepines occurred in the over-50 age group.

A major drawback of the National Household Survey was that it focused entirely on nonmedical use. The survey is based on personal interviews with a representative sample of persons over the age of 12 who live in households in the continental United States. Benzodiazepines were clearly the most common "tranquilizer" used. About 6.5 million Americans 12 years old and over used a tranquilizer at least once during a designated month before the survey. The interpretation of medical and nonmedical use was left to the interviewee and not established by objective criteria applied by a physician knowledgeable in drug abuse and addiction.

Although objective, systematically obtained data on the actual prevalence of tranquilizer use in medical populations is not available, estimates are that about 25 million persons in this country fall into this category (2,14). During 1985 in the United States, a total of 3.7 billion benzodiazepine pills were purchased consequent to the total of 81 million filled prescriptions for benzodiazepines. Simple division reveals that the number of pills equals 16 per person per year, based on a population of 225 million. The actual number of users was 25 million for an average "sale" per person of 148 pills (2,14). Incidentally, the prevalence rate of alcohol dependence is approximately 15% of the general population, or 37 million based on a population of 250 million (33).

Another indication of medical and nonmedical use of benzodiazepines comes from DAWN, which obtains data from emergency room records on clinical observations and self-reported information. Although DAWN does not clearly distinguish between nonmedical and medical users of the benzodiazepines, interesting data regarding medical interventions for drug-related problems result. DAWN was established to detect new drug problems and monitor trends in drug-associated medical emergencies throughout selected U.S. emergency rooms. In 1985 data were collected on drug use during patient visits to emergency rooms from 733 hospitals and from cases of 73 medical examiners located in 27 metropolitan areas throughout the United States. During 1985, 13,501 people produced cocaine "mentions"; 14,696 people produced combined morphine and heroin "mentions"; and 18,492 people yielded benzodiazepine "mentions," a mention being a visit or case where the drug was cited. Important in the DAWN report is that about half of emergency room episodes involving benzodiazepines occur because of a suicide attempt or actual suicide. Moreover, 7 of all the top 50 drugs mentioned in DAWN emergency room statistics for 1985 were benzodiazepines. Diazepam was the most common, and 27% of the time diazepam was mentioned without other drugs; 38% of the time another drug was also mentioned; 22% of the time 2 other drugs were mentioned; and 13% of the time 3 or more other drugs were mentioned in addition to diazepam. In 1985, 49% of diazepam mentions were from legal prescriptions, 3% were stolen, 7.7% were illegal purchases, and 0.1% were from forged prescriptions; 38.8% gave no information at all about their sources (2,14).

In contrast, among young adults 18 to 25 years of age, the lifetime prevalence for use decreased from 15.1% in 1982 to 12.2% in 1985; among youth aged 12 to 17, a slight decrease occurred from 4.9% to 4.8%. These trends in decreasing drug use in these age groups correspond to those trends for other drugs of abuse in this age group, according to surveys of high-school seniors supported by NIDA (2,14). A caution is urged in interpreting these findings in school-age populations as the school "dropouts" are not included in the survey so that the prevalence rates may be falsely "low." Many of these school dropouts were probably drug users, and premature termination from school may have been related to drug use.

These findings, in conjunction with others, indicate that the most common source for the benzodiazepines for both nonmedical and medical use is the physician. This suggests that the practice of distinguishing between nonmedical and medical use is subject to considerable error, because origins of benzodiazepine use ultimately are frequently attributable to physicians.

What presents considerable challenge to the physician is that the signs and symptoms for which benzodiazepines are commonly prescribed can also be consequences of drug dependence and addiction, as stated earlier. Furthermore, if benzodiazepine use evolves into abuse and then pharmacological dependence, as it apparently does with considerable frequency, this means that many benzodiazepine users are, by definition, using benzodiazepines for nonmedical purposes because "medical use" does not ordinarily apply to supporting dependence on a drug with its attendant consequences.

Intoxication

Central Nervous System

Although the benzodiazepines are classified as tranquilizers, they act more as sedatives/hypnotics. For a drug to be a tranquilizer, it must calm or induce tranquility without producing any sedation. The benzodiazepines as a class are clearly sedating and readily induce hypnosis. Tolerance develops to the sedation and hypnosis only partially and after chronic administration. Also, disturbances in mood, sleep, memory, and psychomotor performance occur from acute and chronic use of the benzodiazepines.

The acute effects of the benzodiazepines are similar qualitatively to the classical sedatives such as barbiturates. All the benzodiazepines calm and sedate, and in large enough doses can induce sleep. Some are used clinically as tranquilizers to calm and sedate in usual doses. Other members are used clinically as hypnotics to induce sleep in usual doses. Impairment in psychomotor performance with an increase in reaction time, interruption in hand–eye coordination, and motor ataxia correlates with the degree of sedation.

Although the benzodiazepines induce muscle hypotonia in animals, clinical trials have failed to demonstrate superiority of benzodiazepines over placebos. Triazolam, clonazepam, bromazepam, and diazepam are more selective anticonvulsants than other benzodiazepines. Only diazepam has analgesic effects that are mild—and only transient.

The effects of benzodiazepines on sleep and the electroencephalograph (EEG) are predictably and stereotypic and resemble other sedative/hypnotic drugs. Alpha activity is decreased. Increased low voltage, fast activity in the beta range, predominate. The shift and appearance of activity occurs more in the frontal temporal areas of the brain (34).

Most benzodiazepines decrease sleep latency and time spent awake before falling asleep, and diminish the number of awakenings before tolerance and dependence occur. Stage one of sleep (drowsiness) is decreased by flurazepam, lorazepam, nitrazepam, and temazepam, but increased by chlordiazepoxide, diazepam, and oxazepam. Time spent in stage two is increased by all benzodiazepams, and time spent in stages three and four (slow-wave sleep, SWS) is decreased. The period of rapid eye movement (REM) sleep is usually shortened.

Tolerance is more pronounced to the effects on the REM sleep than to the non-REM sleep parameters. The number of dreams may double during chronic use. After only 3 to 4 weeks of nightly use of many benzodiazepines, there is considerable "rebound" in the amount and density of REM sleep on cessation of the drug. The exceptions are withdrawal from chlorazepate, lorazepam, or nitrazepam that cause a rebound decrease in REM sleep time that may persist for a long period of time. There is also usually rebound increase in SWS that may exceed the rebound in REM sleep. These sleep and EEG changes are more evident with the short-acting (shorter half-life) benzodiazepines (34–36).

The typical signs and symptoms of withdrawal from benzodiazepines are anxiety, depression, tremors, and malaise. Vital signs are often normal, although blood pressure and pulse may be elevated somewhat. More severe withdrawal may include generalized tonic clonic seizures, delirium with disorientation, clouding of sensorium, hallucinations and delusions, myalgia, muscle cramps, and paresthesias, particularly in the extremities. A severe and incapacitating tension headache (band around the head) may be a persistent symptom over months (37–39).

Anxiety is a pronounced effect from withdrawal, and its presence is often confused with the original symptoms of anxiety for which the benzodiazepine was prescribed. Guides to differentiate between the two are the following: anxiety from withdrawal tends to (1) be persistent and pervasive, (2) gradually and imperceptibly subside over weeks and months, (3) not vary with external or environmental factors, and (4) be of different character than the original anxiety problems; anxiety from other sources tends to (1) be discrete, stereotypic, and patterned, (2) occur intermittently, and (3) vary more with outside stimuli. Administration of more benzodiazepines will not easily differentiate between the two as the best anecdote for symptoms of withdrawal, particularly anxiety, is the same drug that is responsible for the initial withdrawal and anxiety was the original symptom for which the benzodiazepine was given (40).

The cardiovascular and respiratory effects are minimal. The benzodiazepines may decrease respirations, blood pressure, and left ventricular work mildly after an acute dose (41).

Diagnosis

In recent years, the concept of "abuse" has undergone significant change. By historical definition, abuse is use of a drug that outside the usual or accepted standard as determined by a given population. An example of such abuse would be infrequent, transient nonmedical use of a benzodiazepine, with some personal or medical consequence in the absence of a pattern of addictive use. In the past, abuse did not ordinarily include the development of addiction, tolerance, or dependence, which are terms that have definite behavioral and pharmacological criteria. However, in ordinary recent usage, the term abuse has acquired these other parameters of abnormal drug use, for reasons that remain unclear, and this practice has led to confusion and critical misuse of diagnostic terminology in clinical practice and research.

The addiction to benzodiazepines is characterized by a preoccupation with the acquisition of benzodiazepines and their compulsive use with a pattern of relapse after abstinence or an inability to reduce use. Addiction implies a loss of control over the use of benzodiazepines, generated by a drive to use the benzodiazepines in spite of adverse consequences. Addiction to a drug, by definition, extends beyond abusive use into pathological dimensions with persistent consequences from the pervasive loss of control. Abuse may be a prelude to addiction as it indicates some inappropriate exposure to the drug and, perhaps, evidence already of some loss of control in a manner that is not deemed normal according to societal definitions. Addictive use, however, not only exceeds standards of use and transcends social norms, but has characteristics that allow it to be identified in medical and nonmedical populations regardless of other diagnoses (12,42).

Tolerance and Dependence

Tolerance to a drug is defined as a loss of a particular drug effect at a constantly administered dose. To maintain the same drug effect, the dose must be increased. Tolerance is an expected accompaniment of regular drug use that reflects the adaptation of the receptor site to the presence of the drug. Teleologically, the function of tolerance is to maintain homeostatic balance so that physiological functioning continues within a normal range despite the effects of the foreign agent.

The case of development of tolerance reflects individual and group differences in pharmacokinetics and pharmacodynamic parameters (12,43,44). Pharmacokinetic variables include rate of absorption, extent of distribution, and rate of elimination of the drug. Larger individuals have more tolerance for a drug because they have greater volumes of distribution; drug metabolism can also be affected by other factors such as drug induction of microsomal enzymes by one drug that enhances the elimination of another drug. For instance, alcohol induces microsomal enzymes to increase the metabolism of the benzodiazepines. Pharmacodynamic tolerance is determined by the action of the drug at the receptor site and the response of the receptor site to the drug. The longer the drug persists at the receptor site, the greater the tolerance to the drug because of the adaptation of the receptor site to the presence of the drug (34).

The relationship of tolerance to addiction is another area that historically has been a major source of confusion. The use of established definitions for tolerance and addiction will serve substantially to clarify their relationship. Tolerance to benzodiazepines occurs as rapidly as one dose in animals and weeks in humans, according to controlled studies (7,9,18). The development of tolerance to benzodiazepines is clinically similar to that for alcohol and vastly different from that for opiates in that only a mild-to-moderate increase in the dose of a benzodiazepine is usually clinically tolerated, although some larger doses are tolerated in multiple drug addicts with chronic use. Similarly, the acquired tolerance to alcohol is modest in most cases, even in chronic alcoholics, as twofold blood-level increases in alcohol are not usually tolerated.

The capacity to develop tolerance to opiates is as much as 10 times greater than for alcohol in humans and animals, but data are not available for comparisons to benzodiazepines. The use of tolerance as a measure of addictive potential probably arose from the opiate model of addiction, which required the development of dependence to opiates. Acquired tolerance to benzodiazepines is not a particularly precise measure of degree of addiction because, as with alcohol, the requirement for continued escalating doses (as occurs with opiate addictive use) is not commonly necessary (12,35,45).

Significant cross-tolerance between alcohol and benzodiazepines exists; this is utilized in the clinical practice of using the benzodiazepines to suppress the signs and symptoms of alcohol withdrawal. The lack of cross-tolerance between the opiates and alcohol, and between opiates and benzodiazepines, is clinically conspicuous because benzodiazepines cannot be used to suppress the signs and symptoms of opiate withdrawal. The principal observation that supports the separation of tolerance and addiction is that tolerance occurs in the absence of addictive use to a variety of drugs, including benzodiazepines, and vice versa.

However, the development of tolerance is not otherwise specific for addictive use because tolerance only marks the adaptation of the receptor to the frequent presence of the agent. An illustrative example is that opiates are given frequently for analgesia, and that tolerance develops readily, requiring greater doses to maintain the same level of analgesia. Usually, however, there is no continued addictive drug-seeking behavior in the majority of the patients to whom narcotics have been medically administered. Moreover, tolerance to the toxic and therapeutic effects of psychotropic medication, that is, antidepressants and neuroleptics, commonly occurs without addictive pursuit of the drugs (36).

The development of pharmacological drug dependence is also not a specific indicator of addictive use for essentially the same reason pertaining to tolerance. Pharmacological dependence is defined as the occurrence of signs and symptoms that are stereotypic and predictable on the cessation of the drug in question. Pharmacological dependence is thus the withdrawal syndrome that occurs typically and specifically after terminating a particular drug. The confusion of pharmacological dependence with addictive use is illustrated in the nosology of substance-dependence disorders in DSM-III-R, which does not necessarily require the withdrawal syndrome to make a diagnosis of "dependence." The diagnostic criteria for "dependence syndrome" in DSM-III-R include preoccupation, compulsivity, and relapse, which are the defining behaviors of addiction; in addition, pharmacological tolerance and dependence (or withdrawal) may be present but are not mandatory to make a diagnosis of a substance-dependence disorder. The popular clinical use of "pharmacological dependence" (withdrawal) interchangeably with a "diagnosis of dependence" (addiction) has been a source of serious error in clinical diagnosis and in the published studies on benzodiazepine dependence and withdrawal (15,16).

Hence, although pharmacological dependence on benzodiazepines develops rapidly and readily, it is not a specific indicator of addictive use of benzodiazepines. In some users, a withdrawal syndrome develops after discontinuing use of benzodiazepines without further drug-related behaviors such as a preoccupation with or a relapse to compulsive use of the drugs. As with other drugs, although withdrawal syndromes are regular occurrences in opiate use and there is commonly development of tolerance, addiction to the opiates after use for analgesia does not automatically develop and more frequently it will not. Although pharmacological dependence frequently accompanies the development of addictive use of benzodiazepines, the development of dependence is a parallel development and independent of, and not specific for, addictive behavior.

One method of distinguishing between dependence with and without addictive use is to note when the patient fails in his attempt to discontinue the benzodiazepines on the recommendation of the physician or at his own discretion. If the patient is unable to discontinue benzodiazepines, confirmation of addiction to benzodiazepines is possible by the identification of a preoccupation with the acquisition and compulsive use of the agent (in spite of the adverse consequences of continued use), as well as a recurrent pattern of relapse after abstinence or an inability to reduce benzodiazepine use.

What may be contributing confusion to the clinical picture is that pharmacological dependence alone may produce the symptoms of anxiety and insomnia, and these symptoms can be mistaken for the original symptoms that evoked the initial use of the benzodiazepine. One can distinguish between dependence and "underlying disorders" by observing that the symptoms of the pharmacological dependence are often more intense and more varied than the original symptoms, and will gradually subside or at least ameliorate after the benzodiazepines have been discontinued for a sufficient period of time. Moreover, the symptoms of dependence do not explain relapse after a period of abstinence has occurred in the absence of significant withdrawal symptoms. The patient's willingness to attempt to discontinue benzodiazepine use, the lack of other drug or alcohol use, and the lessening of the symptoms of withdrawal over time favor an explanation of the symptoms of withdrawal rather than the presence of an addiction.

Pharmacokinetics: Disposition

The clinical effects of the benzodiazepine withdrawal are usually observed to reach a peak intensity within a range of 2 days to 2 weeks, depending on whether the benzodiazepine has a short or long half-life. The short-acting benzodiazepines have a peak withdrawal that begins within 1 day, with a peak intensity at 4 to 5 days; the withdrawal from the longer acting benzodiazepines begins on the third day, with a peak intensity at 10 days after abrupt discontinuation of use. The withdrawal is more protracted than generally appreciated as the symptoms of anxiety and depression may persist in a subacute and chronic course for months and perhaps years before gradually subsiding to imperceptible levels and finally resolving (6,8,11).

The basis for the protracted withdrawal are probably a result of pharmacokinetic and pharmacodynamic properties of benzodiazepines. The benzodiazepines tend to be highly lipophilic, which promotes uptake by the fat stores and muscle depot to be slowly released into the blood stream as the equilibrium shifts back to the blood compartment. The persistence of benzodiazepines in the fat and muscle may produce low-grade symptoms that are experienced for weeks and months from the prolonged release. Urine determinations for benzodiazepines may be positive for weeks after chronic use in humans. Although not clearly documented, studies suggest that the receptor changes that are induced by chronic benzodiazepine stimulation may take prolonged periods to reverse to the prebenzodiazepine state. Models for prolonged and sometimes persistent receptor changes are provided by the known drug-induced receptor changes with neuroleptic and cocaine use. Hypersensitivity or upregulation of postsynaptic dopamine receptors are purported to develop after chronic administration of these drugs (15,16,18,19).

Chemistry

The term benzodiazepine is based on the chemical structure that is composed of a benzene ring (A) fused to a seven-membered diazepine ring (B). Most of the chemically important benzodiazepines contain a 5-aryl substituent ring (C) and a 1,4-diazepine, so that the term has come to mean the 5-aryl-1,4-benzodiazepines. The different types of benzodiazepines are formed by substitution in various positions in the three rings A, B, and C at R_1, R_2, R_3, R_7, and R_8.

The benzodiazepines have essentially the same mechanism of action and chemical effect for all members of the class. The constancy of the effects is attributed to the A, B, and C rings that are present in all members of the class. The benzodiazepines differ from one another only in pharmacokinetic action (33,42,43).

Pharmacokinetics: Metabolism

Absorption

Chlordiazepoxide (Librium), oxazepam (Serax), lorazepam (Ativan), alprazolam (Xanax), and halazepam (Paxipam) are absorbed relatively slowly following oral administration, so that peak concentrations in the plasma may not be attained for hours. Diazepam is rapidly absorbed, to reach peak concentrations in about 1 hour in adults and 15 to 30 minutes in children. Chlorazepate is quickly decarboxylated in the gastrointestinal tract, and the product *N*-desmethyldiazepam (nordazepam) is rapidly absorbed. Prazepam is absorbed slowly and is transformed primarily to nordazepam by the liver through the enterohepatic circulation before reaching the systemic circulation.

All the benzodiazepines are completely absorbed with the exception of chlorazepate, pazepam, and fluazepam, and reach the systemic circulation in the form of their active metabolite. After oral administration the time of peak concentration in plasma ranges from 0.5 to 8 hours for the different benzodiazepines. Those used for their hypnotic effects are absorbed rapidly to reach peak concentrations within 1 hour for triazolam, and in a slower and more variable time for temazepam. Peak concentrations for flurazepam are attained in 1 to 3 hours.

Except for lorazepam, the benzodiazepams are unpredictably absorbed following intramuscular injection. Most of the benzodiazepines are bound to plasma proteins to a large extent (85%–95%). The apparent volumes of distribution for most benzodiazepines are high—about 1 to 3 liters per kilogram. Secondary peaks in the plasma concentrations that have been described for several benzodiazepines such as 6 to 12 hours after an oral dose of diazepam most likely result from enterohepatic recirculation.

The physiochemical and pharmacokinetic properties of benzodiazepines determine their clinical utility. All members of the class have high lipid–water distribution coefficients in the nonionized form. (The nonionized form favors lipid solubility.) The various substituents cause the lipid solubility to vary 50 fold, according to the polarity and electronegativity induced by the substitutions.

The benzodiazepines and their active metabolites bind to plasma proteins. The extent of protein binding correlates strongly with the lipid solubility; the greater the lipid solubility, the greater the protein binding. For example, protein binding is 70% for alprazolam and 99% for diazepam. The concentration in the cerebrospinal fluid is approximately equal to the concentration of free drug in plasma. It is not clear whether clinically significant competition between benzodiazepines and other protein-bound drugs occurs.

There is an initial rapid uptake of benzodiazepines into the brain and other highly perfused organs after either intravenous or rapid oral absorption. Subsequently, there is a phase of redistribution into tissues that are less well perfused, especially muscle and fat. The redistribution phase is quickest for drugs with higher lipid solubility. Further, redistribution is responsible for an accumulation of drug in muscle and fat depot for later, more gradual release back into the systemic circulation. Highly lipid-soluble drugs such as benzodiazepines persist in the body for prolonged periods of time—perhaps months, depending on the amount of muscle mass at the fat storage site.

Enterohepatic circulation further increases the duration so that the effects of active metabolites persist as they pass from the gut through the liver and back into the gut for reabsorption to the liver. Benzodiazepines cross the placental barrier and are secreted in the breast milk of lactating females.

The benzodiazepines are metabolized extensively by several different systems of microsomal enzymes. The active metabolites are biotransformed more slowly than the parent compound. Because of the disparity in metabolic rates between the parent compounds and active metabolites, the duration of action of many benzodiazepines is often longer than the half-time elimination of the parent drug that had been administered initially. For example, the half-life of flurazepam in plasma is 2 to 3 hours, and the half-life of a major active metabolite (N-desalkylflurazepam) is 50 hours or more. Some benzodiazepines that do not have active metabolites are inactivated by the initial reaction. The drugs oxazepam, lorazepam, temazepam, and triazolam have half-lives that correspond to the rate of their biotransformation. Because the benzodiazepines do not induce the synthesis of the hepatic microsomal enzymes significantly, their chronic administration usually does not result in the accelerated metabolism of other substances or of the benzodiazepines themselves.

The metabolism of the benzodiazepines proceeds in three basic stages. The various members are involved in one or more of these stages that determine their duration of action. Some of the benzodiazepines are interrelated by having common intermediary metabolites. Chlordiazepoxide is ultimately biotransformed to the N-disalkylated compound nordazepam, as are diazepam, chlorazepate, prazepam, and halazepam, directly. Nordazepam is biotransformed to the 3-hydroxylated compounds oxazepam and lorazepam, as is temazepam, directly.

The first stage, and most rapid reaction, is the removal of the subtituents to form N-desalylated compounds. These are biologically active compounds, except for triazolam and alprazolam, which contain a fused triazolo ring.

The second stage involves hydroxylation at position number three and yields an active derivative, oxazepam. The rates of these reactions are much slower than those for the first reaction so that there is an appreciable accumulation of hydroxylated products that are biologically active.

The third major stage is the conjugation of the 3-hydroxyl compounds, principally with glucuronic acid; the half-times of those reactions are usually between 4 and 12 hours and the products of the reactions are invariably inactive. Conjugation with glucuronide is the only major route of metabolism available for oxazepam and lorazepam, and it is the preferred pathway for temazepam. Trazolam and alprazolam are metabolized principally by initial hydroxylation of the methyl group on the fused triazolo ring. The products are referred to as 2-hydroxylated compounds (33,42,43).

Neurochemistry

On a continuum with tolerance, pharmacological dependence can be viewed as the deadaptation of the receptor sites to the absence of the drug after the adaptation occurred during the development of tolerance. The withdrawal state from benzodiazepines reflects a hyperaroused state of the central nervous system (CNS) that is the opposite of the sedative and inhibitory state produced by the drugs in the CNS. According to studies, the enhancement of gamma-ammobutyric acid (GABA) receptors by the benzodiazepines promotes a generalized inhibitory effect, to which the development of tolerance represents an adaptation by a decrease in the number of the receptors in response to and in the opposite direction from the suppressant effect. On withdrawal, the receptors deadapt and probably increase in number to return to the normal level of functioning; this dynamic process is expressed as an excitable state produced by the discharging neurons in the CNS.

The manifestations of withdrawal from benzodiazepines that may reflect receptor changes consist of a broad spectrum of signs and symptoms that occur predictably and sequentially, but in varying frequency and severity as the full spectrum occurs only infrequently. The more commonly observed signs and symptoms are intense, pervasive anxiety with superimposed panic attacks, hyperactivity, agoraphobia, agitation, insomnia, and depression; also possible are perceptual abnormalities, such as feelings of depersonalization and unreality, and frank visual hallucinations and paranoid delusions. These symptoms are qualitatively indistinguishable from withdrawal from alcohol and other sedative/hypnotic drugs, and differ only in time course and frequency of occurrence depending on the dose and duration of use and half-life of the benzodiazepines. Other less commonly reported symptoms of benzodiazepine withdrawal are the neurological symptoms of paresthesia and numbness, tremor, muscle stiffness, myalgia, fasciculation, ataxia, blurred vision, and hypersensitivity, especially to sound, light, taste, and smell. Headache and tinnitus are common, with formication and pruritus being less so. Gastrointestinal symptoms may include nausea, vomiting, constipation, diarrhea, abdominal pain, and dysphagia; an irritable bowel syndrome may be diagnosed in benzodiazepine withdrawal. Cardiovascular and respiratory symptoms may include palpitations, shortness of breath, and chest pain. Other assorted symptoms that may be present are hyperventilation, urinary frequency and urgency, actual incontinence, loss of libido, and generalized malaise (8,11,30,41,46).

Other Drug Use

Important to note also is that a substantial amount of the medical use of benzodiazepines occurs in populations of alcoholics and drug addicts who appear to be particularly vulnerable to the development of addiction and dependence. The studies evaluating tolerance and dependence of benzo-diazepines in medical populations often do not use criteria that clearly distinguish between alcoholics and nonalcoholics. Many of the "dropouts" (those who withdraw from the study) appear to be alcoholics and drug addicts who possibly because of addiction did not complete the withdrawal (20,21,23,24). Mistakenly, these addicted individuals may be dismissed as having a severe primary psychiatric disorder that prevented their completion of the withdrawal from benzodiazepines. Dropouts who are not included in the outcome diminish the numbers of patients with addictions and dependence in the studies of medical use of benzodiazepines (20,21,23,24).

Alcoholics and drug addicts constitute 25% of general medical populations and 50% of general psychiatry populations according to many surveys (47,48). The contemporary alcoholic is a polydrug user and addict; as many as 80% of the alcoholics under the age of 30 are addicted to at least one other drug (47,48). Benzodiazepines are drugs frequently used by alcoholics as indicated by clinical practice and studies revealing that as many as up to 50% of alcoholics use benzodiazepines (47,48). Opiate addicts frequently use high-dose benzodiazepines; studies indicate that 30% to 50% are regularly addicted users (48). Cocaine addicts also frequently use benzodiazepines in compulsive patterns of addiction. Physicians are the largest source of benzodiazepines for all populations whether for medical or nonmedical use. Although the presumption is that the physician is, in most instances, prescribing the benzodiazepines for a medical reason, benzodiazepine prescriptions clearly reach both medical and nonmedical populations (37–40,47).

Intervention and Treatment

The treatment of the abuse, addiction, tolerance, and dependence to benzo-diazepines is systematic and effective. No one need suffer morbidity and mortality from benzodiazepines. The first step is to identify which of these is present. The correct diagnosis will determine the efficacy of the treatment.

Abuse usually requires an evaluation and treatment of the precipitating events for the deviant use of the drug. A situational crisis, a chronic condition such as anxiety, insomnia, or pain, a hysterical behavior or misinformed user are some of the more common explanations for abusive use. Information regarding the adverse effects of the benzodiazepines, particularly those leading to the abusive use, and instruction for an alternative treatment may be sufficient to end the abusive use.

Addiction usually requires a more complex set of steps although the conceptual approach is simple. Usually, all that needs to be identified is the preoccupation, compulsive use, and a recurrent pattern of relapse. Denial for accurate use and consequences is a major obstacle that accompanies an addiction. Denial is an inherent feature of an active addiction to anything,

including benzodiazepines. Confrontation with the evidence of the consequences of the addiction is effective in dissipating the denial. A one-to-one
interview is ordinarily not sufficient to obtain a full history of the extent and
complications to identify the criteria of addiction. Corroborative history
from family, physician, and employer is often necessary and helpful to make
the diagnosis of addiction.

Effective outpatient and inpatient programs are available to treat alcohol
and drug addiction. Benzodiazepine addiction lends itself to these programs, particularly if other drugs and alcohol are used by the benzodiazepine addict. The severity of the addiction is the indicator of whether outpatient or inpatient treatment is needed. The inability to remain abstinent and
physical conditions that require close medical evaluation and treatment are
the major criteria for selection of inpatient treatment. The supervised environment with protective structure of an inpatient setting may be required for
the achievement and maintenance of abstinence (49).

Outpatient detoxification is possible in the patient is addicted to benzodiazepines who can tolerate the protracted and gradual taper over an extended period of time. A prolonged detoxification may be unrealistic because it
demands an exercise of control over the drug that the addict often does not
possess. Also, a more integrated and effective personality and cohesive social, family, and employment support may favor outpatient treatment because it provides some external control for the addict and implies some
adaptive ability and strength in interpersonal relationships.

The detoxification from benzodiazepines can be simplified and easily
applied if basic principles are applied. First, benzodiazepines have cross-
tolerance and dependence with each other and with alcohol and other seda-
tive/hypnotic drugs. Any benzodiazepine can be substituted for other benzodiazepines and with barbiturates, so that conversion for equivalent doses
can be calculated. Second, a long-acting benzodiazepine is more effective in
suppressing the withdrawal symptoms and producing a gradual and smooth
transition to the abstinent state. Greater patient compliance and less morbidity will result from the use of the longer acting benzodiazepines (50).

Third, select a benzodiazepine with lower euphoric properties such as
chlordiazepam, avoiding diazepam as much as possible. Fourth, do not
leave p.r.n. doses as this will give the addict a choice that is beyond his
control and will reduce drug-seeking behavior. Withdrawal from benzodiazepines is not usually marked by hypertension and tachycardia as with
alcohol, so that p.r.n. doses are not needed. The anxiety of withdrawal
should be controlled with the prescribed taper unless objectively it appears
that the doses are too low. Caution is urged at this point as drug-seeking
behavior needs to be differentiated from anxiety of withdrawal and the
anxiety of another disorder. Only the anxiety of withdrawal, when severe,
need be treated with increased doses of benzodiazepines although this condition is unusual with the long-acting benzodiazepines. Methods other than
benzodiazepines for treating the anxiety of another disorder and drug-seek-

ing behavior are indicated. The prescriber must be in control of the dispensing of the benzodiazepines for withdrawal as the addict, by definition, is out
of control and cannot reliably negotiate in the schedule for tapering.

Fifth, the duration of the tapering schedule is determined by the half-life
of the benzodiazepine that is being withdrawn. For short-acting benzodiazepines such as alprazolam, 7 to 10 days of a gradual taper with a long-acting
benzodiazepine or barbiturate is sufficient; 7 days for low-dose use and 10
days for high-dose use. For the long-acting benzodiazepines, 10 to 14 days

TABLE 12.1. Dose conversions[a] for sedative/hypnotic
drugs equivalent to Secobarbital 600 mg and Diazepam 60 mg.

Drug	Dose (mg)
Benzodiazepines	
Alprazolam	6
Chlordiazepoxide	150
Clonazepam	24
Clorazepate	90
Flurazepam	90
Halazepam	240
Lorazepam	12
Oxaxepam	60
Prazepam	60
Temazepam	90
Barbiturates	
Amobarbital	600
Butabarbital	600
Butalbital (in Fiorianal)	600
Pentobarbital	600
Secobarbital	600
Phenobarbital	180
Glycerol	
Meprobamate	2400
Piperidinedione	
Glutethimide	1500
Quinazolines	
Methaqualone	1800

[a]For patients receiving multiple drugs (e.g., flurazepam 30
mg/d, diazepam 30 mg/d, phenobarbital 150 mg/d), each
drug should be converted to its diazepam or secobarbital
equivalent. In preceding example patient is receiving equivalent dose of diazepam 100 mg/d or secobarbital 1000 mg/d.
Adapted from Perry PJ, Alexander B (1986). Sedative/hyp-
notic dependence: Patient stabilization, tolerance testing,
and withdrawal. *Drug Intell Clin Pharm* 20:532–537.

of a gradual taper with a long-acting benzodiazepine or barbiturate is sufficient; 10 days for low dose use and 14 days for high dose use. The doses
should be given in a Q.I.D. interval. Exact numerical deductions are not
needed as the long-acting benzodiazepines accumulate to result in a self-
leveling effect of the blood level of the benzodiazepines over time (50,51)
(Table 12.1).

References

1. Anon (1988). Top 200 drugs of 1987. *Am Druggist* 197(2):36–52.
2. DuPont RL, ed. (1988). Abuse of benzodiazepines: The problems and the solutions. A report of a committee of the Institute for Behavior and Health, Inc. *Am
   J Drug Alcohol Abuse* 14(Suppl 1):1–69.
3. Noyes R, Garvey MJ, Cook BL, et al. (1988). Benzodiazepine withdrawal: A
   review of the evidence. *J Clin Psychiatry* 49(10):382–389.
4. American Medical Association (1987). *Drug Evaluations, Antianxiety and Hypnotic Drugs*, 6th Ed., pp. 86–103. Chicago: American Medical Association.
5. Owen RT, Tyrer P (1983). Benzodiazepine dependence: A review of the evidence.
   Drugs 25:385–398.
6. Ashton H (1987). Benzodiazepine withdrawal: Outcome in 50 patients. *Br J
   Addict* 82:665–671.
7. Lader M (1983). Dependence on benzodiazepines. *J Clin Psychiatry* 44:121–127.
8. Ashton H (1984). Benzodiazepine withdrawal: An unfinished story. *Br Med J*
   288:1135–1140.
9. Griffiths RR, Sannerud CA (1987). Abuse of and dependence on benzodiazepines and other anxiolytic/sedative drugs. In *Psychopharmacology*, Meltzer HY,
   ed., pp. 1535–1541. New York: Raven Press.
10. Clinthorne MA, Cisin IH, Balter MB (1986). Changes in popular attitudes and
    belief about tranquilizers. *Arch Gen Psychiatry* 43:527–532.
11. Ashton H (1986). Adverse effects of prolonged benzodiazepine use. *Adverse
    Drug Reac Bull* 118:440–443.
12. Miller NS, Dackis CA, Gold MS (1987). The relationship of addiction, tolerance
    and dependence: A neurochemical approach. *J Subst Abuse Treat* 4:197–207.
13. National Institute on Drug Abuse (1982). *National Household Survey on Drug
    Abuse (1979-1981)*. Washington, DC: US Govt. Printing Office.
14. National Institute on Drug Abuse (1985). *National Household Survey on Drug
    Abuse (1982-1984)*. Washington, DC: US Govt. Printing Office.
15. Mellinger GD, Balter MB, Uhlenhuth ET (1984). Antianxiety agents: Duration
    of use and characteristics of users in the USA. *Curr Med Res Opin* 8(Suppl):4.
16. Mellinger GD, Balter MB, Uhlenhuth ET (1984). Prevalence and correlates of
    the long-term regular use of anxiolytics. *JAMA* 251(3):375–379.
17. Smith DE, Wesson DR, eds. (1985). *The Benzodiazepines: Current Standards for
    Medical Practice*. Lancashire, UK: MTP Press Limited.
18. Smith DE, Wesson DR (1983). Benzodiazepine dependence syndromes. *J Psy-
    choact Drugs* 15(1-2):85–95.
19. Rosenberg HC, Chiu TH (1985). Time course for development of benzodiaze-
    pine tolerance and physical dependence. *Neurosci Biobehav Rev* 9:123–131.
20. Rickels MD, Case G, Schweizer EE, et al. (1986). Low-dose dependence in

chronic benzodiazepine users: A preliminary report on 119 patients. *Psychopharmacol Bull* 22(2):407–415.

21. Busto U, Sellers EM, Claudio NA, et al. (1986). Withdrawal reaction after long-term therapeutic use of benzodiazepines. *N Engl J Med*, 000:854–869.

22. Juergens SM, Morse RM (1988). Alprazolam dependence in seven patients. *Am J Psychiatry* 145(5):625–627.

23. Murphey SM, Tyrer P (1988). The essence of benzodiazepine dependence. In *The Psychopharmacology of Addiction*, Lader M, ed., pp. 157–166. New York: Oxford University Press.

24. Tyrer PJ, Seivewright N (1984). Identification and management of benzodiazepine dependence. *Postgrad Med J* 60(Suppl 2):41–46.

25. Tyrer P, Rutherford D, Huggett T (1981). Benzodiazepine withdrawal symptoms and propranolol. *Lancet* 1:520–522.

26. Lader M, Olajide D (1987). A comparison of buspirone and placebo in relieving benzodiazepine withdrawal symptoms. *J Clin Psychopharmacol* 7(1):11–15.

27. Pertusson H, Lader MH (1981). Withdrawal from long-term benzodiazepine treatment. *Br Med J* 283:643–645.

28. Greenblatt DJ, Harmatz JS, Zinny MA, Shader RI (1987). Effect of gradual withdrawal on the rebound sleep disorder after discontinuation of triazolam. *N Engl J Med* 317:772–728.

29. Mellman T, Uhde TW (1986). Withdrawal syndrome with gradual tapering of alprazolam. *Am J Psychiatry* 143(11):1464–1466.

30. Lader M (1988). The psychopharmacology of addiction: Benzodiazepine tolerance and dependence. In *The Psychopharmacology of Addiction*, Lader M, ed., pp. 1–13. Cambridge: Oxford University Press.

31. Hallstrom L, Lader M (1981). Benzodiazepine withdrawal phenomena. *Int Pharmacopsychiatry* 16:235–244.

32. Fyer A, Liebowitz MR, Gorman JM, et al. (1987). Discontinuation of alprazolam treatment in panic patients. *Am J Psychiatry* 144:303–308.

33. Robins LN, Helzer JE, Przybeck TR, et al. (1988). Alcohol disorders in the community: A report from the epidemiological catchement area. In *Alcoholism: Origins and Outcome*, Rose RM, Barrett J, eds., pp. 15–29. New York: Raven Press.

34. Greenblatt DJ, Shader RI, Divoll M, et al. (1981). Benzodiazepines: A summary of pharmacokinetic properties. *Br J Clin Pharmacol* (Suppl) 11:11S–16S.

35. Haefely W (1986). Biological basis of drug-induced tolerance, rebound and dependence. Contribution of recent research on benzodiazepines. *Pharmacopsychiatry* 19:353–361.

36. Jaffe JH (1985). In *The Pharmacological Basis of Therapeutics*, 7th Ed., Gilman AG, Goodman LS, Rall TW, Murad F, eds., pp. 532–581. New York: Macmillan.

37. Sellers EM, Marshman JA, Kaplan HL, et al. (1981). Acute and chronic drug abuse emergencies in metropolitan Toronto. *Int J Addict* 16(2):283–303.

38. Grantham P (1987). Benzodiazepine abuse. *Br J Hosp Med* 37:999–1001.

39. Perera KMH, Tulley M, Jenner FA (1987). The use of benzodiazepines among drug addicts. *Br J Addict* 82:511–515.

40. Schuster CL, Humphries RH (1981). Benzodiazepine dependency in alcoholics. *Conn Med* 45(1):11–13.

41. Cappell H, Busto U, Kay G (1987). Drug deprivation and reinforcement by diazepam in a dependent population. *Psychopharmacology* 91:154–160.

42. American Psychiatric Association (1987). Psychoactive Substance Use Disorders. In *Diagnostic and Statistical Manual of Mental Disorders*, 3d Ed. (revised), pp.165-186. Washington, DC: American Psychiatric Association.
43. Busto U, Sellers EM (1986). Pharmacokinetic determinants of drug abuse and dependence: A conceptual perspective. *Clin Pharmacokinet* 11:144-153.
44. Perry PJ, Alexander B (1986). Sedative/hypnotic dependence: Patient stabilization, tolerance testing and withdrawal. *Drug Intell Clin Pharm* 20:532-536.
45. Harrison M, Busto U, Naranjo CA (1984). Diazepam tapering in detoxification for high-dose benzodiazepine abuse. *Clin Pharmacol Ther* 36(4):527-533.
46. Griffiths RR, Bigelow GE, Liebson I (1983). Differential effects of diazepam and pentobarbital on mood and behavior. *Arch Gen Psychiatry* 40:865-873.
47. Chan AWK (1984). Effects of combined alcohol and benzodiazepine: A review. *Drug Alcohol Depend* 13:315-341.
48. Miller NS, Mirin SM (1989). Multiple drug use in alcoholics: Practical and theoretical implications. *Psychiatr Ann* 19(5):248-255.
49. Greenblatt DJ, Shader RI, Divoll M, et al. (1981). Benzodiazepines: A summary of pharmacokinetic properties. *Br J Clin Pharmacol* (Suppl) 11:11S-16S.
50. Perry PJ, Alexander B (1986). Sedative/hypnotic dependence: Patient stabilization, tolerance, testing and withdrawal. *Drug Intell Clin Pharm* 20:532-536.

CHAPTER 13

The Pharmacology of Cocaine

History

Cocaine has enjoyed a special mystique in the history of medicine, literature, and civilizations. The fathers of modern surgery and psychiatry were proponents of the use of cocaine (1–3).

William Halstead became dependent on and addicted to cocaine himself with the expectant consequences (3) after he self-administered it while performing surgery and developing new techniques in anesthesia at the Johns Hopkins Hospital.

Sigmund Freud used cocaine for "depressions" during his training years as a physician at the University of Vienna. Freud used cocaine to endure the long and lonely hours of medical training away from his beloved wife. He later prescribed it to a close colleague and friend who had a morphine addiction from chronic pain. Freud also proposed that cocaine be a therapeutic treatment for digestive disorders, cachexia from any cause, morphine and alcohol addictions, and asthma, and be used as a stimulant, a local anesthetic, and an aphrodisiac. Freud was eventually criticized when the toxic and addictive consequences of cocaine became evident after widespread use. Cocaine achieved the status as the "scourge of the world" because of the adverse effects that became apparent to the scientific community when Freud's anticipated intentions did not materialize (1,2).

Sir Conan Doyle wrote many of the episodes of Sherlock Holmes mysteries under the influence of cocaine. The intricate plots were possibly a result of the exalted awareness, rapid pace of thought, and paranoid delusions of persecution and grandiosity that are characteristically produced by the acute and chronic use of cocaine.

The smoking of cocaine dates back to the 5000-year-old practice of the Andean Indians to burn and smoke parts of the coca leaf for religious and medicinal purposes. The Spaniards who had acquired the knowledge of cocaine use from the conquered Andean Indians introduced cocaine to Europe in the fifteenth century. Nieman, an Australian chemist, extracted co-

caine from the coca leaf in 1860. Not long after, Freud became intrigued by
the excitement and euphoria that arose from the effects of cocaine.

Prevalence

Epidemics

The first clearly documented epidemic of cocaine use waxed and waned in
the late nineteenth and early twentieth centuries. In the mid-twentieth century, cocaine use began a gradual comeback to the present peak of a second
epidemic. In the late 1800s others as well as Freud emphasized the medical
and therapeutic possibilities of cocaine. The untoward toxic and costly consequences emerged gradually to produce a vigorous reaction against the
drug by the 1920s. Cocaine was made illegal in 1914 by inclusion in the
Harrison Narcotic Act (4).

The use of cocaine remained "underground" until the 1960s when many
drugs gained popularity among the people of the United States. As the use
of cocaine increased, reassurance from the medical profession that cocaine
use was benign appeared in spite of earlier warnings in history. *The Comprehensive Textbook of Psychiatry*, by Friedman and Saddock (71), contained
the quotation, "If it is used no more than two or three times per week,
cocaine creates no problems." Another article in *Scientific American* (72)
claimed that cocaine was "no more habit forming than potato chips."

Although the general use of cocaine in the United States has decreased
from 1985 to 1988, the prevalence of the addictive use of cocaine has increased over the same time period. The 1988 National Household Survey on
Drug Abuse surveyed the nature and extent of drug abuse among Americans
aged 12 and older. The number of "current" cocaine users decreased from
5.8 million in 1985 to 2.9 million in 1988, or a 50% reduction in overall
cocaine use. Current use is defined as cocaine use within the last 30 days.
Those who used cocaine in the past year decreased from 12 million to 8
million (5).

Unfortunately, the 1988 survey found that more frequent use increased
from 1985 to 1988. Frequent use, defined as once a week or more, of cocaine
was 862,000 in 1988, compared to 647,000 in 1985. Cocaine use of once a
week or more represents addictive use in most instances (5).

Other characteristics of national cocaine use were that cocaine use was
highest among the unemployed (4.6%) and those aged 18 to 25 years (4.5%).
Among the young (aged 12 to 17 years) were 600,000 who had used within
the past year. The survey also found 0.5 million current crack users among
the 2.9 million current cocaine users (5).

Cocaine now ranks as the third most common drug to which individuals
become addicted, alcohol and marijuana being first and second most common, respectively. Users in the United States consume billions of dollars
worth of cocaine annually. The cost in lives, in lost income to industry and

individuals, and in danger and disruption to society is staggering. The debate over whether cocaine is addictive is left to academicians as practitioners treat millions of new cases of cocaine addiction yearly (6).

Patterns of Use

Names

Cocaine has many names that reflect its appearance and effects. Coca paste is known as "base," "pasta," "pitillo," and "buscuso." The hydrochloride powdered form is known as "snow" or "coke," and the freebase rock form as "crack" because of the sound it makes burning in the pipe.

Source

Cocaine is an alkaloid present in the leaves of *Erythroxylon coca*, a "tree or shrub" indigenous to western South America. Abundant amounts are found in the wild state in Peru, Colombia, Ecuador, and Bolivia. The coca leaf bears no pharmacological relationship to the cocoa (cocoa or chocolate) bean or to the kola nut, although confusion between them is reflected in the medical literature (7).

Cocaine Paste

Coca paste is derived from dried coca leaves dissolved in a solution of kerosene or gasoline, alkaline bases, potassium permanganate, and sulfuric acid. The coca paste contains cocaine, sulfate, other coca alkaloids, diluents, and adulterants (8,9). The salt form of cocaine hydrochloride is prepared from coca paste mixed with hydrochloric acid and is water soluble.

Freebase Cocaine

Cocaine exists in the plant as a base; thus, it is relatively insoluble in water. Cocaine as a weak base is rapidly absorbed through membranes in an alkaline environment (7,10). The "free" cocaine base is freed from the powder or salt form of cocaine hydrochloride by extraction with a base such as sodium hydroxide or ether.

Crack

Crack is not a new drug, but represents a new strategy in the sale and marketing of street cocaine. Crack is a "rock" form of cocaine that is sold as ready-made "freebase" cocaine in tiny pellets. Crack is 25% to 100% pure freebase and does not require further chemical processing, as does cocaine hydrochloride. Crack is immediately and completely absorbed when smoked in a water pipe. The introduction of "cheap" crack packaged in small vials that sell for about $20 has increased its availability to lower-income and younger adolescent users (8,11–13).

Adulterants

Many of the adulterants and diluents that are added to the coca paste and cocaine hydrochloride are not removed by ordinary extraction procedures for freebase preparation. Some of the preparations contain manganese carbonate, which can produce a Parkinson syndrome, lidocaine, which looks and numbs like cocaine and causes seizures, and ephedrine and weak stimulant properties to enhance potency (8,11).

Routes of Administration

Oral Route

Oral ingestion (powder or leaf) was the common route of administration in Freud's time, but absorption is limited by the acidic environment of the stomach where the pH does not favor absorption of a weak base. The bioavailability of oral cocaine is similar to the intranasal route (IN), but the effects are experienced sooner and are more intense by the IN than by oral administration, perhaps because the vasculature of the nose is closer to the brain than is the gastrointestinal tract (14,16).

Intranasal and Intravenous Routes

The common routes of administration today for cocaine are intranasal, intravenous, and smoking. Intranasal remains the most popular method of cocaine use although smoking is rapidly gaining in popularity (15). The majority of consumers "sniff" the cocaine hydrochloride powder through the capillary-rich mucosa of the nose. The intravenous route is preferred often by those who inject other drugs such as opiates.

Inhalation Route

The inhalation route of cocaine is the method for the most rapid delivery to the brain, two to three times faster than the intravenous route. The volatile cocaine freebase is inhaled as smoke through the bronchial tree to reach the capillary-rich alveoli in the lungs that provide a vast surface area (72 m^2 of membranes) for instantaneous absorption with the gaseous exchanges. The inhalation route also bypasses the venous system because the pulmonary venous (arterial blood) blood flow from the lungs to the heart is pumped directly through the aorta into the cerebral circulation in the brain. The intravenous circulation is a longer route for cocaine because it follows the systemic return of venous blood through the vena cavae into the heart and eventually to the lungs before returning to the heart for distribution to the brain. The intranasal route is an even slower route that requires passage of cocaine through the tiny capillaries and venules before entry into the systemic venous circulation (8,11).

Comparative Onset for Routes of Administration

The intensity and duration of the acute effects correlate well with the rate of rise and height of the peak level of cocaine obtained in the blood, which in turn determine the levels of cocaine reaching the brain. The route of administration determines the rate and peak of blood levels achieved.

It only takes 5 to 10 seconds by smoking, 30 to 120 seconds intravenously, and 1 to 3 minutes intranasally for cocaine to reach and produce the onset of effects in the brain. Clinical histories of cocaine addicts suggest that the incidence is greater and the course quicker for addiction to cocaine to occur with inhalation because the onset of addictive use is measured in weeks for inhalation rather than months as for the intranasal route. The addiction potential correlates with the faster and higher peak blood levels obtained with inhalation.

Intoxication

Acute Intoxication

The psychological and physiological effects depend on the delivery and distribution of the drug to the target organs. The brain is the major organ affected by cocaine. The psychological and physiological effects are direct manifestations of the chemical interaction between cocaine and the brain. Neurochemical events are initiated by the interaction between cocaine and the brain to produce predictable and stereotypic changes in mind and behavior.

Acute Physiological Effects

Peripheral Effects

The acute physiological effects are manifestations of sympathetic nervous system discharge. The peripheral effects of sympathetic stimulation mediated by the neurohormones norepinephrine and epinephrine include tachycardia, hypertension, sweating, hyperpyrexia, urinary and bowel retention, muscular contractions, and cutaneous flushing (17–20). Following acute intoxication in usual doses, the physiological effects are transient and short lived. No adverse sequelae ordinarily result unless underlying medical conditions exist that are worsened by an acute increase in tone of the sympathetic nervous system.

Central Effects

In higher doses and with chronic use, amnesia, delirium, seizures, stupor, and coma may result paradoxically from this stimulant in large enough doses. The seizures, usually of the generalized toxic-chronic type, may lead to sustained convulsions that arrest respiration and induce fatal cardiac arrhythmias. Cardiac effects that are induced directly by cocaine are atrial and ventricular tachyarrhythmias, which are more likely to be fatal if an underlying, predisposing heart problem already exists. Blood pressure may be severely elevated to produce stroke with cerebral infarction and hemorrhage in a susceptible individual.

Idiosyncratic reactions or individual variability in psychological and physiological responses are important factors, in addition to dosage, in determining the severity and type of any toxicity from cocaine (21,22).

Acute Psychological Effects

Mood

The acute psychological effects begin soon after cocaine reaches the brain. The major areas of brain function affected are mood, cognition, drive states, and level of awareness. An immediate and intense euphoria, analogous to a sexual orgasm, occurs and may last seconds to minutes depending on the route of administration. Other alterations arising from elevation in mood include giddiness and enhanced self-confidence. The subsequent, more prolonged level of mood is a milder euphoria mixed with anxiety, which lasts from minutes to hours followed by a more protracted and persistent anxious and dysphoric state over a span of hours to days.

Arousal

The thoughts may race and the speech becomes loquacious, even garrulous. An enhanced self-awareness with a heightened level of self-arousal often occurs. The heightened arousal may lead to insomnia. Motor activity is often increased with agitated, fidgety, and stereotypic behavior accompanying subjective sensations of restlessness.

Cognition

Concentration and attention may be improved initially in low doses, but both become impaired with increased doses.

Appetite and Libido

Appetite is suppressed as it is with most central nervous system (CNS) stimulants. In low doses, the libido is stimulated and sexual performance is enhanced by a retardation in ejaculation. In larger, acute intravenous doses, spontaneous orgasm may occur.

Craving or Drive for Cocaine

The craving or drive to use cocaine is the most intense after recent use and diminishes with continued abstinence. The craving or drive to use cocaine usually does not completely disappear and tends to recur spontaneously even after prolonged abstinence, especially if addictive use has occurred at anytime (10,23).

Chronic Intoxication

Chronic, persistent, and regular intoxication with cocaine by any route of administration has identifiable and characteristic consequences. The dependence syndrome or withdrawal from chronic cocaine use also has a typical and predictable protracted course (24–26).

Chronic Psychological Effects

Euphoria

The euphoria of intoxication wanes, becoming less intense and shorter in duration as tolerance develops with continued chronic use. An extremely interesting phenomena is that many cocaine addicts report that the very first or initial trial of cocaine yields the greatest euphoria ever experienced. Subsequent episodes of cocaine-induced euphoria are not as intense or as long, because the euphoria diminishes increasingly with further cocaine use over the months and years. In a sense, the addict continues to futilely chase the initial high. Furthermore, the users experience less euphoria with successive use within a short time, such as a binge over hours and days. Subsequent use of cocaine after a period of abstinence will result in a transient return of euphoria followed by a rapid redevelopment of tolerance to the euphoria.

Depression and Anxiety

Anxiety and depression that accompany repeated cocaine use increase to an intense level. The addict may experience profound depression with sensations of helplessness, hopelessness, and suicidal thinking. Intense anxiety, insomnia, and depressed appetite combine to produce fatigue and eventual exhaustion. The addict is typically anxious, irritable, fearful, apprehensive, suspicious, dysphoric, and guarded in less severely intense intoxicated states and in short periods of abstinence between episodes of chronic intoxication (21,27,28).

Delusions and Hallucinations

Delusions of paranoia are common and quite distressing to the addict who believes others are "spying on him" or "out to get him." A less intense but pervasive paranoia is persistently felt by the addict between episodes of use. Derogatory auditory hallucinations and bizarre visual hallucinations are less commonly present in the chronic user.

Libido

The libido is depressed, and actual sexual performance is impaired with impotency in males and inorgasmia in females. Men have difficulty with erections and ejaculations whereas females are sexually unresponsive and inorgasmic.

Chronic Physiological Effects
Medical

Muscular twitches, positional tremors, and generalized weakness are common in chronic use. Malnutrition, weight loss, and susceptibility to superimposed infections follow heavy, chronic use. Cardiac angina, systemic hypertension, palpitations, tachyarrhythmias, and myocardial infarction may occur from repeated cocaine intoxication.

Eventually, nasal ulcer and bleeding and chronic sinusitis are inevitable consequences of chronic intranasal use and chronic pharyngitis and bronchitis from chronic inhalation. AIDS (acquired immune deficiency syndrome), viral hepatitis, and endocarditis are sequelae of intravenous cocaine use.

Withdrawal

The acute and prolonged withdrawal from cocaine in the abstinent state following chronic, regular intoxication is dramatic. The initial acute phase of the withdrawal (hours to days) is termed the "crash." During the crash, an intense depression, fatigue, hypersomnolence, hyperphagia, and drive for repeated cocaine use are present. The later phase (weeks to months) is characterized by mood lability with anxiety and depression, anhedonia, low energy, sleep disturbances, and suspiciousness. Recurring "urges" or "drive" to use cocaine appear spontaneously or in response to cues in the environment at any time and indefinitely in the future in the addict's life (26,29,30).

Diagnosis

Addiction

The criteria for the diagnosis of cocaine addiction are similar to those required for an addiction to any other drug, including alcohol (31). The criteria for an addiction to drugs are descriptions of addictive behavior. The underlying mechanisms subserving an addiction to drugs and alcohol are attributable to neurochemical changes in particular locations in the brain (26,32).

The behavioral criteria are the preoccupation with acquisition of cocaine, the compulsive use of cocaine in spite of adverse consequences from the drug, and the relapse or return to cocaine after a period of abstinence. The diagnosis of a cocaine addiction cannot be made unless all the criteria are satisfied. Loss of control regarding cocaine use is pervasive throughout the three criteria (33). Responsible for the loss of control is the relentless drive to pursue, use, and repeatedly return to cocaine (26,33–35).

Preoccupation

The preoccupation with cocaine is identified by the pursuit of cocaine. The acquisition of cocaine entails great expense in money, time, energy, and planning for the addict. Cocaine assumes a high priority in the repertoire in the addict's life. The preeminence of cocaine use is evident in the impairment of interpersonal relationships with others, particularly family, friends, and in employment (36,37).

Compulsivity

The compulsive use of cocaine is often but not necessarily manifested by regular use. *The essential feature of compulsive use is continued use of cocaine in spite of adverse consequences.* The adverse consequences may be medical, legal, financial, and psychosociological, and often involve the interpersonal relationships between the user and those with whom he is in contact. The addict may become profoundly depressed and even suicidal from cocaine use but continues to use cocaine illogically as the depression worsens. The depression is chemically induced from cocaine's action on the brain, probably through manipulation of the neurotransmitters. The depression often lifts with abstinence from cocaine so the elimination, not institution, of cocaine is indicated (31,38,39).

Relapse

A persistent pattern of loss of control with relapse or return to cocaine is confirmatory of addiction. The diagnosis of addiction is made longitudinally over time by identifying the recurrent pattern of the drive to use cocaine with loss of control (40–42).

Tolerance and Dependence

Tolerance

Pharmacological tolerance is defined as the diminishing drug effect to a particular dose or, conversely, the need to increase the dose to maintain the same drug effect. The development of pharmacological tolerance to many of the effects of cocaine does occur. The basis of the development of the tolerance is neurochemical (26,43).

Tolerance represents a neuroadaptation by the brain in response to the presence of cocaine. The adaptation is the brain's attempt to maintain homeostasis in spite of the drug effect, to achieve a new balance within normal physiological function. The brain "resists" the action of cocaine by the development of tolerance.

Acute Tolerance

The neurochemical basis for tolerance may involve the neurotransmitters, dopamine, norepinephrine, and serotonin. Development of acute tolerance is reflected by changes in both presynaptic and postsynaptic neurons designed to regulate and maintain dopaminergic, noradrenergic, and serotonergic function within the normal range by (1) increasing the rate of neurotransmitter production, (2) inhibiting the enzymes that degrade the neurotransmitters, and (3) decreasing the number of neurotransmitter receptor sites.

Chronic Tolerance

The development of chronic tolerance appears to involve depletion of the neurotransmitters in the presynaptic neurons. The development of chronic tolerance is based on the phenomenon of supersensitivity. The number of receptor sites on the postsynaptic neuron is increased as a compensatory response to depletion of the neurotransmitter in the presynaptic neuron that follows chronic use of cocaine.

Course of Tolerance

Tolerance develops to many of the effects of cocaine. A dramatic illustration of tolerance is reduction in euphoria induced by cocaine. Most addicts report that the most intense euphoria experienced is the initial trial of the drug, after which the intensity of the euphoria diminishes with each use over weeks, months, and years. Also, during a cocaine "binge" or "run," the euphoria felt decreases as use increases because of the development of tolerance.

Other effects to which tolerance to cocaine develops are tachycardia, hypertension, anorexia, arousal, and an increase in libido. Tolerance is dependent on other factors such as individual responses, body size, genetic predisposition, and other drug use. Tolerance to many effects may often return after a period of abstinence; however, the redevelopment of tolerance occurs rapidly with continued use of cocaine (26,43).

Dependence

Pharmacological dependence to cocaine is defined by the withdrawal syndrome. Depression, hypersomnia, and hyperphagia are signs and symptoms of neurochemical changes that are cocaine induced in the brain during the development of pharmacological dependence. The drive states, sleep-wake cycles, and mood are neurochemical in origin, altered by cocaine during intoxication and readjust as a part of withdrawal from cocaine.

Addiction

The relationship between tolerance, dependence, and addiction is not necessarily one to one and bilateral. Tolerance and dependence represent predictable adaptations by the brain to the presence of cocaine. Tolerance and dependence may occur in the absence of addictive behavior. On the other hand, addictive behavior often includes the development of tolerance and dependence because of frequent, regular use of cocaine. Furthermore, the detection of the "signs and symptoms" of tolerance and dependence may be difficult because of their sometimes subtle character and resemblance to other conditions; that is, anxiety, depression, sleep, and appetite disturbances require subjective report and resemble variations in normal functions and other psychiatric diagnosis. Finally, denial is inherent in addiction and frequently makes the acquisition of historical information regarding tolerance and dependence in cocaine use difficult (26,43).

Pharmacokinetics

Absorption

Rate and Dose

The rate and amount of absorption depend on the route of administration and dose of cocaine. The height of the peak determines the intensity of the effect and in turn is determined by the route of administration. Inhalation with rapid absorption results in the highest peak blood level, followed by the intravenous route. The intranasal route is slower, provides a lower peak blood level, and the effects are more prolonged. The dose determines the duration of the effect so that the larger the dose, the longer the effect of cocaine; that is, a larger dose taken orally will have a less intense but longer effect than an intravenous dose, which will have a more intense but shorter lasting effect. Acute effects, such as euphoria and seizures, are more likely to occur following large doses and a more rapid route of administration (44–46).

Vasoconstriction

The vasoconstrictive effects of cocaine reduce the rate of absorption from capillaries by inhibiting its own uptake into the blood vessels as in the intranasal and intravenous routes.

Metabolism

Enzymes and Metabolites

The metabolism of cocaine involves enzymes in both blood and liver. Cocaine is rapidly metabolized to a number of water-soluble metabolites that are excreted in the urine. The major metabolites in the urine are benzoylecgonine (BE) and ecognine methyl ester (EME), which result from hydrolysis of cocaine by the action of esterases in the liver and in the blood. Some benzoylecgonine may be formed nonenzymatically in vitro (46).

In humans, the distribution of recovered cocaine in unchanged and changed forms in the urine is cocaine, 10%; BE, 46%; and EME, 41% (of the cocaine dose) during the first 12 hours. Plasma concentrations of cocaine fall rapidly within hours after absorption from any rate of administration to amounts detected by only highly sophisticated analytical methods. Benzozlecgonine concentrations have a slower rate of excretion over days so that it is detectable in the urine longer than cocaine and EME, which are excreted over hours. Consequently, most analytical tests measure BE (47).

A demythylated product of benzoylecgonine, norcocaine, is found in low levels in humans. Norcocaine has properties of a local anesthetic, inhibits norepinephrine reuptake, and alters drug-taking behavior in animals (48).

Elimination Half-Life

Following administration of cocaine by the intranasal, intravenous, or inhalation routes, peak blood levels are reached in seconds to minutes depending on the route and purity of cocaine. The half-life contributes to the rapid administration of cocaine during binges in which an inhalation may be repeated as often as every 5 minutes (49).

Neurochemistry

Brain Effects

Stimulant

Individuals use cocaine to alter brain function. The effects in subjective sensation and objective behavior are a direct result of the CNS stimulation and depression. Cocaine's actions are similar to those produced by other CNS stimulants—amphetamines, meythlphenidate, caffeine, etc. (43). The stimulant action is mediated by the catecholamine effects that are enhanced by cocaine; norepinephrine for arousal, epinephrine for anxiety, and dopamine for euphoria and motor activity.

Electroencephalographic Findings

Human electroencephalographic (EEG) effects of cocaine are to desynchronize the background activity with diffuse, fast beta waves that resemble the arousal state. The generalized discharge rate may reach seizure threshold levels to produce generalized spike and wave patterns. The origin of the seizure focus appears to be the limbic system, as indicated by neurophysiological recording techniques with implanted electrodes (50–52).

Depressant

Cocaine in large enough doses depresses the CNS by producing stupor, coma, and respiratory depression. A frequent cause of sudden death from cocaine may be depression of the medullary centers for respiration. Furthermore, cardiovascular arrhythmias and hypertension may be induced by depression of the cardiovascular centers in the medulla. The action of cocaine to suppress CNS activity may be a function of its local anesthetic properties to stabilize neuronal membranes. Large doses may diminish the propagation of electrical impulses in the polysynaptic fibers within the medullary centers for respiration and cardiovascular function (43).

Neurotransmitters

Several neurotransmitter systems in the brain may contribute to the effects of cocaine. Evidence for the involvement of various neurotransmitters in the brain is indirect, and has been obtained from animal studies and extrapolation from clinical effects of cocaine in humans (26,32).

Dopamine

Many cocaine effects are attributable to the dopamine (DA) system.

Mechanism of Action

Specifically, cocaine rapidly blocks the reuptake of the dopamine (DA) neurotransmitter into its presynaptic nerve terminal. Reuptake by the vesicles in the presynaptic neuron is the principal means of elimination of action of the neurotransmitter. The neurotransmitter is initially released by the vesicles into the synaptic cleft to act at its receptor on the postsynaptic neuron. Other mechanisms of termination are enzyme degradation by catecholmethyltransferase (COMT) in the synapse (53–56).

Acute Reuptake Blockade. The acute effect of cocaine on dopamine neurons is to stimulate dopamine activity by dopamine reuptake blockade, by increased DA synthesis, and by downregulation of postsynaptic receptors. The postsynaptic receptors are downregulated as the number of receptor sites is reduced by acute administration of cocaine.

Chronic Reuptake Blockade. Chronic administration of cocaine produces an "upregulation" of postsynaptic receptor sites as repeated cocaine stimulation results in the appearances of greater numbers of receptors in the postsynaptic neuron. The proposed mechanism is a compensatory response of the postsynaptic neuron to a deficiency in dopamine stimulation. The chronic blockade of dopamine reuptake results in an exhaustion of dopamine in the mechanism of action. The effects of cocaine on noradrenergic neurons resemble its effects on dopaminergic neurons. Cocaine inhibits the reuptake of norepinephrine (NE) similarly to dopamine into the presynaptic neuron. The reuptake mechanism is the major means of termination of released NE into the synaptic cleft. Cocaine stimulates an acute compensatory increase in tyrosine hydroxylase activity to increase the biosynthesis of NE in the same pathway as for the synthesis of dopamine (19,57,58). Repeated cocaine administration depletes brain NE concentrations.

Functions of Neurons

Central nervous system NE neurons originate from the locus ceruleus neurons that are located in the pons, hypothalamus, and midbrain. The axons of the neurons in the locus ceruleus ascend to supply the cerebral and cerebellar cortices, the thalamus, and the hypothalamus. Norepinephrine-containing neurons subserve the autonomic nervous system in the hypothalamus. Released NE reacts with the postsynaptic neurons that innervate peripheral target organs to increase heart rate and contractibility, increase blood pressure, produce muscle contractions, increase blood glucose, dilate pupils, and produce piloerection and sweating. Arousal and vigilance seen in cocaine users originates in the NE-containing neurons in the reticular activating system located in the midbrain (59,60).

Serotonin

Mechanism of Action

The reuptake of 5-hydroxytryptamine (5-HT) is inhibited to increase 5-HT levels in the synaptic cleft after acute administration to enhance the serotonin effect. Both 5-HT synthesis and turnover are reduced, and 5-HT concentrations depleted, after chronic stimulation with cocaine. Uptake of tryptophan, the precursor to serotonin syntheses, is also inhibited so that less 5-HT is synthesized (61,62).

Location of Neurons

Serotonin neurons in the CNS are located in the raphe regions of the pons and upper brainstem. The caudal neuronal clusters project axons down to the medulla and spinal cord. The rostral neuronal clusters course through the median forebrain bundle to innervate the encephalus and telencephalus, including the corpus striatum and cerebral cortex. The stimulation of central 5-HT neurons produces inhibitory effects on neurons innervated by the fibers. Disruption of 5-HT transmission results in increased motor behavior, presumably from a release of 5-HT inhibition on dopamine neurons in the basal ganglia. The acute effect by cocaine is to enhance the inhibitory effect on the medullary neurons where the respiratory center is located. Arrest of respiration induced by cocaine may be a function of increased inhibition by 5-HT because the cocaine is blocking the reuptake mechanism (63–65).

Other Drug Use

Use of Other Drugs

Most cocaine users have used other drugs before and during their cocaine use. Both cannabis and alcohol appear to be gateway drugs to cocaine; 98% of cocaine addicts have used marijuana several years before their initial cocaine use, and 90% of cocaine addicts have used alcohol several years before trying cocaine. The average age of initial cannabis and alcohol use is that of early adolescence, whereas cocaine use typically begins in the early twenties. However, the onset of "crack" use in adolescence is lowering the average age of introduction to cocaine (66–69).

Many cannabis and alcohol users qualify for DSM-III-R criteria for cannabis and alcohol dependence before and during cocaine addiction. Other common combinations include cocaine and heroin, cocaine and other sedatives such as benzodiazepines, barbiturates, and quaaludes, and cocaine with hallucinogens such as phencyclidine (PCP). A classical "speedball" is the simultaneous use of cocaine with heroin or a barbiturate, often by intravenous administration (69,70).

Hierarchy of Drug Use

Another interesting phenomena is the hierarchy of drug use among cocaine addicts. Many cocaine users will decrease their consumption of marijuana as they increase their cocaine intake. Conversely, alcohol intake and use of tranquilizers and sedative/hypnotics closely follow cocaine use, ostensibly to enhance the cocaine effect or to sedate the cocaine-induced anxiety. The hallucinogenic properties of marijuana and PCP, with the tendency to arousal, may discourage their use with cocaine which has similar effects.

Common explanations offered by cocaine addicts for other drug use are the following: (1) to substitute when cocaine is not available, (2) to sedate a cocaine-induced anxiety, (3) to relieve a cocaine-induced depression, (4) to enhance or complement a cocaine-induced euphoria, and (5) because other drugs and alcohol are the primary drugs of choice and the addiction occurs to the other drugs as well as cocaine.

Generalized Vulnerability

The sequential and simultaneous use of a variety of different classes of drugs suggests a universal susceptibility or vulnerability to drug use and/or addiction. Stimulants and sedatives or "uppers and downers" may share more similarities than differences in their effects on the brain. A final common pathway in the reward center and changes in the limbic system may underlie a general mechanism for alcohol/drug addiction (26).

Common Mechanisms of Action

Many drugs of different pharmacodynamic actions may affect common neurotransmitters such as dopamine, serotonin, and gamma-aminobutyric acid. Both alcohol and cocaine raise dopamine levels acutely, although alcohol alters membrane fluidity of the neurons and cocaine blocks the reuptake of neurotransmitters. The psychological and physiological symptoms produced by different classes of drugs are similar; alcohol (a sedative) and cocaine (a stimulant) produce similar changes in mood, cognition, and behavior. The intoxicated and withdrawal states in low to moderate doses are alike as both produce euphoria, hyperactivity, arousal, and in higher doses, delirium, stupor, and coma. Important differences are present, as excitement

and seizures occur in the intoxicated state with cocaine and during withdrawal from alcohol (26).

Intervention and Treatment

General Principles

Acute detoxification or "crashing" from cocaine often does not require more
than supportive psychological treatment. The withdrawal syndrome of depression, somnolence, hyperphagia, anxiety, paranoia, and "craving" subsides gradually over days and weeks. No significant alterations in vital signs
usually occur.

Acute hospitalization may be indicated for special consequences of chronic cocaine use that include suicidal risk, inability to abstain from cocaine,
and other associated drug use such as alcohol, tranquilizers, and sedatives/
hypnotics that may require detoxification.

Pharmacological Treatment

The pharmacological interventions may include benzodiazepines (Librium)
for the anxiety and agitation that is especially intense the first few days.
Librium given on an as-needed basis for agitation in 25- to 50-mg doses
every 4 to 6 hours is usually sufficient. Tricyclic antidepressants, desipramine, and imipramine may be employed to neutralize the signs and symptoms of the withdrawal or "crash." The doses used are similar to those
employed in the treatment of major depression. Initial doses of 50 to 100 mg
may be given, with an increase of 50 mg to 100 mg per day for 3 to 5 days to
a total dose of 150 to 250 mg for desipramine and 150 to 300 mg for
imipramine.

These agents may reduce the relapse to cocaine in the ensuing weeks in
individuals with a severe withdrawal reaction, particularly if combined with
other group and individual therapies and self-help groups such as Alcoholics
Anonymous, Narcotics Anonymous, and Cocaine Anonymous. The tricyclic antidepressants alone will not significantly promote abstinence from
cocaine. The tricyclics are usually withdrawn sometime during the first 6
months in a gradual taper over 2 to 3 weeks. Early reports of bromocriptine
and amantadine that suggested efficacy have not been confirmed by larger
studies (26–28).

Programmatic Treatment

Group Therapy

The long-term management of cocaine addiction rests with the group and
individual therapies, and with self-help groups based on the disease concept
of cocaine addiction. Typical treatment approaches utilized by inpatient and
outpatient therapy are structured programs that emphasize abstinence as a

primary goal. The group process is employed as the primary modality of treatment. Identification of members with other members is an essential step in therapeutic transformation. Dissipation of the denial and an acceptance of the cocaine addiction by the addict is achieved by group interaction and confrontation.

A commitment to recovery is gradually established in the addict. Attendance at meetings of Alcoholics Anonymous (AA) or Narcotics Anonymous (NA) is strongly encouraged during the course of treatment and after discharge. Weekly attendance at AA or NA is associated with significant abstinence rates — between 50% to 90% — after 1 year post discharge.

Individual Therapy

Individual therapy may be useful in selected cases. Supportive, cognitive, "here-and-now" psychotherapy is the most effective for cocaine addicts, especially in the earlier stages of recovery. Direction and guidance of the cocaine addict are toward personal responsibility for their cocaine addiction and its consequences.

Family Therapy

Cocaine addiction is a family illness. The family is severely affected by the cocaine addiction (and the alcoholism that is commonly associated with cocaine addiction). The family also is an important source of enabling for the cocaine addict to continue the cocaine addiction. Treatment directed at the family is to encourage an end to the enabling and to establish a commitment to a personal recovery for them. Attendance at Alanon and Naranon by the family is strongly encouraged.

References

1. Burnfeld S (1974). Freud's studies on cocaine. In *Cocaine Papers: Sigmund Freud*, Byck R, ed. New York: Stonehill.
2. Petersen RC (1983). Cocaine: The lessons of history. In *Cocaine: A Second Look*. Rockville, MD: American Council on Marijuana and Other Psychoactive Drugs.
3. Byck R, ed. (1974). *Cocaine Papers: Sigmund Freud*. New York: Stonehill
4. Cohen S (1984). Recent developments in the abuse of cocaine. *Bull Narc* 35:3–14.
5. National Institute on Drug Abuse (1988). *National Household Survey on Drug Abuse*. Washington, DC: U.S. Govt. Printing Office.
6. Kleber HD, Gawin FH (1984). A review of current and experimental treatments. In *Cocaine: Pharmacology, Effects and Treatment of Abuse, NIDA Research Monograph, Vol. 50*, Grabowski J, ed., pp. 111–129. Washington, DC: U.S. Govt. Printing Office.
7. Jones R (1985). The pharmacology of cocaine. In Grabowski J, ed., *NIDA Res Monogr Ser* 50:182–192.
8. Smith DE (1986). Cocaine-alcohol abuse: Epidemiological, diagnostic and treatment considerations. *J Psychoact Drugs* 18(2):117–129

9. Gold MS (1987). Crack abuse: Its implications and outcomes. *Resid Staff Physician* 33:45–53.
10. Gold MS, Washton AM, Dackis CA (1985). Cocaine abuse: Neurochemistry, phenomenology and treatment. In Adams EH, Kozel NJ, eds., *NIDA Res Monogr Ser* 61:130–150.
11. Gold MS (1987). The cocaine epidemic: What are the problems, insights and treatments? *Pharmacy Times*, 53:36–42.
12. Perez-Reyes, Diguiseppi BS, Ondrusek G, et al. (1982). Freebase cocaine smoking. *Clin Pharmacol Ther* 32:459.
13. Siegel RK (1982). Cocaine smoking. *J Psychoact Drugs* 14:271.
14. Siegel RK (1985). New patterns of cocaine use: Changing doses and routes. *NIDA Res Monogr Ser* 61:204–220.
15. Van Dyke C, Ungerer J, Jatlow P, et al. (1982). Intranasal cocaine dose relationships of psychological effects and plasma levels. *Int J Psychiatry Med* 12:1–13.
16. Washton AM, Gold MD, Pottash ALC (1983). Intranasal cocaine addiction. *Lancet* 2:1374.
17. Bose KC (1976). Cocaine intoxication and its demoralizing effects. *Br Med J* 1902; 1:1020–1022. In *Cocaine — Summaries of Psychosocial Research*, pp. 66–67. Rockville, MD: National Institute of Drug Abuse (NIDA).
18. Fischman MW, Schuster CR, Resnekov L, et al. (1976). Cardiovascular and subjective effects of intravenous cocaine administration in humans. *Arch Gen Psychiatry* 33:983–989.
19. Muscholl E (1961). Effect of cocaine and related drugs on the uptake of noradrenaline by heart and spleen. *Br J Pharmacol* 16:352–359.
20. Taylor D, Ho BT (1977). Neurochemical effects of cocaine following acute and repeated injection. *J Neurosci Res* 3:95–101.
21. Gay GR (1982). Clinical management of acute and chronic cocaine poisoning. *Ann Emerg Med* 11:562–572.
22. Kilbey MM, Ellinwood EH (1977). Chronic administration of stimulant drugs: Response modification. In *Cocaine and Other Stimulants*, Ellinwood H, Kilbey M, eds., pp. 410–429. New York: Plenum Press.
23. Millman RB (1986). Drug dependence: General principles of diagnosis and treatment. In *Psychiatry Update, Vol. 5*, pp. 122–136. Washington, DC: American Psychiatry Press.
24. Brower KJ, Paredes A (1987). Cocaine withdrawal (letter). *Arch Gen Psychiatry* 44:298–299.
25. Kleber HD, Gawin FH (1987). Cocaine withdrawal (reply). *Arch Gen Psychiatry* 44:298–299.
26. Miller NS, Dackis CA, Gold MS (1987). The relationship of addiction, tolerance and dependence: A neurochemical approach. *J Subst Abuse Treat* 4:197–207.
27. Lasagna L, Von Felsinger JM, Beecher HK (1955). Drug-induced mood changes in man: I. Observations on healthy subjects, chronically ill patients, and post-addicts. *JAMA* 157:1066–1120.
28. Gawin FH, Kleber HD (1986). Abstinence symptomatology and psychiatric diagnosis in chronic cocaine abusers. *Arch Gen Psychiatry* 43:107–113.
29. Gold MS, Pottash ALC, Annitto WJ, et al. (1983). Cocaine withdrawal: Efficacy of tyrosine. *Soc Neurosci Abstr* 9:157.
30. Gold MS, Dackis CA (1984). New insights and treatments: Opiate withdrawal and cocaine addiction. *Clin Ther* 7(1):6–21.

31. Keller MB, Shapiro RW, Lavori PW, et al. (1982). Recovery in major depressive disorder: Analysis with the life table and regression models. *Arch Gen Psychiatry* 39:905–910.
32. Dackis CA, Gold MS (1985). New concepts in cocaine addiction: The dopamine depletion hypothesis. *Neurosci Biobehav Rev* 9:469–477.
33. Edwards G, Arrif A, Hodgson R (1981). Nomenclature and classification of drug and alcohol related problems. *Bull WHO* 59:225–242.
34. American Psychiatric Association (1980). *Diagnostic and Statistical Manual of Mental Disorders*, 3d Ed. Washington, DC: American Psychiatric Association.
35. Kuehnle J, Spitzer R (1981). DSM-III classification of substance use disorders. In *Substance Abuse: Clinical Problems and Perspectives*, Lowinson JH, ed., pp. 19–23. Baltimore: Williams & Wilkins.
36. Fischman MW, Schuster CR (1982). Cocaine self-administration in humans. *Fed Proc* 41:241–246.
37. Runsaville BJ, Spitzer RL, Williams JBW (1986). Proposed changes in DSM-III substance use disorders: Description and rationale. *Am J Psychiatry* 143:468.
38. Gawin FH, Kleber HD (1986). Abstinence symptomatology and psychiatry diagnosis in cocaine abusers: Clinical observations. *Arch Gen Psychiatry* 43:107–113.
39. Keller MB, Shapiro RW (1982). "Double depression": Superimposition of acute depressive disorders. *Am J Psychiatry* 139:438–442.
40. Gold MS (1984). *800-COCAINE*. New York: Bantam.
41. Jellinek EM (1960). The disease concept of alcoholism. New Haven, CT: Hillhouse Press.
42. Verebey K, Gold MS (1984). The psychopharmacology of cocaine. *Psychiatr Ann* 14(10):714–723.
43. Goodman L, Gilman AG, eds. (1980). *The Pharmacological Bases of Therapeutics*, 6th Ed. New York: Macmillan.
44. Spiehler VR, Reed D (1985). Brain concentrations of cocaine and benzoylecgonine in fatal cases. *J Forensic Sci* 30:1003–1011.
45. Van Dyke C, Jatlow P, Barash PG, et al. (1978). Oral cocaine: Plasma concentrations and central effects. *Science* 100:211–213.
46. Lesse H (1980). Prolonged effects of cocaine on hippocampal activity. *Commun Psychopharmacol* 4:247.
47. Misra AL, Nayak PK, Block R, et al. (1975). Estimation and disposition of [3H]benzoylecgnonine and pharmacological activity of some cocaine metabolites. *J Pharm Pharmacol* 27:784–786.
48. Borne RG, Bedford JA, Buelke JL, et al. (1977). Biological effects of cocaine derivatives: I. Improved synthesis and pharmacological evaluation of norocaine *J Pharm Sci* 66:119–120.
49. Wilkinson P, Van Dyke C, Jatlow P, et al. (1980). Intranasal and oral cocaine kinetics. *Clin Pharmacol Ther* 27:386–394.
50. Kilbey MM, Ellinwood EH, Easler ME (1979). Effect of chronic cocaine pretreatment in kindled seizures and behavioral stereotypes. *Exp Neurol* 64:306–314.
51. Post RM, Kopanda RT, Lee A (1975). Progressive behavioral changes during chronic lidocaine administration: Relationship to kindling. *Life Sci* 17:943.
52. Striplig JS, Gramlich CA, Cunningham MG (1983). Effect of cocaine and lidocaine on the development of kindled seizures. *Soc Neurosci Abstr* 9:486.

53. Wise RA (1984). Neural mechanisms of the reinforcing action of cocaine. *NIDA Res Monogr Ser* 50:15–33.
54. Taylor DL, Beng TH, Fagan JD (1979). Increased dopamine receptor binding in rat brain by repeated cocaine injections. *Commun Psychopharmacol* 3:137–142.
55. Ross SB, Renyi AL (1967). Inhibition of the uptake of tritiated catecholamines by antidepressant and related agents. *Eur J Pharmacol* 2:181–186.
56. Cooper JR, Bloom FE, Roth RH (1982). *The Biochemical Basis of Neuropharmacology*. New York: Oxford University Press.
57. Langer SZ, Enero MA (1974). The potentiation of responses to adrenergic nerve stimulation in the presence of cocaine: Its relationship to the metabolic fate of released norepinephrine. *J Pharmacol Ther* 191:431–443.
58. Whitby LG, Hertting G, Axelrod J (1960). Effect of cocaine on the disposition of noradrenaline labelled with tritium. *Nature* 187:604–605.
59. Roberts DC, Corcoran ME, Fibiger HC (1977). On the role of ascending catecholaminergic systems in intravenous self-administration of cocaine. *Pharmacol Biochem Behav* 6:615–620.
60. Banerjee SP, Sharma VK, Kung-Cheung LS, et al. (1979). Cocaine and D-amphetamine-induced changes in central beta-adrenoceptor sensitivity: Effects of acute and chronic drug treatment. *Brain Res* 175:119–130.
61. Ross SB, Renyi AL (1969). Inhibition of the uptake of 5-hydroxytryptamine in brain tissue. *Eur J Pharmacol* 7:270–277.
62. Freidman E, Gershon S, Rotrosen J (1975). Effects of acute cocaine treatment on the turnover of 5-hydroxytryptamine in the rat brain. *Br J Pharmacol* 54:61–64.
63. Knapp S, Mandell AJ (1972). Narcotic drugs: Effects on the serotonin biosynthetic systems of the brain. *Science* 177:1209–1211.
64. Pradhan SN, Battachargya AK, Pradhan S (1978). Serotonergic manipulation of the behavioral effects of cocaine in rats. *Common Psychopharmacol* 2:481–486.
65. Schubert J, Fryo B, Nyback H, Sedvall G (1970). Effects of cocaine and amphetamine on the metabolism of tryptophan and 5-hydroxytryptamine in mouse brain in vivo. *J Pharm Pharmacol* 22:860–862.
66. National Commission on Marijuana and Drug Abuse (1973). Drug use in America: Problems in perspective. In *Second Report of the National Commission on Marijuana and Drug Abuse*. Washington, DC: National Institute of Abuse.
67. Adams EH, Kozel NJ, eds. (1985). Cocaine use in America: Introduction and overview. *NIDA Res Monogr Ser* 61:45–49.
68. Miller NS, Gold MS, Klahr AL, et al. (1988). Alcohol use in cocaine addicts. *Subst Abuse* 9(4):216–221.
69. Miller NS, Gold MS, Klahr AL, et al. (1990). Cannabis diagnosis of patients receiving treatment for cocaine dependence. *J Subst Abuse* 2:107–111.
70. Grinspoon L, Bakalar JB (1985). *Cocaine: A Drug and Its Social Evolution*. New York: Basic Books.
71. Freedman AM, Kaplan HI, Saddock BJ (1975). *Comprehensive Textbook of Psychiatry*, 2nd Ed., Vol. 2, Baltimore, MD: Williams and Wilkins.
72. Van Dyck C, Byck R (1982). Cocaine. *Sci Am* 246:128–141.

CHAPTER 14

The Pharmacology of Hallucinogens and Designer Drugs

History

The hallucinogens represent a broadly defined class of drugs that cross pharmacological boundaries. These drugs are grouped together as much for historical reasons as for psychological effects. By strict definition, the hallucinogens alter and distort perceptions in space and time. An hallucination is a false perception, and these drugs produce exaggerated sensory phenomena including visual, auditory, and tactile hallucinations. These perceptions originate internally from drug-induced changes in the brain, and as in hallucinations, project onto an external reality.

These fantasy-producing drugs became popular in the 1960s, particularly among the "hippie generation." The youthful users justified their chemically medicated expansion of reality as a search for inner reality, uncovering the deepest experiences and profound intuitive truths. Ironically, as research has shown, these drugs induce psychological artifacts by stimulating neurotransmitters involved in the sensory centers for vision, audition, and touch (1).

At any rate, a biochemical scheme will be used in this chapter that is commonly found in writings on hallucinogens. There are three groups: indoelamines, phenyl ethylamines, and isopropylamines.

The first group, indoelamines, which contain more than one ring includes LSD (D-lysergic acid diethylamide), psilocin, psilocybin, and DMT (*N, N*-dimethyl tryptamine). These are substituted tryptamines and the karma alkaloids, which are beta-carboline derivatives. The second group, the phenyl ethylamines, which contain one ring, includes mescaline. The third group are the phenyl isopropylamines, which are methoxylated amphetamines and are all "designer drugs." They have six possible substitutions on the 6-carbon ring, which determines differences in properties. Included in this group are 2,5-dimethyl-4-methyl amphetamine (DOM or STP), 3,4-methylene-dioxy amphetamine (MDA), 2,5-dimethoxy-4-ethyl amphetamine (DOET), 3-methoxy-4,5-methylenedioxy amphetamine (MMDA), 0, 3, 4, 5-trimethoxy amphetamine (TMA), 3,4-methylenedioxy methamphetamine (MDMA), "Adam" or "ecstasy," and *N*-monoethyl (MDA) – "Eve" (2). (See Table 14.1.)

TABLE 14.1 The chemical formulae of psychedelic drugs.[a]

Indoles (indolealkylamines)

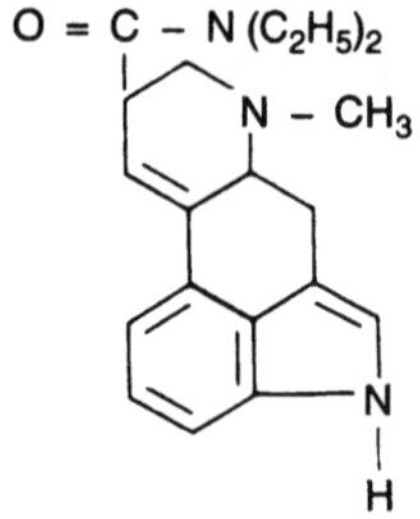

D-lysergic acid diethylamide
LSD

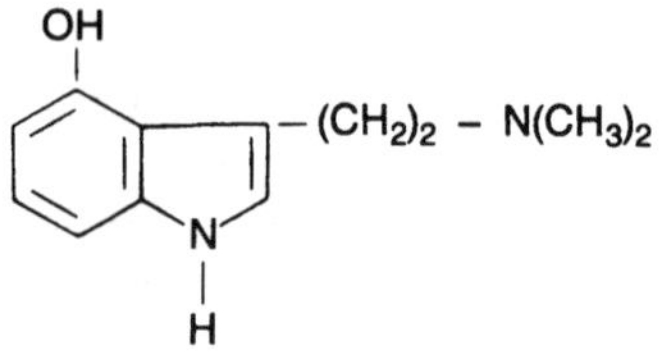

psilocin

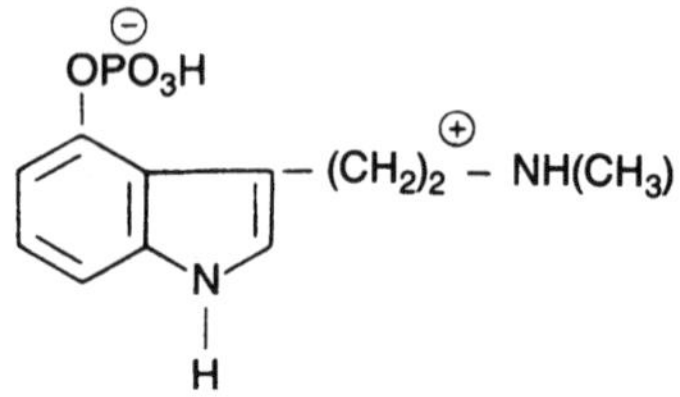

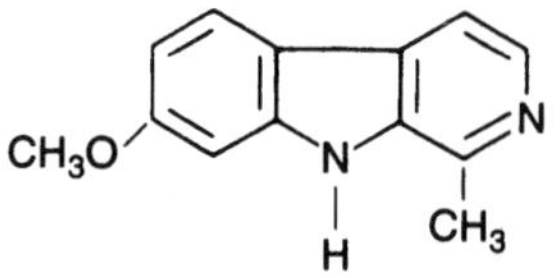

harmine
(harmala alkaloids)

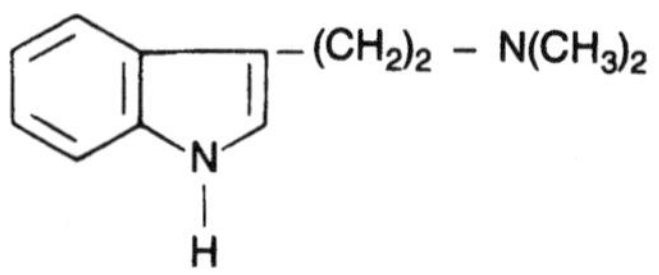

psilocybin

DMT
N, N-dimethyltryptamine

DET, DPT
N, N-diethyltryptamine
N, N-dipropyltryptamine

Phenylalkylamines

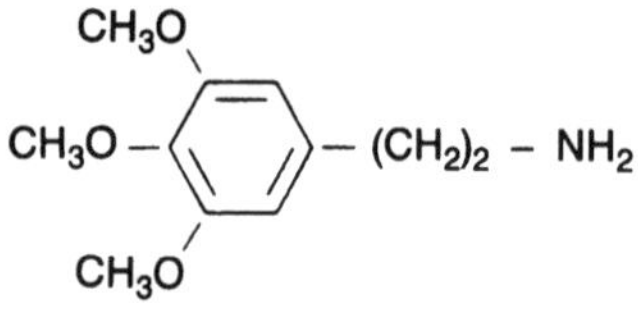

mescaline
3,4,5-trimethoxyphenylethylamine

Phenylisopropylamines (PIA)

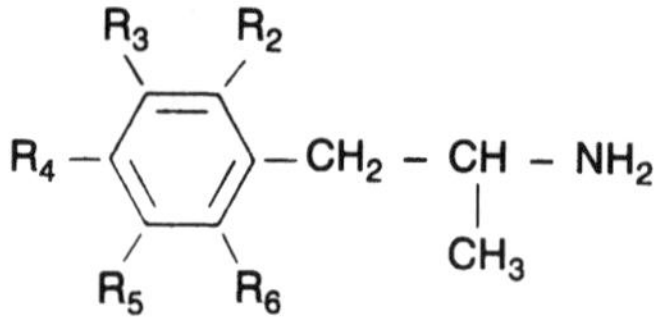

MDA: 3,4-methylenedioxyamphetamine
MMDA: 3-methoxy-4,5-MDA
DOET: 2,5-dimethoxy-4-ethylamphetamine
DOM: 2,5-dimethoxy-4-methylamphetamine
TMA: 3,4,5-trimethoxyamphetamine
MDMA: 3,4-methylenedioxymethamphetamine

[a]From Ref. 1.

Prevalence

No one knows for sure the exact prevalence of the use of the hallucinogens. Most would agree that their current frequency and magnitude of use do not match the epidemic proportions of the 1960s in the United States. As then, and more so now, the hallucinogens are found to have a geographic distribution that has clear historical roots. These drugs have always predominated and still do in the western United States. They are found elsewhere, particularly in large urban areas, but do not appear to be present in any proportion similar to that in California and the southwestern states (3–5).

The widely cited study of high-school seniors indicates that hallucinogens are still used, as 10% and 22% of high school seniors have used hallucinogenic stimulants in the past year and 2% and 5% in the past 30 days. Daily use is less than 1%. Recent surveys suggest that the overall trend is for decreasing use of these drugs as well as other drugs (6).

Patterns of Use

Youth remains the overwhelming consumer of these drugs. However, an occasional overzealous and ill-advised investigator or practitioner may use these drugs on themselves, subjects, and patients. The use may continue into adulthood in some cases, although clinical experience and some research suggest that many users whether addicted or not will "burn out" or progress beyond these drugs to other drugs (5).

Hallucinogens are strictly illicit drugs that are Schedule I, that is, they have a high addictive potential without medicinal benefit. Physicians cannot prescribe these drugs for clinical indications; they may be employed for approved investigative purposes (2).

The drugs may be smoked (inhaled), injected (intravenous, i.v.), snorted (intranasal), and ingested (oral). The current popular routes of administration include smoking and intravenous injection. The recent trend of inhaling stimulants and other drugs such as sedatives has introduced a practice that appears to be increasing the addictive use of these drugs. The inhalation route provides for the quickest delivery and highest concentration of drug to the brain. The path of the inhaled drug is to the lungs, then to the heart where it is pumped directly into the brain. The intravenous route is longer because the drug must circulate through the venous system to the heart, then to the lungs and back to the heart before entering the brain. The other routes are slower and result in a lower blood concentration (7).

Because of the rapid rise of concentration of the drug in the brain, the addiction potential may be greater. Self-administration studies suggest that the reinforcement potency of a drug correlates with the latency and amount of drug reaching the brain centers, that is, the shorter duration and the greater blood level, the greater addiction. The smoking of "crack" freebase cocaine is an illustration of a highly addicting power of cocaine (7).

The practice of concurrent and simultaneous use of other drugs is very common among hallucinogen users. Although hallucinogens may be the predominant drug used by the addict, other drugs are used as well, with or in substitution for, the hallucinogens. Alcohol, marijuana, cocaine, sedatives/hypnotics (benzodiazepines), barbiturates, quaaludes, etc. are drugs frequently used by the hallucinogen users. The occurrence of multiple drug addiction is far more the rule than the exception by today's contemporary alcoholic and drug addict (8), including the hallucinogen addict.

The hallucinogens contained in mushrooms are in the form of naturally occurring nitrogen-containing compounds. There are several hundred varieties that have been used since ancient times for religious, recreational, literary, and addictive purposes over the years. The first hallucinogens may have originated from the mushroom, *Amanita muscaria*. The LSD contained in ergot alkaloid from plants is believed to have been used in pre-Colombian times. Divine mushrooms containing psilocybin were known to Indians populations for centuries. The bullous of the cacti *Lipophore williamsii* and *L. diffusa* is the source of mescaline. Nutmeg, which contains myristicin, a compound similar to mescaline, is readily available. Satrale, the principal component of oil and sassafras, is similar to myristicin and has similar effects in larger amounts (1).

Intoxication

LSD is one of the most powerful psychoactive drugs known. Ten milligrams produces euphoria and decreased inhibition; 50 to 100 mg is the minimal hallucinogenic dose, whereas 400 to 500 mg produces full hallucinogenic effects. LSD is well absorbed orally. Sympathomimetic effects begin within 30 minutes, and the hallucinogenic phase peaks at 2 to 3 hours with a duration of 8 to 12 hours. LSD, psilocybin, and mescaline have similar clinical effects and duration of action (Table 14.2).

These drugs, as indicated by their name, produce hallucinations. The most common with acute and chronic use is visual. The visual hallucinogens may be poorly formed as with LSD or well formed as with methamphetamines. They frequently involved vivid colors and array of forms and sometimes as specific as images of people. Contrary to popular belief, these hallucinogens, especially with LSD are not typical of schizophrenia (9,10).

All the hallucinogens have sympathomimetic effects in addition to the euphoria. The methamphetamine derivatives in particular produce an intense euphoria greater than experienced with many other drugs. The general state of arousal includes hyperactivity, increased alertness, and exaggerated responses to external stimuli. The most constant psychological effect is the perceptual distortions and hallucinations. Objects undulate, their boundaries are lost and merge; people's faces are distorted as well as self-body parts (11,12).

TABLE 14.2. Classes of psychedelic drugs.[a]

Drug (Class and common name)	Psychedelic dose range	Time of effects (peak/duration)	Physiological and psychological effects
Indolealkylamines			
LSD (acid)	50–150 mg	2–3 hr/8–12 hr	Sympathomimetic
Psilocybin (mushrooms)	10–20 mg	1½ hr/4–6 hr	Gentler than LSD More visual and euphoric Less panic and less paranoia
Harmala alkaloids	200–400 mg (oral)	4–8 hr	Nausea, vomiting, sweating, dizziness, lassitude, tremor, numbness, trance with intense imagery
DMT (businessman's trip) (mind blowing)	50 mg (smoked, injected)	5–20 min/30 min	More intense Sympathomimetic (bp, pulse, dilated pupils) Sudden, more intense thoughts and visions
Phenylalkylamines			
Mescaline (cactus, peyote buttons, mesc)	200 mg 3–5 peyote buttons	2–3 hr/8–12 hr	Bitter taste, nausea, vomiting ↑ sympathomimetic ↑ sensual and perceptual
Phenylisopropylamines (PIA) (Designer drugs)			
DOM (STP, after the oil derivative)	5–8 mg 10–30 mg (street dose)	6–8 hr 16–24 hr	Low dose like LSD High dose ↑ sympathomimetic ↑ flashbacks, ↑ psychosis Chlorpromazine adverse reaction
MDA (love drug)	100–150 mg (low) > 200 mg (high)	1–2 hr/8–12 hr	Low-empathic, insight with little perceptual change High-↑ sympathomimetic, jaw tension, sweating, psychedelic with hallucinations
DOET	2–5 mg	5–6 hr	Low dose like MDA
MDMA (ecstasy, Adam)	100–150 mg (low) > 200 mg (high)	1–2 hr/8–12 hr	Low dose like MDA High dose ↑ sympathomimetic and psychedelic
TMA	500–100 mg (low) > 250 mg (high)	2–3 hr/8–12 hr	Low dose like mescaline High dose ↑ anger and hostility

[a]From Ref. 1.

The sensory acuity is heightened for all modalities. Perceptions are more vivid. There is an acute attentiveness to details with overvalued attribution of meaning, and ordinary objects, events, and thoughts are novel and profound (13,14).

Cognitive effects are to disrupt concentration, decrease recent memory, and impair insight and judgment. Depersonalization and derealization are common occurrences. At times, a fragmentation or loss of self-identity may promote mystical experiences. Suspiciousness and frank paranoid delusions may occur, particularly with chronic use (15,16).

The effects in mood are predictable; these include a intense euphoria, followed by anxiety, panic, and depression alternating in an intense mood lability and irritability. Suicidal actions are prominent, particularly with STP, mescaline, and methamphetamine. The expression "speed kills" is an outgrowth of the intense feelings of depressions with despair, hopelessness, helplessness, and paranoid delusions that may accompany chronic use of these drugs (17,18).

The paranoid delusions may provoke the urge to "strike out" in retaliation, and as a result homicides have been reported (19). The violent behaviors that have been associated with these drugs are numerous, and as mentioned involve acts directed at self and others. Also, because of the illicit nature of the drugs and at times the antisocial personality of the users, criminal activity involving violence may occur (20).

Toxicity

There are two types of toxicity associated with hallucinogenic amphetamines and their analogues: acute and chronic toxicity. Hallucinogenic drugs do not cause respiratory depression as do opiates and sedatives/hypnotics. Most deaths have been induced with paramthoxy amphetamine (PMA) and 3,4-methylene dioxyamphetamine (MDA). The acute toxic manifestations are expressions of excessive CNS stimulation that result from the discharging sympathetic nervous system and include restlessness, agitation, sweating, rigidity, convulsions, hypertension, tachycardia, and hyperpyrexia. Vasoconstriction and vasospasm have also been reported. The causes of death may be related to any of these manifestations, including cardiovascular arrhythmias and cerebrovascular accidents (1,2).

Other Drugs

Crystal Metaphetamine ("Ice")

"Ice" is not a designer drug or new analogue of methamphetamine. Ice derives its name in the United States from its appearance of large crystals. Ice is imported from the Far East into Hawaii and to a Hiropon. We have now interviewed ice users who have called 1-800-COCAINE. Prices for "ice" at the retail level are comparable to those for heroin. Ice is D-methamphetamine, which is an analogue of amphetamine, a CNS stimulant. The primary route of administration is inhalation (smoking), but it can be injected, snorted, or taken orally, similar to "crack" or freebase cocaine. The drug has a rapid onset of action (approximately 7 seconds), which is also similar to crack but differs in having a much longer duration of action, 12 to 24 hours compared to 20 to 30 minutes. Smoking provides a direct delivery of "ice" to the brain, bypassing the venous system. The pharmacological effects reported by users include intense euphoria, hyperactivity, delusions and paranoid hallucinations, anorexia and weight loss, anxiety, depression, acute hypertensive crises, violence, trauma and accidents, irritability, nervousness, insomnia, and palpitations. These people often complain of anger and irritability and demonstrate violent and destructive behavior. Unlike the acute paranoid disorder of cocaine users, these psychotic symptoms do not appear to resolve during a few hours, and may persist for days after cessation of use. Calls to 1-800-COCAINE about ice increase after each national media mention.

MDMA

MDMA (3,4-methylenedioxy methamphetamine, or "ecstasy" as it is known on the streets, is a controlled substance and an analogue of the hallucinogenic amphetamine type. MDMA was patented in 1914 but never marketed. MDA (3,4-methylenedioxyamphetamine) is a structurally related to MDMA. MDA produces degeneration of serotonin nerve terminals in rat brain.

Ecstasy is currently a major street drug in the western United States, although its actual prevalence is unknown. Large-scale use in the eastern United States has not been verified. Ecstasy produces intense euphoria and dramatic and vivid hallucinations, and replaced MDA in 1970s and 1980s because of these superior effects. MDMA also has less stimulating effects than MDA. MDA use still persists, however (1,2).

Other psychological symptoms include bizarre and poorly formed geometric patterns and complex visual images, especially with closed eyes, similar to other hallucinogens. Physical symptoms are common and include jaw-clenching, bruxism, sweating, ataxia, nausea, and dizziness in addition to the sympathomimetic effects of tachycardiac, hypertension, hyperflexia, and tremor. Other adverse effects include residual withdrawal effects that last for weeks, including exhaustion, depression, fatigue, nausea, and numbness. Because of the sympathomimetic effects, certain medical conditions may be aggravated by MDMA, MDA, and other hallucinogens. These include diabetes mellitus, liver disease, seizure disorders, glaucoma, cardiovascular disease, hypertension, hypoglycemia, hyperthyroidism, and pregnancy. The adverse psychological reactions are similar to those of classic hallucinogens, and include panic dissociative and psychotic reactions, insomnia, rage reactions, and delusions. Other toxic manifestations include ataxia, nystagmus, emotional lability, vomiting, and parethesias. Overdose reactions include tachycardia, palpitations, hypertension, hypotension, hyperthermia, renal failure, disseminated intravascular coagulation, and rhabdomyoyses (1,2).

MPTP (1-methyl, 4-phenyl, 1,2,6-tetral hydropyridine, I) is a designer drug in the classical sense. A designer drug is defined as the replacement of an illegal, controlled substance with a similarly acting but slightly modified compound that is legal. MDTP is a meperidine and fentanyl analogue. Both are synthetic opiates. MPTP is an analogue of meperidine, and has been implicated as a cause of irreversible drug-induced parkinsonism. Numerous research publications have appeared describing the pharmacological and toxicological effects of MPTP in various animal species. The psychological effects of MPTP are similar to those of the synthetic opiate meperidine (1,2).

Tolerance and Dependence

Tolerance and dependence to the various hallucinogens do occur. The observable measurements regarding this development of tolerance and dependence are similar to those for stimulants. The tolerance may vary from individual to individual and from one pharmacological effect to another; that is, the tolerance to the euphoria and sedative may be greater than to the hypertension and tachycardia. The degree of tolerance may be mild to marked. Because most hallucinogen users are users of multiple drugs, other drugs and alcohol will affect the development of tolerance of dependence to these drugs (21,22).

The dependence syndrome is similar to other stimulants and rather constant across hallucinogens. The withdrawal effects include anxiety, depression, hypersomnia, hyperphagia, suicidal impulses, ideation, feelings of derealization, depersonalization, and other manifestations of sympathetic nervous system exhaustion. The dependence syndrome may be protracted over days, weeks, or even years (1,2).

Diagnosis

The diagnosis is made by applying the same criteria for addiction, tolerance, and dependence that are used for all drugs. Addiction is defined as a preoccupation with acquiring the drug, compulsive use of the drug, and a pattern of relapse over time. Tolerance is the need to increase a dose to maintain an effect or the loss of an effect at a particular dose. Dependence is the onset of predictable signs and symptoms of withdrawal for a particular drug.

The hallucinogen addict is commonly a multiple drug addict who uses and is addicted to a variety of drugs, including alcohol. The user is typically youthful and uses hallucinogens concurrently and simultaneously with other drugs. Hallucinogens are rarely the first drugs used. It usually is a progression of use from other drugs. Alcohol is most often the first drug used, and frequently in combination with the hallucinogens.

Neurochemistry

These drugs affect the catecholamine system. LSD alters primarily the serotonin system. These are two serotonin receptors (S1 and S2), and LSD has a high affinity for both. Also, there are both inhibitory and excitatory postsynaptic serotonin effects as well as inhibitory presynaptic autoreceptors. LSD-type hallucinogens have both serotonin agonist and antagonist effects in different brain areas. The postsynaptic effects on serotonin contribute to the distinct behavioral syndromes. The presynaptic effects do not seem to be critical in the production of the behavior effects. Furthermore, serotonin antagonists may hold certain LSD-induced effects (23,24).

The mechanism of action of the amphetamine analogues, such as MDA and MDMA is similar to the amphetamines. The amphetamines are indirect, acting as catecholamine agonists by promoting the release of norepinephrine, dopamine, epinephrine, and serotonin from presynaptic storage sites. The net effect is to enhance the catecholamine nerve transmission by increasing the synaptic and postsynaptic concentrations of the neurotransmitters. The correlation between these demonstrated laboratory effects and the clinical effects is significant (23,24).

Because MPTP is an analogue of meperidine (a synthetic opiate), the clinical effects correlate with predictable activity at the opiate receptors. The actions are agonistic. The exact mechanism involved in the selective toxicity in the basal ganglia that produces the severe extrapyramidal syndrome has yet to be clarified (2).

Intervention and Treatment

The treatment of the withdrawal is frequently supportive. The medical sequelae from the withdrawal are benign and usually do not require pharmacological therapy. The practice of talking a patient "down" is common with some of the hallucinogens and arose from its effectiveness in treating LSD. "Talking down" is basically reassuring and supporting an individual who is on a bad trip or in a frightening intoxicating state. This method may be employed for any of the hallucinogens, which may inspire fear that at times may be terrifying.

It is important to recognize that most hallucinogenic users are multiple drug addicts/alcoholics who must be assessed for their other drug addictions and their medical complications. These patients may be referred for traditional inpatient and outpatient treatment for drug and alcohol addiction as well as long term participation in Alcoholics Anonymous and Narcotics Anonymous.

References

1. Moreines R (1989). The psychedelics. In *Drugs of Abuse*, Giannini AJ, Slatry AE, eds., pp. 207–241. Oradel, NY: Medical Economic Books.
2. Redda KK, Walker CA, Barnet G (1989). *Cocaine, Marijuana, Designer Drugs: Chemistry, Pharmacology and Behavior*. Boca Raton, FL: CRC Press.
3. Cohen S (1985). LSD: the varieties of psychotic experience. *Psychoact Drugs* 17: 291–296.
4. Nicols DE, Glennon RA (1984). Medicinal chemistry and structure activity relationships of hallucinogens. In *Hallucinogens: Neurochemical, Behavioral and Clinical Perspectives*, Jacobs B, ed. New York: Raven Press.
5. Hollister L (1984). Effects of hallucinogens in humans. In *Hallucinogens: Neurochemical, Behavioral and Clinical Perspectives*, Jacobs B, ed. New York: Raven Press.
6. NIDA (1988). *NIDA Capsules. National High School Seminar Health Survey*. Washington, DC: U.S. Department of Health and Human Services, Public Health Services.
7. Miller NS, Gold MS, Millman RB (1989). Cocaine: General characteristics, abuse in addiction. *NY State J Med* 89:390–395.
8. Miller NS, Mirin SM (1989). Multiple drug use in alcoholics: Practical and theoretical implications. *Psychiatr Ann* 19(5):248–255.
9. Glass GS, Bowers MB, Jr. (1970). Chronic psychosis associated with long-term psychotomimetic drug abuse. *Arch Gen Psychiatry* 23:97–103.
10. Tucker GJ, Quinlan D, Harrow M (1972). Chronic hallucinogenic drug use and thought disturbance. *Arch Gen Psychiatry* 27:443–446.
11. Bowers MB Jr., Freedman DX (1966). "Psychedelic" experiences in acute psychoses. *Arch Gen Psychiatry* 15:240–248.
12. Houston J (1969). Phenomenology of the psychedelic experience. In *Psychedelic Drugs*, Hicks R, Fink P, eds., New York: Grune & Stratton.
13. Yensen R (1985). LSD and psychotherapy. *Psychoact Drugs* 17:267–277.
14. Smith DE, Seymour RD (1985). Dream becomes nightmare: Adverse reactions of LSD. *Psychoact Drugs* 17:297–303.
15. Bowers MG, Jr. (1972). Acute psychosis induced by psychotomimetic drug abuse. *Arch Gen Psychiatry* 27:437–442.
16. Tsuang MT, Simpson JC, Kronfol Z (1982). Subtypes of drug abuse with psychosis. *Arch Gen Psychiatry* 39:141–147.
17. Hayner GN, McKinney H (1986). MDMD: The dark side of ecstasy. *Psychoact Drugs* 18:341–347.
18. Robbins E, Robbins L, Frosch W, et al. (1967). Implications of untoward reactions to hallucinogens. *Bull NY Acad Med* 43:985–999.
19. Reich P, Hepps RB (1972). Homicide during a psychosis induced by LSD. *JAMA* 291:869–871.
20. NIAD (1985). Patterns and trends in drug abuse. A national and international perspective. Rockville, MD: National Institute Drug Abuse.

21. Downing J (1986). The psychological and physiological effects of MDMS on normal volunteers. *Psychoact Drugs* 18:335–340.
22. Greer G, Tolbert R (1986). Subjective reports of the effects of MDMA in a clinical setting. *Psychoact Drugs* 18:319–327.
23. Hamon M (1984). Common neurochemical correlates to the action of hallucinogens. In *Hallucinogens: Neurochemical, Behavioral and Clinical Perspectives*, Jacobs B, ed. New York: Raven Press.
24. Aghajanian GK, Sprouse JS, Rasmussen K (1987). Physiology of the midbrain serotonin system. In *Psychopharmacology: The Third Generation of Progress*, Metzler H, ed. New York: Raven Press.

CHAPTER 15

The Pharmacology of Inhalants and Volatile Solvents

History

The term "organic solvent" is derived from the basic chemical structure of hydrocarbons of the aliphatic, aromatic, and halogenated forms. Because many of these hydrocarbons are volatile, the route of administration is typically by inhalation as a volatile gas or aerosol through the nose or mouth. The volatile solvents and aerosols are subject to significant liability for abuse and addiction as well as toxicity (1).

The inhalation of organic solvents or gases dates back in recorded history to the ancient Greeks. In the oracle of Delphi, the Pythoness would sit over an opening in a rock emitting carbon dioxide to inhale the gas so that she could induce a trance state to deliver the prophecy. When carbon dioxide was no longer available, the Pythoness inhaled fumes generated by scorching the laurel leaves in a copper bowl (2).

Further history of inhalation of these drugs is lacking until the advent of the anesthetic agents nitrous oxide and ethyl ether in the nineteenth century, when their efficacy in clinical medicine was appreciated. In Ireland, ether was popularized as a means of reducing alcoholism, but the addictive use of ether became so widespread that it was necessary to reintroduce alcohol use (2).

Reports of gasoline sniffing first appeared in the medical literature in the early 1930s, and contemporary use of volatile substances was recorded in the literature in 1951 with a description of gasoline use by two boys. By the early 1960s, solvent use was pervasive in the United States. The organic solvents are available in a wide variety of forms for administration from glue and model cement sniffing, to inhalation of antifreeze, paint thinner, lighter fluid, cleaning solutions, typewriter correction fluid, and, more recently, propellant gases of aerosol products (1).

Prevalence

The true prevalence of use is not known, nor are adequate estimates for use available. However, it is generally agreed that the age of introduction and most common use is adolescence although users may be found at any age. The most common example of solvent inhalation is sniffing of airplane glue or model cement among the young. Many states and cities have restrictions on the sale of glue such as requiring the purchase of a model kit to be used with the cement, and the prices of the kits are included with the price of the cement. The practice of using aerosols to produce excellent highs began with their introduction in 1967, with deaths being reported from the aerosol use (3–5).

The association of volatile solvent use and other drug use including alcohol is very significant. Many solvent addicts also have a substantial history of alcohol and drug use and addictions. This finding is in keeping with the characteristics of the contemporary alcoholic and drug addict who uses multiple drugs far more often than not (6).

As with other drugs, the practice of inhaling glue in a paper or plastic bag (bagging) in a group is preferred, although solitary use is not uncommon. Another form of self-administration is "huffing," which is to inhale through the mouth and nose from a cloth soaked with the solvent, such as gasoline and paint thinners. Liquids such as typewriter fluid are inhaled directly from the container, and aerosols are sprayed into a bag to be inhaled (7,8).

The toxicity from the volatile organic solvents has been well known in the medical literature for years. The volatile substances are pursued for their ability to produce central nervous system (CNS) effects such as intoxication and addiction. The clinical effects are similar to alcohol ingestion but most closely resemble general anesthetics, corresponding to the first phase of excitation and euphoria, followed by progressive CNS depression and confusion, and stupor, seizures, and cardiopulmonary arrest in sufficient doses. Unfortunately, the volatile solvents are not controlled similarly to other psychoactive substances nor is the potential for abuse and addiction adequately known although the toxicity is appreciated somewhat more (9,10).

Patterns of Use

Volatile solvent sniffers typically are young males between 10 and 15 years old. Use often begins as young as 7 or 8 years of age, and many females and some adults are known to use organic solvents for abuse and addiction. Solvent inhalation, as with other forms of drug abuse and addiction, has no other particular social or geographical boundaries and occurs among the poor and the affluent in cities, suburbs, and rural areas alike. As a form of intoxication organic solvents are similar to alcohol and marijuana, and as an expression of abuse and addiction they are equal to the better known drugs of addiction such as alcohol or opiates. Although many users either have or go on to develop an alcohol, marijuana, or opiate addiction, the use of organic solvents by themselves does not necessarily mean other drug use, either concurrently or prospectively, will occur. However, the regular user of only volatile solvents represents a minority of the users of volatile solvents (11,12).

Generally, the solvent use decreases with increasing age as the users go on to use other drugs or cease being interested in the solvents. In a national survey of high-school seniors, 10% to 13% of each senior class reported using inhalants at least once from 1975 to 1982, and 10% to 11% reported using amyl and butyl nitrates. Daily use was reported by 0.1% of the senior classes, which are rates similar to that reported for lysergic acid (LSD) and phenylcyclidine (PCP). The same group of students reported daily use of alcohol or cannabis in 5% to 10% of the seniors (13,14).

Although the use of solvents is relative to other drug use, the frequency of solvent use is probably not as great as with other drugs. A study showed that 72.8% of the student solvent users used solvents once or twice in the previous 12 months, while only 1.5% reported using them 40 or more times in a year. In contrast, 6.4% of cannabis users, 20% of alcohol users, and 7.2% of LSD users reported using these drugs about 40 or more times over the previous 12 months.

Solvent use by adults is less common than by youths but is not rare. The use by physicians, dentists, and nurses who have access to anesthetic gases is significant. Moreover, the use of alkyl nitrates (butyl, isobutyl, and amyl), which are vasodilators, are used as aphrodisiacs and are purported to intensify and prolong orgasm but are also used for the intoxicating effect. In 1980, about 17% of young adults aged 18 to 25 years indicated some experience with inhalants. The use of solvents is also high among populations with a high rate of addiction to other drugs who would use alcohol and drugs if available but may not, such as in prisons (15,16).

Other adults at risk for the development of a solvent problem are those who are exposed to them, such as shoemakers, sandal makers, cabinet makers, and printers. The list may be extended to hairstylists, janitors, maintenance workers, painters, gas station attendants, mechanics, bicycle repairers, dry-cleaning workers, and those involved in petroleum products or the manufacture of products containing solvents. Any workplace that has solvents and medical workers may use ether, chloroform, trichloroethylene, and halothane with fatal results (17,18).

Because organic solvents are readily available in such a wide variety of substances, their use is difficult to control. The range of products employed that contain organic solvents is extensive and includes gasoline, cleaning solutions, lighter fluid, and paint and lacquer thinners, as well as the more commonly used household and plastic model cements and glues. In recent years, aerosols such as spray deodorants, foot powders, spot removers, furniture polish, nonstick frying pan sprays, whipped cream, and other products that contain organic solvents have become increasingly popular.

All these products contain one or more of a wide variety of volatile substances that have a similar, generalized depressant effect on the CNS similar to that of volatile general anesthetics. Toluene (toluol) is highly popular because it lacks the irritant effects that are possessed by others and has a not unpleasant odor; rapid vaporization provides a "high." Many other solvents are represented in the following chemical categories: aliphatic hydrocarbons and gasolines, aromatic hydrocarbons, halogenated hydrocarbons, ketones, esters, alcohols, and glycols. Plastic model cement generally contains toluene; lighter fluid contains naphtha, cleaning solutions and aerosols contain halogenated hydrocarbons, and nail polish removers contain acetone. Aerosols may also be propelled by carbon dioxide, nitrous oxide, or other inert compressed gases as well as fluorocarbons (19–22).

Intoxication

Sniffers of glues and cements generally squeeze the contents of a tube or tubes into the bottom of a paper or plastic bag. The opening of the bag is held tightly over the mouth and sometimes the nose, and the vapors are inhaled. Liquid materials may be inhaled directly from the container or from a saturated cloth, gauze or cotton, which may be placed over the mouth and nose or in a bag and sniffed through the nose (23).

Most aerosol users evacuate the gas from the container directly, or filter the contents through a cloth to inhale the gas or spray the gas into a plastic or paper bag, as with glue sniffing. The volatile solvents are often warmed by holding the bag in the hands or placing near a source of heat to increase the solvent concentration to significant levels (24).

The inhaler continues until satisfied or as long as the supply lasts. Excessive, prolonged, or continuous inhalation of high vapor concentrations will result in sedation, sleep, and perhaps death. If a plastic bag is used and unconsciousness is reached, the bag may become sealed by a vacuum. Under these conditions, hypoxia rapidly develops to result in suffocation and is a common cause of death in solvent users. The sniffer must find a place where the odors are not as noticeable. Sometimes a white powdery ring appears around the mouth where the bag was held and glue contacted the skin. Vapors may also be smelled on the breath from some distance away for an hour or more after the sniffing episode (23,24).

Over-the-counter nasal inhalants are common forms of addictive use by solvent users. Solvents may also be taken by ingestion. Spray disinfectant, hair spray, and chloroform have been diluted and ingested along with beer, liquor, and a mixer (25–27).

Because the materials being inhaled are volatile or gaseous, they act to produce a number of immediate and transient effects such as euphoria, excitement, sedation, lightheadedness, delusions, and visual and auditory hallucinations similar to those that result from other hallucinogens. Continued and higher doses lead to slurred speech, ataxia, frank intoxication, and poor insight and judgment. A variety of types of intoxications are experienced as with any drug, from a feeling of omnipotence and reckless abandon to a "stoned sensation" as being numb. There are distortions of space and time as with hallucinogens, but these vary from user to user; gasoline users however regularly report visual hallucinations. Occasionally, a user will act on a delusion or hallucination such as jumping off a high place in an apparent effort to fly. The inhalation may continue in long runs as prolonged periods of hours alternating with sleep (28).

The period of acute intoxication will vary from 15 to 45 minutes with prolonged periods of drowsiness and stupor for hours. Amnesia, either total or partial, may exist for the period of intoxication. Unpleasant side effects may also be experienced for variable periods after intoxication; these include photophobia, conjunctivitis, diplopia, tinnitus, sneezing, rhinitis, coughing, nausea, vomiting, diarrhea, chest pain, and myalgias and arthralgias (29,30).

Diagnosis

The solvent addict or user can be diagnosed like any other drug addict or alcoholic. The definition of addiction to solvents by any route of administration is a preoccupation with the acquisition of the solvent, compulsive use, and relapse after a period of abstinence or an inability to reduce the amount of use — in this case, no use, because solvents are not intended to be used by inhalation for the purposes of intoxication. Whenever someone is preoccupied with using solvents and especially if the use continues in spite of adverse consequences, then an addiction to solvents is present. Abuse of the solvents is any use short of the addictive use.

Tolerance and Dependence

Tolerance is defined as the need to increase the dose of a solvent to maintain the same effect or the loss of an effect at the same dose. Tolerance to the CNS effects occurs quickly and dramatically, as only weeks of use may be required to produce an escalating dose schedule. It has been reported that eight tubes of glue were necessary to produce the effect that only one tube was able to do. There are few actual data on cross-tolerance in clinical studies, but there are research data that demonstrate cross-tolerance between various general anesthetic agents, and many of the solvents act like and have properties of anesthetics (31).

Pharmacological dependence is defined as the onset of signs and symptoms that are predictable and stereotypic on the cessation of the solvent. There is a definable withdrawal syndrome following the cessation of solvents, depending on the type, dose, and duration of the solvent use. Typical symptoms are fine tremors, irritability, anxiety, insomnia, tingling sensations, seizures, and muscle cramps after stopping the use of the drug. Frank delirium tremens have been reported on withdrawal from toluene. In any assessment of withdrawal in a solvent user, the use of other drugs and their withdrawal syndromes must be considered (32–34).

Toxicities

Toxicities and pathological syndromes resulting from inhalation are given in Tables 15.1 and 15.2, respectively.

TABLE 15.1. Toxicities from inhalation.

Chemicals	Toxicities
Aliphatic hydrocarbons	
Aliphatic nitrates (*n*-butyl, isobutyl, amyl nitrite)	Dizziness, syncope, giddiness, hypotension, cerebral ischemia, headache, tachycardia, increased intraocular pressure, confusion, sudden death (methemoglobinemia, convulsions, myocardial ischemia, coma, cardiovascular collapse, asphyxia/fatal overdose).
Petroleum distillates, naphtha, kerosene, gasoline	Irritation of mucous membranes, nausea, ataxia, dizziness, hallucinations, narcoses, cardiac arrhythmias (ventricular filbrillation), respiratory arrest, syncope, death. Myoclonia, chorea, encephalopathy and tremor, pulmonary hemorrhage and edema, pneumonitis, plumbism, anemia, lead encephalopathy, confusion, dementia, cerebral edema, peripheral and cranial neuropathies, paresthesias, proteinuria, hematuria, fatal overdose.
n-Hexane	Eye and nasopharynx irritation, dizziness, giddiness, nausea, headache, CNS depression, peripheral neuropathy, anemia, basophilic stippling, bone marrow depression, fatal overdose.
Aromatic hydrocarbons	
Benzene	Irritation of conjunctiva and visual blurring, mucous membranes, dizziness, headache, unconsciousness, convulsions, tremors, ataxia, delirium, tightness in chest, irreversible brain damage with cerebral atrophy, fatigue, vertigo, dyspnea, respiratory arrest, cardiac failure and ventricular arrhythmias, leukopenia, anemia, thrombocytopenia, petechiae, blood dyscrasia, leukemia, bone marrow aplasia, fatty degeneration and necrosis of heart, liver, adrenal glands, fatal overdose.
Naphthalene	Irritation and injury of conjunctiva and cornea, perspiration, nausea, vomiting, headache, cataracts, hemolytic anemia (greater in glucose-6-phosphate dehydrogenase deficiency), hepatic necrosis, hematuria, jaundice, proteinuria, oliguria or anemia, excitement, confusion, convulsions and coma, dermatitis, fatal overdose.
Styrene	Irritation of mucous membranes, CNS depression and narcosis, fatal overdose.
Toluene	CNS depression, syncope, coma, cardiac arrhythmias and sudden death, ataxia, convulsions, rhabdomyolysis, increased creatine phosphokinase, abdominal pain, nausea, vomiting, hematemesis, peripheral neuropathy, paresthesias, encephalopathy, optic neuropathy, cerebellar ataxia, distal renal tubular acidosis, hyperchloremia, hypokalemia, azotemia, hypophosphatemia, hematuria, proteinuria, pyuria,

TABLE 15.1. *Continued*

Chemicals	Toxicities
	hepatomegaly, lymphocytosis, macrocytosis, basophilic stippling, hypochromia, esophinophil, EEG abnormalities, decreased cognitive function, fatal overdose.
Xylene	Irritation to eye and mucosa, CNS depression and narcoses, reversible corneal damage, death, pulmonary edema and hemorrhage, fatty degeneration of heart, liver, adrenals and increased LFTs, fatal overdose.
Esters (Methyl-, ethyl-, *n*-propyl-*n*-butyl acetate, methyl, and ethyl formate)	Irritation of eyes, skin and mucous membranes, CNS depression on liver and kidney necrosis, CNS depression, fatal overdose.
Glycols Ethylene glycol	Oxalosis, impaired renal and liver function, stupor, coma, convulsions, irreversible brain damage, pulmonary edema, respiratory failure, nausea, vomiting, headache, tachycardia, hypotension, hypoglycemia, hypocalcemia, intravascular hemolysis, lymphocytosis, proteinuria, hematuria, fatal overdose.
Halogenated inhalants and chlorinated hydrocarbons Trichloromethane Trichloroethylene Methyl chloroform	Decreased myocardial contractility, arrhythmias, cardiac arrest and failure, myocarditis, hepatotoxemia, renal failure, paresthesias, tinnitus, ataxia, headache, narcosis, CNS damage, sudden death, fatal overdose.
Carbon tetrachloride Ethylene dichloride	Nausea, vomiting, confusion, unconsciousness, coma, respiratory slowing, color blindness, blurred vision, memory loss, paresthesias, tremors, dermatitis, CNS edema, congestion and hemorrhage, edema and inflammation of lungs, kidneys, spleen, pancreas, fatty degeneration of liver and cardiac arrhythmias and sudden death, fatal overdose.
Methylene chloride	Cardiovascular death, liver and kidney abnormalities, fatal overdose.
Fluorinated hydrocarbons Trichlorofluoromethane	Cardiac arrhythmia, decreased cardiac contractility and output, fatal overdose.
Alcohols Methyl alcohol	Abdominal discomfort, dizziness, fatigue, headache, nausea, vertigo, CNS depression, coma, vomiting, acidosis, mydriasis, retinal edema and ganglion cell destruction, philophobia, mydriasis, areflexia, hemorrhagic infiltration of basal ganglia, decreased vision and blindness, fatal overdose.

TABLE 15.1. *Continued*

Chemicals	Toxicities
Ethyl alcohol	Irritation of mucous membranes, headache, excitability, narcosis, memory and cognitive impairment, cerebral and cerebellar atrophy, seizures, delirium, coma, peripheral neuropathy, myopathy, Wernicke–Korsakoff's optic neuropathy, ataxia, metabolic acidosis, fatty degeneration of liver, hepatitis, cirrhosis, hepatic splenomegaly, hepatoma, pancreatitis, pancreatic cancer, esophageal ulcers and cancer, Mallory–Weiss syndrome, gastric ulcers and cancer, peptic ulcer, cardiac arrhythmias, cardiomegaly, cardiomyopathy, hypertension, microcytic and megaloblastic anemia, B_6, B_{12}/folate deficiency, bone marrow depression, leukopenia, thrombocytopenia, pulmonary and CNS infections, nasopharyngeal cancer, gonadal and adrenal insufficiency, fetal alcohol effects syndrome, fatal overdose.
Isopropyl alcohol and *n*-propyl alcohol	Irritation of eyes and mucous membranes, nausea, vomiting, abdominal pain, hematemesis, narcosis, coma, areflexia, depressed repressions, oliguria and diuresis, fatal overdose.
Butyl alcohol	Irritation of eyes and mucous membranes, CNS depression, kidney and liver damage, fatal overdose.
Ketones	
Acetone	Irritation of eyes and mucous membranes, dermatitis, dizziness, lacrimation, salivation, nausea, vomiting, dysuria, albuminuria, tachycardia, ataxia, stupor and coma, fatal overdose.
Methyl ethyl ketone	Irritation of mucous membranes, CNS depression, dermatitis, paresthesias, emphysema, liver and kidney congestion, fatal overdose.
Methyl-*n*-butyl ketone	Peripheral neuropathy.
Nitrous oxide	Hallucinations, respiratory depression, paresthesias, seizures, respiratory arrest, brain hypoxia, coma, ataxia, impotence, leg weakness, fatal overdose.

Interventions and Treatment

The treatment of the acute and chronic toxicity is largely supportive and symptomatic, and requires removal or cessation of use of the solvent. The agent must be identified and any specific modalities of treatment may be instituted, for example, chelating agents for lead. Often the toxicities are reversible, although permanent damage to the brain, liver, kidney, and bone marrow, for which there is no treatment, may occur from chronic solvent use (35–37).

TABLE 15.2. Pathological syndromes by inhalation.[a]

Organ systems	Chemicals	
Nervous Systems		
Central nervous system disturbance	Toluene	Aliphatic nitrate
	Trichloroethylene	Petroleum distillate
	Trichloromethane	Naphtha
	Carbon tetrachloride	Kerosene
	Chloroform	n-Hexane
	Ethylene dichloride	Benzene, naphthalene
	Acetone	Styrene, toluene, xylene
	Cyclohexanol	Esters
	Methyl ethyl ketone	Nitrous oxide
	Methyl isobutyl ketone	
	Butyl alcohol (oral)	
	Ethyl alcohol (oral)	
	Methyl alcohol	
	Isopropyl alcohol (oral)	
	Ethylene glycol	
	Leaded gasoline	
Peripheral nervous system	Toluene	Petroleum distillates
	Trichloroethylene	Naphtha, kerosene, n-Hexane
	Methyl alcohol	
	Ethyl alcohol	
	Gasoline	
	Methyl-n-butyl ketone	
Heart	Benzene	Aliphatic nitrates
	Xylene	Petroleum distillates
	Toluene	Naphtha, kerosene,
	Trichlorethylene	Gasoline
	Trichloromethane	Trichlorofluoromethane
	Carbon tetrachloride	
	Chloroform	
	Ethylene dichloride	
	Ketones	
	Ethyl alcohol	
Liver	Benzene	
	Xylene	
	Toluene	
	Trichloroethylene	
	Trichloromethane	
	Carbon tetrachloride	
	Chloroform	
	Ethylene dichloride	
	Ethyl acetate	
	Ethylene glycol	
	Methyl cellulose	
	Ethyl alcohol	
	Esters	

TABLE 15.2. *Continued*

Organ systems	Chemicals	
Kidney	Toluene	Isopropyl alcohol
	Trichlorethylene	
	Trichloromethane	
	Carbon tetrachloride	
	Chloroform	
	Ethylene dichloride	
	Ketones	
	Ethyl acetate	
	Ethylene glycol	
	Methyl cellulose	
Hematological	Benzene	Aliphatic nitrates, petroleum
	Toluene	distillates, kerosene,
	Gasoline	*n*-hexane, ethyl alcohol
	Naphthalene	
Adrenal	Benzene	
	Xylene	
Pulmonary	Trichlormethane	Petroleum distillates, naphtha,
	Carbon tetrachloride	kerosene, benzene, xylene,
	Chloroform	nitrous oxide
	Ethylene dichloride	
	Ethylene glycol	
	Gasoline	
Pancreas	Trichloromethane	
	Carbon tetrachloride	
	Chloroform	
	Ethylene dichloride	
Fatal overdoses	All	

[a]References
Dreisback RH (1987). *Handbook of Poisoning*, 10th Ed. Los Altos, CA: Lange Medical Publications.
Gosselin RE, Smith RP, Hodge HC (1981). *Clinical Toxicology of Commercial Products*, 5th Ed. Baltimore: Williams & Wilkins.
Klaassen CD, Amdur MO, Doull J (1986). *Casarett and Drull's Toxicology*, 3d Ed. New York: Macmillan.
Hodgson E, Levi PE (1987). *A Textbook of Modern Toxicology*. New York: Elsevier.

Of paramount importance is the removal of the offending agent that is producing the adverse consequences. Identification of the solvent as a problem is sometimes sufficient to produce abstinence. At other times, psychotherapy is indicated for additional psychological problems that may be present. If an addiction is detected, as it often might be, then treatment of the addiction is required before lasting cessation of the solvent use is achieved (38,39).

The specific treatment of the addiction to solvents is necessary to prevent relapse or recurrent use of these agents. Because the addiction to solvents is the same as the addiction to any drug, and many of the solvent addicts are addicted to other drugs, the traditional forms of inpatient and outpatient therapies are effective. A thorough physical and medical evaluation is indicated to assess the possible existence of toxicities (40–45).

The mainstay of the treatment is to confront the usual denial of the drug use and to establish a commitment to recovery. These goals may be achieved as an outpatient or inpatient, depending on the ability of the user to maintain abstinence and the magnitude of social and vocational support. Continued involvement in 12-step programs such as Alcoholics Anonymous and Narcotics Anonymous is often desirable, and is indicated to maintain abstinence from the solvents and any other drugs (46).

References

1. Hoffman FG (1983). Generalized depressants of the central nervous system. Volatile solvent and aerosol inhalation ("glue sniffing"). In *A Handbook on Drug and Alcohol Abuse*, 2d Ed., pp. 130–149. New York: Oxford University Press.
2. Cohen S (1977). Inhalant abuse: An overview of the problem. In: *Review of Inhalants: Euphoria to Dysfunction*, Sharp CW, Brehm ML, eds. Washington, DC: U.S. Govt. Printing Office.
3. Sokol J (1965). Glue sniffing among juveniles. *Am J Correction* 27:18.
4. Watson JM (1979). Solvent abuse: A retrospective study. *Community Med* 1:153–156.
5. Nicholl AM (1983). The inhalants: An overview. *Psychosomatics* 21:914–921.
6. Miller NS, Mirin SM (1989). Multiple drug use in alcoholics: Practical and theoretical implications. *Psychiatr Ann* 19(5): 248–255.
7. Press E, Done AK (1967). Solvent sniffing, I and II. *Pedriatics* 39:451–461.
8. Clinger OW, Johnson NA (1951). Purposeful inhalation of gasoline vapors. *Psychiatr Q (NY)* 25:557.
9. Barnes GE, Vulcano BA (1979). Bibliography of the solvent abuse literature. *Int J Addict* 14(3):401–421.
10. Garriott J, Petty CS (1980). Death from inhalant abuse: Toxicological and pathological evaluation of 34 cases. *Clin Toxicol* 16(3):305–315.
11. Balster RL (1987). Abuse potential evaluation of inhalants. *Drug Alcohol Depend* 49:7–15.
12. Jacobs AM, Ghodse AH (1988). Delinquency and regular solvent abuse: An unfavorable combination? *Br J Addict* 83:965–968.
13. Merry J, Zachariadis N (1962). Addiction to glue sniffing. *Br Med J* 2:1448.
14. Smart RG (1986). Solvent use in North America: Aspects of epidemiology, prevention and treatment. *J Psychoact Drugs* 18(2):87–96.
15. Joel E (1928). Aethersucht (Ether addiction). *Dtsch Med Wochenschr* 54:1081–1083.
16. Samples VL (1963). "Sniffing" at McNeil Island. *Am J Correction* 30(3):11, 13, 27.
17. McHugh MJ (1987). The abuse of volatile substances. *Pediatr Clin N Am* 34(2): 333–340.

18. Bowers AJ, Sage LR (1983). Solvent abuse in adolescents: The who? what? and why? *Child Care Health Dev* 9:169–178.
19. Westermeyer J (1987). The psychiatrist and solvent-inhalant abuse: Recognition, assessment and treatment. *Am J Psychiatry* 144:903–907.
20. Ranson DL, Berry PJ (1986). Death associated with the abuse of typewriter correction fluid. *Med Sci Law* 26(4):308–310.
21. Masterton G (1979). The management of solvent abuse. *J Adolesc* 2:65–75.
22. Dinwiddie SH, Zorumski CF, Rubin EH (1987). Psychiatric correlates of chronic solvent abuse. *J Clin Psychiatry* 48:334–337.
23. Garrett G, Johnson S (1967). Plastic-bag asphyxia in glue-sniffer. *Lancet* 1:954.
24. Lawton JJ, Malmquist CP (1961). Gasoline addiction in children. *Psychiatr Q (NY)* 35:555.
25. Storms WW (1973). Chloroform parties. *JAMA* 225:160.
26. Schoelzel EP, Menzel ML (1985). Nasal sprays and perforation of the nasal septum. *JAMA* 253:2046.
27. Pentel P (1984). Toxicity of over-the-counter stimulants. *JAMA* 252:1989–1903.
28. Cohen S (1975). Inhalant abuse. *Drug Abuse Alcohol News* 4:9.
29. Woolfson RC (1982). Psychological correlates of solvent abuse. *Br J Med Psychol* 55:63–66.
30. Mahmood Z (1983). Cognitive functioning of solvent abusers. *Scott Med J* 28:276–280.
31. Massengale ON, Glaser H, LeLievre RE, et al. (1963). Physical and psychological factors in glue sniffing. *N Engl J Med* 269:1340.
32. Tsushima W, Towne W (1977). Effects of paint sniffing on neuropsychological test performance. *J Abnorm Psychol* 86:402–407.
33. Orbaek P, Rosen I, Svensson K (1988). Electroneurographic findings in patients with solvent-induced central nervous system dysfunction. *Br J Ind Med* 45:409–414.
34. Allister C, Lush M, Oliver JS, et al. (1981). Status epilepticus caused by solvent abuse. *Br Med J* 283:1156.
35. Harris WS (1973). Toxic effects of aerosol propellants on the heart. *Arch Intern Med* 131:162.
36. Ackerly WC, Gibson C (1964). Lighter fluid "sniffing." *Am J Psychiatry* 120:1056.
37. Hormes JT, Filley CM, Rosenberg NL (1987). Neurologic sequelae of chronic solvent vapor abuse. *J Clin Psychiatry* 48:8.
38. Jacobs AM, Ghodse AH (1987). Depression in solvent abusers. *Soc Sci Med* 24(10):863–866.
39. Prockop L, Couri D (1977). Nervous system damage from mixed organic solvents. *Natl Inst Res Monogr Ser* 15:185–189.
40. Debarona MS, Simpson DD (1984). Inhalant users in drug abuse prevention programs. *Am J Drug Alcohol Abuse* 10(4):503–518.
41. Hershey CO, Miller S (1982). Solvent abuse: A shift to adults. *Int J Addict* 17(6):1085–1089.
42. Epstein MH, Wieland WF (1978). Prevalence survey of inhalant abuse. *Int J Addict* 13:271–284.
43. Morse JMD, Thomas E (1984). Hepatic toxicity from disinfectant abuse. *JAMA* 252:1904.

44. Blatherwick CE (1972). Understanding glue sniffing. *Can J Public Health* 63:272–276.
45. Gilbert J (1983). Deliberate metallic paint inhalation and cultural marginality: Paint sniffing among acculturating central California youth. *Addict Behav* 8:79–83.
46. Miller NS (1987). A primer of the treatment process for alcoholism and drug addiction. *Psychiatry Lett* 5(7):30–37.

CHAPTER 16

The Pharmacology of Marijuana (Cannabis)

History

The Problem

Many theories exist to explain the etiology of marijuana dependence (1-3). Significant disagreement about the diagnosis and treatment of marijuana dependence (addiction) prevails (4-9), and uncertainty that it is a primary disease that requires medical consideration predominates. Marijuana addiction still remains an often unspeakable, hidden, and provoking subject.

The fact is that more people are using marijuana today than ever before. The medical and psychosocial problems associated with marijuana are larger and more pervasive (8,10-13). The age range of those affected has increased dramatically. Problems with marijuana associated with teenagers and adults have become common (14-17).

Neither social strata, ethnicity, occupation, nor financial status provides barriers to the onset of and complications from marijuana addiction. What used to be considered the providence of only "the other side of the tracks" is now affecting many individuals, families, the workplace, and the community (16-19).

Studies indicate that a substantial number of patients in a typical general medical practice will have significant medical and psychosocial problems associated with marijuana use (10,20-22). These numbers are increased if alcohol and other drug problems are included (8,11,16,23-27).

Other Drug Use

Many marijuana addicts have an additional concurrent drug or alcohol problem. Frequently marijuana is used daily by the addict together with daily or intermittent addictive use of cocaine or alcohol (8,11,16). Without careful and persistent probing during the history, these other drugs may be omitted through denial by the addict (28). Today's addict who is less than 30

years of age commonly uses marijuana daily for years. Marijuana is frequently the first or second drug in the chronological sequence of drugs
eventually used during adolescence. The drug most often used in conjunction with, before, or after marijuana is alcohol (8,11,16,29). This combination will persist with marijuana being used daily and alcohol more intermittently. Interestingly, marijuana use will diminish dramatically for some
addicts who begin to use cocaine addictively, whether the cocaine is administered intranasally, by inhalation, or intravenously (29). The physician should
be skilled not only at the diagnosis of the conditions that are associated with
marijuana use but also at the diagnosis of the cause, which is often a
marijuana addiction.

Intoxication

The effects of marijuana intoxication are hallucinogenic. The sensations of
distortions of space and time are reported frequently by the user. Also,
sedation, ennui, euphoria, increased appetite, and heightened imagination
and creative thinking commonly occur. Memory and concentration impairments are often present even at low doses, along with cognitive confusion
and abstraction difficulties, especially with chronic use (30–32).

The intoxicated user frequently reports that he feels fuzzy, dizzy, sleepy,
and "dreamy." He feels more friendly toward others and finds greater pleasure in others' company; less often, the user becomes quiet and remote. The
users typically have increased awareness of their environment: vision is
sharper, sounds are more distinct, things seem humorous, and laughter
comes easily and frequently. The user not uncommonly feels he has achieved
a novel profundity of thought and an extraordinary acuity of insight that do
not match objective observation.

Perception in time is distorted so that the time passes slowly and feelings
of depersonalization occur. Visual imagery may occur, but sometimes only
with the eyes closed. Larger doses are hypnotic and induce sleep. Paranoid
ideation occurs among users, with intense suspicion at times or, less commonly, with frank paranoid psychosis. The decrements in cognitive and
psychomotor performance appear to be dose related: the larger the dose, the
greater the decrement, although tolerance may occur. Short-term or immediate memory loss is a frequent concomitant of tetrahydrocannabinol (THC)
intoxication and withdrawal; subjects fear completing long sentences because they will forget what they have started to say so that the ending of the
sentence may well be incongruous with its beginning. The specific impairments that are demonstrated include story recall, remembered digits, and the
like. The result may be a "peculiarly disconnected" pattern of speech,
characterized by slightly disjointed sentences and abrupt, irrelevant conver-
sational tangents.

An "acute brain syndrome" or acute psychosis may occur that resembles a
delirium in which the patient is disoriented and confused with clouded

sensorium, has visual and auditory hallucinations, and experiences feelings of depersonalization and derealization (33,34).

The amotivational syndrome (overused and nonspecific term) described in marijuana addicts includes personality changes that develop over time: diminished drive, decreased ambition, lessened motivation, apathy, shortened attention span, distractibility, poor judgment, impaired communication skills, introversion, "magical" thinking derealization and depersonalization, decreased capacity to carry out complex plans or prepare realistically for the future, a peculiar fragmentation in the flow of thought, habit deterioration, and progressive loss of insight. This syndrome may be caused by the chronic effects of THC on brain cells and on long-term storage in the fat with slow subsequent release (35–39).

Tolerance and Dependence

Tolerance and dependence may not be essential to the diagnosis of marijuana addiction (40). These adaptive, homeostatic body functions probably occur in response to marijuana in most individuals who use marijuana whether they are addicted or not (41,42). Tolerance varies according to genetic, dispositional (size), behavioral (learned), and pharmacodynamic mechanisms (receptor) in any given individual (43,44). The tolerance that may develop to cannabis-induced symptoms can be subtle. Tolerance may develop to the mood changes, sedation, distortion in space and time, tachycardia, orthostatic hypotension, skin and body temperature changes, intraocular pressure decrease, electroencephalogram (EEG) slowing, impaired psychomotor task performance, and behavior. After abrupt cessation of chronic cannabis use, signs and symptoms of abstinence that indicate the development of dependence include anxiety, depression, disturbed sleep and appetite, irritability, tremors, perspiration, nausea, muscle convulsions, and restlessness.

The signs and symptoms of tolerance and dependence may be subtle and persist for at least months because a large amount of THC is taken up and stored in fat tissues to be slowly released back into the bloodstream over protracted periods of time (45). Further, these signs and symptoms of tolerance and dependence are subtle and are often confused with and misattributed to states other than drug-induced that also share these signs and symptoms, making their value questionable (35,46,47).

Diagnosis

Morality and Causality

Marijuana addiction remains a moral dilemma for many. That marijuana addiction is a mysterious and metaphysical affliction that originates in an individual who lacks responsibility and motivation is a popular view held by many. From that point of view, only enough inner "willpower" exercised by the addict is needed to overcome "self-inflicted" or abnormal marijuana use. Another common belief is that underlying conditions, either mental or physical, are primarily responsible for the cause of a marijuana addiction. Current medical and psychiatric evidence would support the conclusion that none of the foregoing is true. Recent clinical, neurochemical, and neuropharmacological studies suggest that marijuana addiction is a primary disease of the mind and central nervous system (6,10,42–44,48–50).

The addiction is initiated when marijuana is ingested by individuals with a susceptible predisposition. A pattern of pathological signs and symptoms of a behavioral, psychological, and physical nature ensues from an interaction between cannabis and the brain (48,51). Primary marijuana dependence (addiction) by itself has a characteristic clinical course that is predictable and identifiable. Addiction to marijuana can stand alone and does not need other conditions to support and define it (3,6,10,31,38,49–51).

Denial

A few fundamental points need to be recognized and accepted before the diagnosis can be made successfully. The first and most important point is that denial is essential to the propagation of the marijuana addiction. This denial is present not only in the addict or problem user but also in those associated with the addict. The second point is that the addict and those affected by the addict resist considering that marijuana may be a serious problem or a problem at all for the individual. This is paradoxical, because it is more logical to assume that the knowledge an addiction to marijuana causes related consequences is valuable so that the condition can be treated. The third point is that effective treatment is currently available for marijuana dependence, and may provide a solution to the related medical and psychiatric problems that are produced by the addiction to marijuana (49,51).

Cause and Effect

The important criterion for diagnosing cannabis dependence or problem use is that using marijuana is affecting someone's ability to function, either psychologically or physically (20,48). Caution is urged throughout the process of establishing a diagnosis because abnormal marijuana use is frequently attributed to the effect of the problem rather than to the cause of it (10,51–53).

For instance, someone complaining about having difficulty with sleep and believing that marijuana use is a remedial measure is more likely to be suffering from the effects of cannabis on sleep (54). Cannabis suppresses rapid-eye-movement (REM) sleep so that marijuana use may cause insomnia and disturbed sleep (44,52,55). Electroencephalographic studies have confirmed many characteristic neurophysiological changes in addition to REM suppression that underlie behavioral effects of acute and chronic marijuana use (44). Acute administration of marijuana produces diffuse slowing of background activity, whereas withdrawal from chronic marijuana administration results in diffuse, fast activity, suggestive of an activated or anxious state of arousal (56,57).

Depression is a common consequence of marijuana use (55,58). Rarely does anyone who uses more than one or two "joints" of marijuana on any regular basis escape having a disturbance of cognition and irritability of mood from marijuana. However, the relationship between cannabis and mood is often incorrectly reversed, in that the reason given for smoking marijuana is because of the depression. Studies have demonstrated that initially depressed individuals do not necessarily use more marijuana, and may even use less marijuana. Marijuana addicts appear to use in spite of the depression that is caused and worsened by marijuana, and to report a dysphoric response to marijuana inhalation or ingestion (20,49).

People appear to exacerbate use because of a susceptibility of the reinforcing effects of marijuana. Marijuana addicts may inherit a predisposition to develop marijuana dependence, because alcohol and marijuana dependence often occur together (29,59–61). People do appear to be motivated to use, although not to use excessively, because of stresses and related life problems. Marijuana use in the setting of stress is not abnormal unless the consumption of marijuana is marked by a persistent pattern of loss of control.

Most individuals, whether addicted to marijuana or not, appear to use marijuana for the same reasons, that is, happiness or sadness, success or failure, weddings or divorces, birth or death. Only a casual perusal of using practices is needed to confirm these patterns of apparent motivations for using marijuana abnormally in the presence of these life events that are only incidental. The reasons addicts use marijuana abnormally is because marijuana apparently provides an unusual reinforcement to those with a vulnerability to marijuana not possessed by others (44,49,51,52,62). In short, life problems, emotions, circumstances, and events may lend to marijuana use but do not explain addictive use. Moreover, these conditions may be frequent consequences that result from abnormal marijuana use.

Diagnostic Criteria

Once a personal or social impairment is determined to exist in the setting of active marijuana use, the diagnosis of addictive use or cannabis dependence can be suspected (49,51,58). Abnormal or addictive use is defined by loss of control that is manifested by preoccupation, compulsivity, and relapse regarding marijuana use (49,63).

Preoccupation with marijuana is illustrated in a variety of ways, but the essential feature is the persistent presence of marijuana in the individual's pattern of living and repertoire of choices. Marijuana occupies a high priority in the individual's routine in spite of problems related to its use; other responsibilities in the individual's life are relegated to a secondary status. The addict may give up or postpone important social, occupational, or family responsibilities because of the preoccupation with marijuana use, and the importance of marijuana may be evidenced by its regular or intermittent use. Loss of control regarding the importance of marijuana in the addict's life underlies the preoccupation with it.

Compulsivity is manifested by continued use in the presence of or in spite of marijuana-related consequences. Regular or repetitive use is frequent, but is not a requirement for compulsivity. The distinguishing feature is the continued abnormal use of marijuana when common sense or logic dictates moderation in use or abstinence. The addict may appear at work or in social events in the intoxicated state, unable to perform adequately. The pitfall to avoid is the attribution of consequences as the cause for compulsive marijuana, that is, "I am smoking abnormally because I have marital difficulties." The reverse is more likely to be true. Loss of control of the use of marijuana is particularly evident in the behavior of compulsive use.

Relapse is a critically important and especially revealing feature of addictive behavior. Coincidental associations between abnormal marijuana use and its consequences may occur without addiction to marijuana but usually not repetitively in a recurrent, identifiable pattern. Relapse often confirms a suspected or presumptive diagnosis of a marijuana addiction. A relapse or return after a period of abstinence in spite of previous adverse consequences can confirm the presence of preoccupation and compulsivity with marijuana use.

Need for Historical Corroboration

The nature of the disease of marijuana addiction, with inherent denial by both the afflicted marijuana addict and those associated with the addict, requires a departure from the traditional one-to-one patient–physical assessment for diagnosis and treatment. Often additional, corroborative historical information regarding marijuana intake and related consequences is needed to identify behaviors that suggest an addiction to marijuana. Those who are knowledgeable about the patient suspected of having addiction should be approached with care and concern. Caution is urged even at this state in the diagnostic process, because denial and rationalization may exist even among those who know the addict. Fear, intimidation, and disdain plague many treatment practitioners who attempt to tread the waters of denial and protection within and surrounding the addict. These critical elements represent part of the entire spectrum of the disease of addiction.

Complications

Medical Disorders

Cardiovascular Effects

Marijuana (THC) may produce tachycardia, hypotension, and decrease in peripheral resistance. The sinus tachycardia is dose dependent and may be blocked by propranolol, suggesting a sympathetic nervous system response. Premature arterial contractions, premature ventricular contractions, myocardial infarction, angina, T-wave and S-T segment changes, P-wave change, and second-degree heart block may occur with acute and chronic marijuana use. The actual frequency of these EKG abnormalities is not known (43,44,64).

Pulmonary

Acute administration of marijuana by inhalation produces significant bronchodilation that can last for hours. Chronic marijuana use is destructive to pulmonary tissue and function. Abnormalities in pulmonary function from chronic irritation of marijuana inhalation can occur, and chronic obstructive, pulmonary disease may result (43,44,64,65).

Reproduction

Impaired fertility may occur from decreased testosterone levels, reduced sperm counts, and abnormalities in structure and function in sperm in males (24,66,67). In females, chronic marijuana use may lead to abnormal menstruation, failure to ovulate, and possible teratological abnormalities (68,69).

Immunological

Immunity in marijuana use is a newly explored area. Conclusions are tentative (70).

Neurological Disease

Neurological complications such as dementia syndrome, impaired recent memory (for recent events), hallucinosis, and delirium are relatively common in chronic marijuana consumption (55,71–74). Some degree of dementia, as indicated by a global impairment of intellectual function in areas of concentration, memory, and abstraction abilities, is probably a frequent accompaniment of regular marijuana use (28,44,73,74). As little as one to two "joints" inhaled per day can result in measurable cognitive deficits that are often reversible with complete abstinence from marijuana (43,44). Depressed I.Q. scores in the areas of concentration, memory, and abstraction measured in marijuana addicts continue to show improvement for months following cessation of marijuana consumption and maintenance of abstinence (43,44,71,75).

Cannabis may have an antiepileptic effect similar to that of alcohol in the intoxicated state. Frank structural neurological damage from the chronic use of THC is controversial. Studies indicate that neuroradiographic abnormalities may occur on computerized tomography (CT) scans of the brain, although the concurrent use of alcohol by the subjects confounds interpretation of the study because alcohol is an agent known to produce cellular and structural brain damage, which is reflected on CT scans (73,76–78).

Psychiatric Complications

Marijuana produces a multiplicity of subtle and overt psychiatric symptoms. These symptoms can and do cluster in a constellation to produce psychiatric syndromes (43,62–64), which can have multiple etiologies. The manifestation of any of the psychiatric syndromes can be indistinguishable from or identical to those produced by causes other than marijuana (43,44, 49,51). If marijuana use is not detected in the history or by physical examination or laboratory investigations, then a syndrome can be and commonly is erroneously attributed to causes other than marijuana.

Few syndromes in psychiatry lend themselves to identification of specific etiological agents or pathological processes. Marijuana addiction produces syndromes in which marijuana can be identified as the cause.

Depression

Depression is one of the more common symptoms and syndromes produced by marijuana (33,44,49,51). Depression that is secondarily produced by marijuana can be severe and is associated with high suicide rates. The full-blown picture of disturbances in mood, affect, and cognition, and the presence of neurovegetative signs, can be attributed to marijuana use. Cannabis dependence as a primary disorder represents an important risk factor in suicide. Idiopathic affective disorder as a primary cause of depression is of only low relative importance in a discriminant function analysis of risk factors for suicide in comparison to marijuana and other drugs (79,80).

The spectrum of the depression induced by marijuana that includes the subjective symptoms and objective signs is identical to that required for the diagnosis of a major depression in primary affective disorder. An individual subjectively may complain of sadness, dysphoria, profound hopelessness, a sense of worthlessness, and self-blame, which at times can be of delusional proportions. The chemical effect of marijuana tends to produce poor control of emotions, tearfulness, crying spells, lethargy, poor initiative, lack of energy, and general mental and spiritual demoralization similar to the syndromes of diffuse brain damage of any etiology. Objectively, an individual may demonstrate a depressed affect, psychomotor retardation, disturbance in appetite and sleep (31,44,49,51,72). The initial treatment of the secondarily induced depression is removal of and abstention from the primary etiological agent, which is marijuana (49,51).

Many studies indicate that consumption of marijuana initiates and sustains a depression (33,44,49,51,72). Few studies actually support the popularly held notion that marijuana use is because of or results from depression. Initially depressed individuals may use more of, the same amount of, or less marijuana, and do not show a consistent pattern of use in the presence of depression. An addict continues to use persistently in spite of the drug-induced depression for reasons attributable to marijuana addiction. The motivation for marijuana use appears to be marijuana itself, and not the depression (33,34,51,58,72).

Anxiety

Anxiety is a cardinal manifestation and clinically useful indicator of frequent or excessive marijuana use (43,44,72,81). The symptom of anxiety is produced by the discharge of the autonomic nervous system, largely through the contribution of the sympathetic neurons located in the hypothalamus that are excited during marijuana withdrawal. These symptoms can include apprehension, tension, overreactivity to internal and external stimuli, excessive response to stress, sweating, and tremors. The THC blood level cannot be practically maintained at a steady state, because this would require a constant infusion over time that is achievable by oral intake or by inhalation, especially when tolerance to marijuana has developed. A decline in the blood level of marijuana triggers the firing of the sympathetic nervous system to produce the onset of withdrawal symptoms. The spectrum of the presentation of the anxiety may range from a subtle and mild to a severe and pervasive anxiety during withdrawal. The anxiety may be persistent and long lasting because of the protracted withdrawal from the slowly released THC (cannabis) from the fat stores (32,46,47).

Sexual Problems

Because sexual dysfunctions and various forms of impotency are so commonly associated with marijuana use, complaints in the area of sexual performance should suggest taking a marijuana history. Decreased desire (libido) regularly occurs in men and women who frequently consume marijuana. Paradoxically, marijuana may induce uninhibited, aggressive sexual behavior that may be offensive and even dangerous. More subtly, marijuana use may dull the emotions and impair the ability to experience the intimacy required to mutual satisfaction in sexual performance (24,66,82).

Excessive sympathetic discharge during marijuana withdrawal may lead to failure to maintain an erection and/or premature ejaculation in men. Marijuana intoxication produces difficulty in achieving and maintaining an erection and experiencing ejaculation in men and absence of orgasm in women (82). Chronic, persistent marijuana intake may result in lowered testosterone levels (67–69,83).

Personality

Personality disturbances that result from addiction are also common. The types of maladaptive behaviors, mental disorders, and mood disorders that develop in addicts are many and varied (27,30,32,81). Hysterical and antisocial attitudes and behaviors are often evident in those addicted individuals who might ordinarily manifest them in an abstinent or treated state. Marijuana addicts may become attention-seeking, demanding, aggressive, emotionally labile, immature, and tend to blame others. The defense mechanisms of denial and projection that are operative in marijuana use extend to many other acts of the addict's life. A refusal to admit and accept responsibility for one's action and attribution of one's shortcomings to others are favorite ploys of the addict. Antisocial acts and attitudes of varying types and degrees that are frequently present in the addict include disrespect and lack of concern for others, driving while intoxicated, assault, and other indications of poor judgment and self-centeredness (3,20,49,51,81,84).

It is important to recognize and emphasize that addicts, before the onset of addiction, represented a large variety of personalities. No specific type of personality appears to be predisposing to the development of cannabis dependence. As discussed, a common superimposed pattern of personality in the addicted may develop in the course of cannabis dependence (52,85).

Trauma

Trauma of all kinds is frequently associated with marijuana use. Visible evidence of trauma such as bruises, new and old wounds, and fractures seen on examination are indications of intoxication. The intoxicated state that affects mental judgment and motor coordination lends itself to vulnerability to accidental trauma. Accidents are a leading cause of death at any age. Alcohol and marijuana often may play a prominent role in accidents. At least 50% of all highway fatalities are related to alcohol and/or drug use, including marijuana.

Sociological Complications

Interpersonal relationships are fundamentally and severely impaired in the addict (2,16,32,86). The difficulties in establishing and maintaining productive relationships with others often begin with those close to the addict, particularly family, peers, and significant others. Marital discord, separation, and impending divorce frequently are symptoms of the underlying disturbance in interpersonal relationships. The typical addict will only confide about how "misunderstood" he is by his or her spouse and friends, denying much personal responsibility for the difficulties.

Employment problems may or may not be obvious. The marijuana addict's performance may or may not be significantly affected depending on the degree of impairment. The addict is often dishonest in the history of marijuana use, and capacity or productivity diminishes as the addiction progresses. However, the addict may often be able to meet his or her responsibilities by some relative measures that can prompt rationalization that marijuana is not having a significant effect on the work performance (2,27,32).

Legal problems may exist or develop (14). The offenses are often in the form of theft, assaults, or other expressions of impropriety, indiscretion, and poor judgment that indicate loss of control with marijuana.

References

1. Block RI, Wittenborn JR (1986). Marijuana effects on the speed of memory retrieval in the letter-matching task. *Int J Addict* 21: 281–285.
2. Goodstadt MS, Chan GC, Sheppard MA, Cleve JC (1986). Factors associated with cannabis non-use and cessation of use: Between and within survey replications of findings. *Addict Behav* 1:275–286.
3. Grinspoon L (1986). *Marijuana Reconsidered*. Cambridge: Harvard University Press.
4. Anthony JC (1984). Young adult marijuana use in relation to antecedent misbehavior. *Nat Inst Drug Abuse Res Monogr Ser* 55:238–244.
5. Kaplan H, Martin SS, Johnson RJ, Robbins CA (1986). Escalation of marijuana use: Application of a general theory of deviant behavior. *J Health Soc Behav* 27:44–61.
6. Kaymakcalan S (1981). The addictive potential of cannabis. *Bull Narc* 33(2):21–31.
7. Negrete JC (1988). What's happened to the cannabis debate? *Br J Addict* 83:359–372.
8. O'Donnell JA, Clayton RR (1982). The stepping stone hypothesis – marijuana, heroin and causality. *Chem Depend* 4:229–241.
9. Smith JW, Schmeling G, Knowles PL (1988). A marijuana smoking cessation clinical trial utilizing THC-free marijuana, aversion therapy, and self-management counseling. *J Subs Abuse Treat* 5:89–98.
10. American Medical Association (1981). Council on Scientific Affairs: Marijuana. *JAMA* 246:1823–1827.
11. Goodstadt MS, Chan GC, Sheppard MA (1982). Developmental and generational trends in alcohol, cannabis and tobacco use – A ten-year cohort analysis. *Drug Alcohol Depend* 10:303–320.
12. Goodstadt MS, Sheppard MA, Chan GC (1984). Non-use and cessation of cannabis use: Neglected foci of drug education. *Addict Behav* 9:21–21.
13. Murray GF (1986). Marijuana use and social control: A sociological perspective on deviance. *Int J Addict* 21:657–669.
14. Erickson PG (1986). Cannabis revisited. *Br J Addict* 81(1):81–85.
15. Anon (1985). Recent development in scientific research relating to the control of cannabis (Editorial). *Bull Narc* 37(4):1–2.
16. Rootman I, Smart RG (1985). A comparison of alcohol, tobacco and drug use as determined from household and school surveys. *Drug Alcohol Depend* 16:89–94.
17. Smart R, Adlaf EM (1986). THC consumption among students. Its estimation and log-normality. *Br J Addict* 81:59–62.

18. Schwartz RH (1986). Middle-class adolescent daily marijuana users: Demographic behavioral and scholastic characteristics. *Am J Dis Child* 140:326-327.
19. Smith TE (1985). Ecology of adolescents' marijuana abuse. *Int J Addict* 20: 1421-1428.
20. Gold MS, Pottash ALC, Estroff TW (1985). Substance-induced organic mental disorders. In *Psychiatry Update*, Hales RE, Frances AJ, eds., pp. 227-240. Washington, DC: American Psychiatric Press.
21. Hollister LE (1986). Health aspects of cannnabis. *Pharmacol Rev* 38:1-20.
22. Jones RT (1984). Marijuana, health and treatment issues. *Psychiatr Clin North Am* 7:703-712.
23. Abelson HI, Miller JD (1985). A decade of trends in cocaine use in the household population. *Nat Inst Drug Abuse Res Monogr Ser* 61:35-49.
24. Cone EJ, Johnson RE, Moore JD, Roache JD (1986). Acute effects of smoking marijuana on hormones, subjective effects and performance in male human subjects. *Pharmacol Biochem Behav* 24:1749-1954.
25. Anon (1982). Marijuana and health. Ninth report of the U.S. Congress from the Secretary of Health and Human Services. DHHS Publication No. ADM 82-1516:5. Washington DC: U.S. Gov. Printing Office.
26. O'Malley PM, Johnson LD, Backman JG (1985). Cocaine use among American adolescents and young adults. In *Cocaine Use in America: Epidemiologic and Clinical Perspectives*, Kozel HG, Adams EH, eds. NIDA Research Monograph No. 61. Rockville, MD: National Institute on Drug Abuse.
27. Weckowicz TE, Collier G, Spreng Z (1977). Field dependence, cognitive functions, personality traits and social values in heavy cannabis users and non-user controls. *Psychol Rep* 41:291-302.
28. Fehr K, Kalant H (1983). Long-term effects of cannabis on cerebral functions: A review of the clinical and experimental literature. In *Cannabis and Health Hazards*, Fehr K, Kalant H, eds., Proceedings of an ARF/WHO Scientific Meeting on Adverse Health and Behavioral Consequences of Cannabis Use, 1981. Toronto: The Addiction Research Foundation.
29. Miller NS, Gold MS, Klahr A (1989). The diagnosis of alcohol and cannabis dependence in cocaine dependence (submitted).
30. Foltin RW (1986). *Marijuana effects and behavioral contingencies. Natl Inst Drug Abuse Res Monogr Ser* 67:355-361.
31. Hofmann F (1983). *A Handbook on Drug and Alcohol Abuse.* New York: Oxford University Press.
32. Murray JB (1986). Marijuana's effect on human cognitive functions, psychomotor functions and personality. *J Gen Psychol* 113(1):23-55.
33. Pillard RC (1970). Marihuana. *N Engl J Med* 283:294.
34. Snyder SH (1971). Uses of marijuana. New York: Oxford University Press.
35. Ellis GM Jr., Mann MA, Judson BA, Schramm NT, Taschian A (1985). Excretion patterns of cannabinoid metabolites after last use in a group of chronic users. *Clin Pharmaco Ther* 38:572-578.
36. Keshavin MS, Lishman WA (1986). Prolonged depersonalization following cannabis abuse. *Br J Addict* 81(1):140-142.
37. Negrete JC (1973). Psychological adverse effects of cannabis smoking. A tentative classification. *Can Med Assoc J* 108:195.
38. Onyang RS (1986). Cannabis psychosis in young psychiatric patients. *Br J Addict* 81:419-423.

39. West LJ (1970). On the marijuana problems. In *Psychotomimetic Drugs*, Efron D, ed., p. 45. New York: Raven Press.
40. Miller NS, Dackis CA, Gold MS (1987). The relationship of addiction, tolerance and dependence to alcohol and drugs: A neurochemical approach. *J Subst Abuse Treat* 4:197-207.
41. Hillard CJ, Harris RA, Bloom HS (1985). Effects of the cannabinoids on physical properties of brain membranes and phospholipid vesicles: Florescence studies. *J Pharmacol Exp Ther* 232:579-588.
42. Karler R, Calder LD, Turkanis SA (1984). Changes in CNS sensitivity to cannabinoids with repeated treatment: Tolerance and auxoethesia. *Natl Inst Drug Abuse Res Monogr Ser* 54:312-322.
43. Harris LS, Dewey WL, Razdan RK (1977). Cannabis: Its chemistry, pharmacology and toxicology. In *Drug Addiction*, Martin WR, ed. Berlin: Springer-Verlag.
44. Jones RT, Benowitz N, Backman JA (1976). Clinical studies of cannabis tolerance and dependence. *Ann NY Acad Sci* 282:221-239.
45. Johansson E, Agurell S, Hollister LE, Halldin MM (1988). Prolonged apparent half-life of delta-tetrahydrocannabinol in plasma of chronic marijuana users. *J Pharm Pharmacol* 40: 374-375.
46. Goodman LS, Gilman AG, Rall TW, Murad F (1985). *The Pharmacological Bases of Therapeutics*, 7th Ed. New York: Macmillan.
47. Jones RT, Benowitz NL, Horning RI (1981). Clinical relevance of cannabis tolerance and dependence. *J Clin Pharmacol* 21(Suppl 8-9):1435-1525.
48. Estroff TW, Gold MS (1986). Psychiatric presentations of marijuana abuse. *Psychiatr Ann* 16:221-224.
49. Miller NS (1987). A primer for the treatment process for alcohol and drug addiction. *Psychiatry Lett* 5(7):30-37.
50. Negrete JC (1974). Symptoms of cannabis intoxication in a group of users. *Toxicomanics* 7:7-18.
51. Dackis CA, Gold MS, Estroff TW (1989). Inpatient treatment of addiction. In *Treatment of Psychiatric Disorders: A Task Force Report on the American Psychiatric Association*, Karasy TB, ed. Washington, DC: American Psychiatric Association.
52. Gold MS, Vereby K, Dackis CA (1985). Diagnosis of drug abuse, drug intoxication and withdrawal states. *Psychiatry Lett* 3(5):23-24.
53. Tennant FS, Groesbeck CJ (1972). Psychiatric effects of hashish. *Arch Gen Psychiatry* 27:133-136.
54. Pivik RT, Zarconi V, Dement WC, Hollister LE (1972). Delta-9-tetrahydrocannabinol and synhexyl: Effects on human sleep patterns. *Clin Pharmacol Ther* 13:426.
55. Williams RL, Karacan I (1978). *Sleep Disorders: Diagnosis and Treatment*. New York: Wiley.
56. Barratt ES, Beaver W, White R (1974). The effects of marijuana on human sleep patterns. *Biol Psychiatry* 8:47-54.
57. Low MD, Klonoff H, Marcus A (1973). The neurophysiological bases of the marijuana experience. *Can Med Assoc J* 108:157.
58. Fink M (1976). Effects of acute and chronic inhalation of hashish, marijuana and delta-9-tetrahydrocannabinol on brain electrical activity in man: Evidence for tissue tolerance. *Ann NY Acad Sci* 282:387-397.

59. Cadoret R, Garth A (1978). Inheritance of alcoholism in adoptees. *Br J Psychiatry* 132:252-288.
60. Goodwin DW (1979). Alcoholism and heredity. *Arch Gen Psychiatry* 36:57-61.
61. Goodwin DW (1985). Alcoholism and genetics. *Arch Gen Psychiatry* 42:171-174.
62. Galizio M, Maisto SA (1985). *Determinants of Substance Abuse*. New York: Plenum Press.
63. Jaffe JH (1985). Drug and addiction abuse. In *The Pharmacological Bases of Therapeutics*, 7th Ed., Goodman LS, Gilman AG, Rall TW, Murad F, eds., pp. 532-581. New York: Macmillan.
64. Akens D, Awdeh MR (1981). Marijuana and second-degree heart block. *South Med J* 74:371-373.
65. Laviolette M, Belanger J (1986). Role of prostaglandins in marijuana-induced bronchodilation. *Respiration* 49:10-15.
66. Buffum J (1982). Pharmacology: The effects of drugs on sexual function: A review. *J Psychoact Drugs* 14(1-2):5-44.
67. Markianos M, Stefanis C (1982). Effects of acute cannabis use and short-term deprivation on plasma prolactin and dopamine beta-hydroxylase in long-term users. *Drug Alcohol Depend* 9:251-255.
68. Bloodworth RC (1983). Medical aspects of marijuana abuse. *Psychiatry Lett* 1(2):1-4.
69. Kolodny RC, Masters WH, Kolodner KM, Toro G (1974). Depression of plasma testosterone levels after chronic, intensive marijuana use. *N Engl J Med* 290:872-874.
70. Hollister LE (1988). Marijuana and immunity. *J Psychoact Drugs* 20:3-8.
71. Stevens H, Restak R (1978). Neurological complications of drug abuse. *Ann Clin Lab Sci* 6:514-520.
72. Tunving K (1985). Psychiatric effects of cannabis use. *Acta Psychiatr Scand* 72:209-217.
73. Campbell AMG, Evans M, Thomson JLG, Williams MJ (1971). Cerebral atrophy in young cannabis smokers. *Lancet* 2(7736)1219-1222.
74. Co BT, Goodwin DW, Gado M, Mikhael M, Hill SY (1977). Absence of cerebral atrophy in chronic cannabis users: Evaluation by computerized transaxial tomography. *JAMA* 237:1229-1230.
75. Warma VK, Malholtra AK, Dans R, Das K, Nehra R (1988). Cannabis and cognitive functions: A prospective study. *Drug Alcohol Depend* 21:147-152.
76. Hannerz J, Hindmarsh T (1983). Neurological and neuroradiological examination of chronic cannabis smokers. *Ann Neurol* 13:207-210.
77. Karler R, Turkanis SA (1981). The cannabinoids as potential antiepileptics. *J Clin Pharmacol* 21:4375-4425.
78. Turkanis SA, Karler R (1981). Electrophysiologic properties of the cannabinoids. *J Clin Pharmacol* 21:4495-4635.
79. Littman RE, Fabernow NL, Wold CT, Brown TR (1974). Prediction models of suicidal behavior. In *The Prevention of Suicide*, Beck AT, Resnick HLP, Lettieri DJ, eds., p. 4. Bowier, MD: Charles Press.
80. Martin RL, Cloninger CR, Guze GB, Clayton PJ (1985). Mortality in a follow-up of 500 psychiatric outpatients. *Arch Gen Psychiatry* 42:47-66.
81. Harris DW, Lester D (1986). Marijuana use and personality. *Psychol Rep* 58(1):338.

82. Katchodourian HA, Lunde DT (1975). *Fundamentals of Human Sexuality*, 3d Ed. New York: Holt.
83. Singer R, Ben-Bassat M, Malik Z, Sagin M (1986). Oligozoospermia, asthenozoospermia and sperm abnormalities in exaddicts to heroin, morphine and hashish. *Arch Androl* 16:167–174.
84. American Medical Association (1981). Marijuana: Its health hazards and therapeutic potentials. *JAMA* 246:1823–1827.
85. Goodwin DW (1984). *Psychiatric Diagnosis*, 3rd Ed. New York: Oxford University Press.
86. Edwards G (1983). Psychopathology of drug experience. *Br J Psychiatry* 143:509–512.

CHAPTER 17

The Pharmacology of Multiple Drug and Alcohol Addiction

History

The importance of identifying multiple drug addictions is crucial to clinical diagnosis, prognosis, and treatment as well as to the formulation of the etiology and research models for abuse and addiction to alcohol and drugs. The theoretical implications for the genetic vulnerability and transmission of alcoholism and drug addiction are interesting and far reaching. The traditional understanding of the behavioral principles of addiction and the neurobiology of addiction to individual drugs is challenged by the concept of the multiple addicted, which suggests a universal susceptibility to alcohol and drug addictions.

The contemporary alcoholic usually became addicted to alcohol as the first drug used and progressed to other drug addictions at an alarming rate and to a disturbing magnitude. Most alcoholics under the age of 30 are addicted to at least one other drug and more often to multiple drugs. The addiction to the other drugs is frequently followed by consequences similar to that of the alcohol addiction. Furthermore, the multiplicity of drugs to which addiction develops is not limited to the alcohol; that is, most drug addicts who first become addicted to a drug later develop alcohol addiction. Additionally, alcohol is the first drug used, by the drug addict; and it is used addictively as an adjunct with a drug or in substitution of a drug (1).

The number and variety of drugs the multiple addicted seek has become increasingly extensive and exotic. In addition, the traditional boundaries of addictive use of illicit and therapeutic use of prescribed medications are considerably less distinct. The nonmedical use of medical drugs by drug addicts is widespread. The pure drug addict who is addicted to only one drug is a rare species; it is difficult to find a heroin addict who is not or has not been also addicted to marijuana and/or alcohol, and, more recently, to cocaine. The common practice of adulteration (mixing during preparation) of one illicit drug with another drug makes it difficult and at times impossible for the addict to determine and maintain a monodrug addiction, particularly when the drugs are obtained "on the street."

The effect on the personality development and manifestation of psychiatric symptoms in the personality by multiple drugs is an area that is poorly documented. Although it is a frequent clinical observation that the multiple addicted has greater personality disturbances than the monodrug addict, the impact on the personality by alcohol and multiple drugs has not been measured in any meaningful way. The contemporary alcoholic and drug addict usually becomes addicted at some time in adolescence when the personality is developing and no definite stability or maturity has been established. The result is often a mixture of alcoholism, drug addiction, and an immature personality. The salient clinical observation is that the personality undergoes an arrest of maturation of personality when the onset of addiction occurs.

Moreover, the pharmacological effects of drugs on the brain and behavior critically affect manifestation of personality. Alcohol, marijuana, cocaine, opiates, sedatives/hypnotics, and other drugs produce signs and symptoms of drug intoxication and withdrawal that include disturbances in mood, cognition, and vegetative states. These psychoactive effects on the brain and behavior are often chronic and cumulative in the multiple addicted. The degree of personality disorganization is sometimes marked in the multiple addicted because of the chronic addiction to multiple drugs (2,3).

The natural history of alcoholism is being altered by the emergence of the multiple addiction to drugs. The course of one drug addiction in duration and severity is significantly affected by the addition of another drug addiction. Although not documented and not easily demonstrated, except by retrospective analysis, it is clinically acknowledged that the course of alcoholism is often drastically truncated by the addiction to another drug. From the histories of many alcoholics, interestingly, comes the comment that the course of the alcoholism could have continued uninterrupted if addiction to cocaine or opiates or sedatives had not developed. Review of the histories and clinical presentations strongly suggests that this is likely the case, as in many instances the development of an addiction to another drug motivated the earlier seeking of treatment in spite of a substantial standing addiction to alcohol with already existing significant consequences. A gradual transition from common to uncommon prevalence of drug addiction by alcoholics occurs as age increases, perhaps in roughly a linear progression.

Prevalence

The most complete and cited reference for alcohol and drug "use" is a monitoring survey conducted annually since 1975 by the National Institute on Drug Abuse (NIDA). A nationally representative sample of high-school seniors who are enrolled at the time of the survey are interviewed, usually by telephone. The 20% of the survey who have dropped out or are chronically absent are not polled in this survey. These surveys may underestimate drug use, as many of these "dropout" students probably have alcohol and drug problems that led to their poor success in schools (5).

The results of the survey in 1985 were lifetime use by high-school seniors of alcohol, 93%; of marijuana, 59%; of cocaine, 16%; of other stimulants, 16%; and of tranquilizers, 14%. The use in the last month for the same drugs was 70%, 29%, 5%, 14%, and 2%, respectively (5). Another national survey also sponsored by NIDA surveys households in the United States for drug use by young and old. Similar figures are obtained for the young, and the inverse relationship between age and other drug use among alcoholics is illustrated in this survey (4).

The Drug Abuse Warning Network (DAWN) that records visits to hospital emergency rooms in the United States has found that alcohol used in combination with other drugs was the most frequently cited occurrence and accounted for 24% of all drug-related episodes, excluding those episodes related to alcohol alone for which data were not collected (4).

A national accounting of youths with alcohol and drug problems in the National Youth Polydrug Study revealed that the mean number of drugs regularly used by the alcoholic youths was 4.4. Marijuana and alcohol were the drugs most frequently used on a regular basis, 86% and 80%, respectively, of the sample of 2,750 youths. Amphetamines had the third highest prevalence at 45%, followed by hashish (42%), barbiturates (40%), hallucinogens (40%), and phenylcyclidine (PCP) (32%) (6,7).

As far back as 1930, extending to 1940, 1950, 1960, and 1970, alcoholics used other drugs in alarming frequency. Freed (8) reviewed 15,447 cases in 46 studies during those years and found 3,046 alcoholics who were also addicted to another drug or a 20% rate of drug addiction among alcoholics. Some of the same drugs prevalent today were used then, such as barbiturates, opiates, benzodiazepines, and marijuana.

There have been few studies available that have established the actual prevalence of multiple drug addictions. Curiously, until recently the prevalence of alcoholism was based on "estimates" of consumption rates of alcohol or medical consequences of alcohol use. The prevalence of alcoholism was only recently based on the actual diagnosis of alcoholism (alcohol abuse and dependence) in the Epidemiological Catchment Area (ECA) study. The ECA study is the first national account of the prevalence of alcoholism collected according to the standardized diagnostic criteria contained in DSM-III (9,10).

The study was performed by a team of researchers assigned to sites in five U.S. cities—St. Louis, Los Angeles, Baltimore, New Haven, and Durham. The study was conducted in a standardized fashion with methods that were employed consistently from site to site. The subjects were actually administered structured diagnostic questions in a personally conducted interview, as opposed to other surveys of drug use prevalence that employ written self-administered questionnaires or telephone interviews with a limited number of criteria.

The findings are informative as they indicate that alcoholism is a common disorder. The lifetime prevalence of alcoholism in the total population in the

ECA sample was 13.4%. The lifetime prevalence for alcoholism for men is even more dramatic, with almost a quarter (23.8%) meeting the criteria for alcoholism. The rate for women was much lower at 4.6%, but that figure is increasing steadily. Almost 7% of the total sample who met lifetime criteria for alcoholism had active alcoholism in the past year. The 1-year to lifetime prevalence ratio for the total sample is 0.49%; that is, half of those who have been alcoholic have had active alcoholism in the past year. Another important finding is that the prevalence of alcoholism is significantly higher in men and women under the age of 45 years. For men, lifetime prevalence for ages 18 to 29 was 27%, and for ages 30 to 44 and 45 to 65 was 45%. For women, lifetime prevalences were 7%, 6%, and 3%, respectively (9,10). Alcoholism is established as a youthful disorder, because almost 40% of the cases began between the ages of 15 to 19 years and 80% of the cases have begun by the age of 30 years. A greater number of men had an earlier onset of alcoholism than women. More than half (54%) had a duration of alcoholism of 5 years or less (9,10).

The association of drug addiction among alcoholics was reasonably high in the ECA study; as many as 30% of the alcoholics qualified for a drug addiction. Marijuana addiction was the most common. The reverse, the prevalence of alcoholism among drug addicts, was also illuminating: alcoholism among marijuana addicts was 36%; among barbiturate addicts, 71%; among amphetamine addicts, 62%; among hallucinogen addicts, 64%; among opiate addicts, 67%; and among cocaine addicts, 84%. Of interest is that less than 1% of the total sample admitted to cocaine addiction at some time in their lives, but of these, 84% also had alcoholism. Clearly in a survey that examined the general population, alcoholism is a common complicating factor in the majority of those addicted to drugs (9,10).

When a select population such as those entering a treatment program are examined, the overlap of alcoholism and drug addiction is intensified and the occurrence of the multiple addicted increases significantly, although it parallels the patterns found in the general population.

In large-scale studies of inpatient populations of adult and adolescent alcoholics and drug addicts in various treatment facilities, the number of cocaine addicts with the diagnosis of alcohol dependence was in the 70%–90% range. Similar studies of methadone and heroin addicts show rates of alcohol dependence between 50% and 75%. Approximately 80% to 90% of cannabis addicts are addicted to alcohol. The prevalence of polydrug use and addiction that includes alcohol is the rule for the contemporary drug addict. The monodrug user and addict is a vanishing species in the American culture (11,12).

Patterns of Use

Most studies of both alcoholics and drug addicts indicate that alcohol is the first drug used, and often addictively. The natural history of alcohol dependence is highly variable and age dependent. Older alcoholics who are over the age of 30 years typically began drinking in adolescence and progressed to diagnosable alcohol dependence in their early twenties. A certain proportion, perhaps 10% to 20%, began using cannabis in their twenties. Another 10% may begin use of stimulants, including cocaine and amphetamines, while 20% may use sedatives/hypnotics, predominately benzodiazepines, barbiturates, and meprobamates. About 50% may continue their alcohol dependence without significant use of any additional drugs to alcohol.

The alcoholic under the age of 30 has progressed by a different timetable according to the general increase in drug use in our culture. More than 80% of these alcoholics are addicted to at least one other drug, usually more than one. A triad of alcohol, marijuana, and cocaine addiction is a regular occurrence among the alcoholics being admitted to inpatient and outpatient facilities. Typically, the younger alcoholic begins using alcohol in early teen-aged years, about 13 to 15 years old, and progresses to addictive use of alcohol by 15 to 16 years old. A year or two after the onset of alcohol use other drugs are tried with some being used addictively. These include marijuana, then cocaine, followed by hallucinogens (e.g., PCP), benzodiazepines, and barbiturates in the more common frequency. The pattern of cocaine use has changed dramatically and continues to do so to the present day, most remarkably by an earlier age of onset of use. The skillful marketing techniques for the cheaper form of cocaine, "crack," have lured younger individuals to addictive use (12,13).

Intoxication

The medical and psychiatric complications from multiple drug addiction are attributable to the effect of the respective drug singly as well as to the combination of the effects of multiple drugs used simultaneously or sequentially. The medical complications are numerous but not nearly as common as the psychiatric complications with the exception of intravenous (i.v.) drug use, which is associated with a substantial morbidity and mortality. The proportion of alcoholics who develop the severe gastrointestinal, cardiovascular, and neoplastic sequelae is a distinct minority of the total population of alcoholics. Accidental, suicidal, and homicidal deaths remain common, especially among the young where multiple drug use is significantly more predominant.

The i.v. drug addict is highly prone to develop the acquired immune deficiency syndrome (AIDS). Approximately 50% to 75% of AIDS cases in the United States are among or are attributable to intravenous drug use. The intravenous drug addicts who themselves have AIDS readily transmitted the virus to other drug addicts by sharing syringes and needles, sexual contact, and other means that involve an exchange of blood between donor and recipient. As many as 50% of the i.v. drug addicts are seropositive (HIV-positive) for AIDS in some cities, such as New York. Intravenous drug addicts represent about 1% of the population or 250,000 individuals.

Other relatively common sequelae from i.v. drug use are viral and toxic hepatitis, endocarditis, lethal overdoses, pulmonary infections and allergic reactions, meningoencephalitis, brain abscesses, accidents, and trauma (3).

Virtually any psychiatric syndrome can be caused by alcohol and drugs. The drug-induced psychiatric syndromes are clinically indistinguishable from the idiopathic psychiatric disorders they mimic. Personality disorders, mania, depression, schizophrenia, anxiety disorders, and eating disorders are caused by alcohol and drugs, especially when used addictively.

One of the most devastating effects of alcohol and drugs is the impact on the personality, particularly that of the younger developing adolescent. The fundamental disturbance in personality from alcohol and drug addiction is in interpersonal relationships. This disturbance in interpersonal relationships occurs in many arenas of the addict's life, including family, friends, school, employment, legal, and social. The characteristic personality that develops after chronic use has many features, but a narcissistic, antisocial, depressive, dependent, immature, and histrionic core appears to predominate the personality. This core personality appears to be more pronounced and prominent in the multiple addicted.

This core personality appears to develop as a result of the addictive process from reacting to the sense of loss of control over alcohol and drug use, specifically the preoccupation with acquiring multiple drugs and using them compulsively to the exclusion of others. Furthermore, the toxic effects of alcohol and drugs on the brain produces an organic syndrome that impairs insight and judgment, fosters impulsivity, disturbs mood and affects memory and cognitive functions. These mental functions are expressed in the various personality traits. These adverse effects on the mental structure and life of the addict are more evident in the multiple addicted as a result of the multiple drug effects and the lifestyle required to obtain expensive, illicit drugs.

The existence of a personality that predisposes to alcoholism and drug addiction or the addictive process has not been confirmed. No one personality seems to determine the biological development of alcoholism and drug addiction. However, some personalities appear to promote exposure to alcohol and drugs, especially for the development of multiple drug addiction. The antisocial personality in adults and the conduct disorder in children enhance the potential for exposure to alcohol and drugs, particularly at a young age. Because of the early and significant exposure to multiple drugs, in these personality types in which the vulnerability exists, the addictive process is likely to develop from the use of the drugs.

Another less documented phenomenon in research studies, but readily accepted in clinical experience, is the arrest of personality development and maturation at the time of onset of addiction. Whether the onset of the addiction is in adult life or, especially, in childhood, the delayed maturation of the personality is frequently obvious. It is not uncommon for the "multiple addicted" with previously well-integrated personalities to undergo a deterioration with the appearance of narcissistic, antisocial, and depressive characteristics that increase with the progression of the addiction. The developing personality in childhood may not only be delayed but may be supplanted by the core personality of the multiple addictive process. The dilemma between which came first, the multiple drug use or the personality, may be a moot issue because the core personality of the multiple addicted may be integrated into the basic personality of the individual so that it is impossible to make the distinction between the two. This dilemma is present in the adult as well, but is more an issue of deterioration in personality than a delay in maturation of the adolescent from multiple drugs as the basic personality is formed by the age of 18 years.

A possible composite personality that illustrates the problems of the multiple addicted is derived from examining the individual characteristics from each drug effect on personality. The drugs including alcohol have "typical" effects on the personality, which are manifested with different emphasis to form a core personality for the multiple addicted. For instance, the antisocial traits of the violence associated with cocaine addiction and the criminal activity associated with heroin addiction are combined with narcissistic traits of the alcoholic to produce a perverse combination of effects on the personality.

The effect of the various drugs also produce other psychiatric syndromes. Virtually any psychiatric syndrome can be caused by alcohol and drugs.

Diagnosis

Investigations into the utility of the DSM-III-R criteria for substance-dependence disorders have confirmed what is occurring among alcoholics. The dependence syndrome as defined in DSM-III-R is used to diagnose all types of alcohol and drug dependence (14). The findings of an important study supported a common dependence syndrome for alcohol and drugs, particularly alcohol, opiates, and cocaine (15).

The practice of multiple drug use by today's addict has many practical implications for diagnosis. The identification of only alcohol in a patient is often tenuous and misleading. Because denial is a part of the addictive process, underreporting and underestimation of drug use is to be expected in a clinical interview, especially if only the alcoholic is interviewed. Corroborative sources increase the likelihood of obtaining a more accurate history but still may not reveal the total pattern and amount of alcohol and drug use. These sources may be family, employer, legal agencies, and urine and blood testing for drugs (16).

Questions regarding the essentials of diagnosis are difficult to have answered in the reticent multiple addicted in even the most obvious cases. The criteria for addiction that include a preoccupation with, compulsive use of, and relapse to alcohol and drugs are candidly denied by many alcoholics and drug addicts who are actively using the alcohol and drugs. Questions regarding the development of tolerance and dependence to alcohol and drugs are equally difficult to have adequately answered. Persistent pursuit of the patient in subsequent interviews and a knowledge of the natural history of alcohol and drug use and addiction, particularly in the multiple addicted, will often yield rewarding results (17).

The differential diagnosis of the multiple addicted is especially troublesome because of the multiple drug effects on the mind and behavior. Alcohol produces significant depression that is indistinguishable from major depression defined in DSM-III-R. The severe disturbance in mood and effect can be associated with mood-congruent psychotic delusions, psychomotor retardation, vegetative symptoms, and suicidal actions. Alcohol withdrawal with its hyperexcitable and hyperaroused state and alcohol intoxication with its episodes of euphoria, poor judgment, and poor insight with consequent behaviors have been confused with mania. Alcohol hallucinosis with auditory and sometimes visual hallucinations is to be differentiated from schizophrenia. The anxiety produced by repeated stimulation of the sympathetic nervous system in alcohol intoxication and withdrawal is indistinguishable from the anxiety disorders of generalized anxiety, panic attacks, and phobias. In fact, phobias such as agoraphobia are quite common in alcoholics. The older terminology of alcoholic paranoia describes a syndrome that fits well into the criteria for agoraphobia, only caused by alcohol.

Cocaine and other stimulant intoxication produces effects that fulfill the criteria for mania, that is, the triad in mania of euphoria, hyperactivity, and distorted self-image are principal pharmacological effects of cocaine intoxication. The withdrawal from cocaine, particularly in chronic use, is characterized by severe depression with the attendant signs and symptoms that fulfill criteria for major depression. The chronic effects of cocaine are to induce delusions, particularly paranoia and hallucinations, both visual and auditory, that are indistinguishable from schizophrenia. Furthermore, the anxiety generated from the pharmacological effects of addictive chronic cocaine use is in the form of generalized anxiety, panic attacks, and intense agoraphobia.

Marijuana, PCP, and other hallucinogens are drugs that produce intense distortions of mood, affect, thinking, and perceptions with the development of depression, mania, delusions, and hallucinations. The chronic effects of marijuana are similar to both alcohol and cocaine in that marijuana appears to have psychopharmacological effects somewhere between sedative and stimulant properties. Other hallucinogens such as LSD, methamphetamine, and psilocybin share properties with marijuana.

All these drugs have the aforementioned effects on personality when used chronically in an addictive mode. The deterioration in personality and the delay in maturation in personality are produced by all the drugs, including alcohol. The multiple addicted is more severely affected and experiences a more pronounced effect on the personality.

The combined effects of the multiple addiction of drugs and alcohol are commonly seen in the contemporary drug addict, and the penchant to become addicted to multiple drugs and alcohol is clearly established. The difficulty in sorting out and attributing various drug effects to the correct drug and a combination of drugs is significant and at times impossible, as is the differentiation of the effect of acute and chronic drug use and addiction from other psychiatric disorders. However, some guidelines may be employed that aid in differentiating between the possible diagnoses.

Foremost, an important aspect is maintaining a differential diagnosis and not being compelled to make a single final diagnosis. Further, it is essential to keep in mind that alcohol and drug addiction are primary disorders that produce these symptoms and syndromes. The treatment of the multiple addiction with detoxification and abstinence will frequently be sufficient to establish the definitive diagnosis. However, occasionally the drug effects, particularly in the multiple addicted, will persist for protracted periods so that prolonged drug effects may be present.

Intervention and Treatment

The complete knowledge of all drugs used in the multiple addicted has important implications in treatment in the acute detoxification period as well as the sustaining of recovery in relapse prevention. Different drugs including alcohol may require individualized detoxification schemes that do not always overlap. The physiological withdrawal from alcohol is treated with benzodiazepines, whereas the delusional and hallucinatory symptoms of PCP are treated with a neuroleptic and opiate withdrawal with clonidine or methadone. Furthermore, the protracted withdrawal from hallucinogens, cannabis, and stimulants may require prolonged pharmacological intervention with neuroleptics and antidepressants if psychotic and depressive symptoms persist.

The treatment modalities for the addiction are affected by other drug use, particularly if alcohol exists as an addiction. Individualized education and support are indicated for specific drugs such as cocaine and opiates. The principles of the abstinence-based treatment program that includes Alcoholics Anonymous will work for the alcoholic who has additional drug addictions. The similarities among the multiple drug and alcohol addictions are greater than the differences, so that recovery in self-help groups such as Alcoholics Anonymous and Narcotics Anonymous by the multiple addicted is not only possible but is now more the rule than the exception. Individual psychotherapy may be directed at the personality core of alcohol and multiple drug addiction and its effects on the mind and behavior.

The management of overdose or intoxication should include a thorough history and physical examination and drug screens for blood and urine. Because of the typical denial that is present in the multiple addicted as well as in those who know and are associated with the multiple addicted, a reliable account of type and severity of drug is difficult and sometimes impossible to obtain. For these reasons, it is desirable to assess the clinical condition frequently with an open mind and always to maintain a differential diagnosis regarding the drugs involved in the overdose or intoxication.

In the case of overdoses, the stomach should always be emptied by inducing vomiting or using activated charcoal. If the clinical condition does not improve, other drug states should be considered. It is a matter of routine for emergency rooms to give naloxone to attempt to reverse opiate drugs in all overdoses. The respiratory and cardiovascular systems need support in cases of multiple drug overdoses from common drugs such as alcohol, opiates, sedatives/hypnotics, and antidepressants. The drugs have a consistent synergistic depressant effect on respirations and generate arrhythmias in the cardiovascular systems. Psychotropic medications such as antidepressants are frequently involved in overdoses with other drugs, particularly alcohol. Constant monitoring of the vital signs in intensive care units may be required in cases of overdose.

The physician should treat objective signs of intoxication and withdrawal and consider the self-report of the multiple addicted with skepticism. The drug-seeking behavior of the addicted can be confused with signs and symptoms of withdrawal so that iatrogenic overuse of medications may occur in a population where the use of drugs needs to be minimized. The drug-seeking behavior of the multiple addicted may be particularly strong because the potential interchangeability of drugs is high.

Examples of these omissions of drug reports by the multiple addicted occur often in clinical practice in the alcoholic and multiple drug addict. The alcoholic frequently denies the use of other drugs such as marijuana and sedative/hypnotic drugs. The cocaine addict frequently denies the use of alcohol and marijuana. The opiate addict denies the use of alcohol, marijuana, and benzodiazepines. The need to obtain corroborative history and drug screens is especially significant in the multiple addicted populations to adequately diagnose and treat the detoxification syndromes.

Because of the generalized vulnerability to alcohol and drugs of the multiple addicted, the use of any drugs or medications renders a risk of reactivating the alcohol and drug addiction. The use of anticholinergic and antihistaminic drugs often becomes addictive in the multiple addicted. Even aspirin or Tylenol may be used addictively, particularly by the multiple drug addict.

The clinical use of "anticraving" or blocking drugs in the multiple addicted is not a common practice. They are used most often in the acute withdrawal period and not administered on a continuous basis. Abstinence from drugs should be the ultimate goal in this vulnerable population. However, bromocriptine and antidepressants have been used in treating the craving for cocaine. Bromocriptine is a dopamine agonist and desipramine enhances dopamine transmission for the purported effect of neutralizing the dopamine depletion that is believed to underlie the cocaine craving. Only modest experimental success has been achieved with these drugs in treating the multiple addicted in the acute withdrawal period.

Antabuse (disulfiram) is a drug that has been used with limited efficacy over the years. Antabuse is a competitive inhibitor of alcohol dehydrogenase, an enzyme that is responsible for degrading acetaldehyde, the breakdown product of the action of the enzyme alcohol dehydrogenase on alcohol. Acetaldehyde is a noxious intermediary that produces an unpleasant syndrome of nausea, vomiting, lightheadedness, and, unfortunately, cardiovascular collapse in severe reactions. The more alcohol consumed and the higher the dose of Antabuse, the more severe the adverse reaction. A major difficulty is that the alcoholic must continue to take Antabuse daily so that the reaction will take place when alcohol is imbibed. It only takes a day or two for the Antabuse to be washed out before alcohol can be consumed without significant interactive effect. At times, the alcoholic is able to drink "through" or in spite of the Antabuse reaction.

The use of methadone maintenance for opiate addicts is controversial. The intent of the methadone maintenance program is to provide under legal and controlled conditions an oral opiate to avoid the use of needles and illicit heroin. The goal is to reduce the morbidity and mortality from intravenous drug use and the criminal practices required to obtain the heroin. The major drawbacks are that it is not clear that methadone significantly reduces intravenous drug use, as methadone addicts appear prone to use intravenous heroin and methadone. Furthermore, other drugs such as cocaine, marijuana, and benzodiazepines, continue to be used by the methadone addict.

References

1. Galizio M, Maisto SA (1985). *Determinants of Substance Abuse.* pp. 383–424. New York: Plenum Press.
2. Miller NS (1987). A primer of the treatment process for alcoholism and drug addiction. *Psychiatry Lett* 5(7):30–37.
3. Hoffman FG (1983). *A Handbook on Drug and Alcohol Abuse*, 2d Ed. New York: Oxford University Press.
4. Richards LG (1981). *National Institute on Drug Abuse Demographic Trends and Drug Abuse, 1980-1995.* Research Monograph Series, No. 335. Rockville, MD: U.S. Department of Health, Education and Welfare; Public Health Service; Alcohol, Drug Abuse, and Mental Health Administration.
5. U.S. Department of Health and Human Services (1986). Drug use among American high school students, college students, and other young adults: National trends through 1985. *DHHS Publication No. (ADM)*, pp. 86–1450.
6. Santo Y, Farley EC, Friedman AS (1980). Highlights from the national youth polydrug study. In *Drug Abuse Patterns among Young Polydrug Abusers and Urban Appalachian Youths*, pp. 1–16. DHHS Publication No. 80-1002, Washington, DC: US Department of Health and Human Services; Public Health Service; Alcohol, Drug Abuse, and Mental Health Administration.
7. Watkins VM, McCoy CB (1980). Drug use among urban Appalachian youths. In *Drug Abuse Patterns among Young Polydrug Abusers and Urban Appalachian Youths*, pp. 17–34. DHHS Publication No. 80-1002.

8. Freed EX (1973). Drug abuse by alcoholics: A review. *Int J Addict* 8(3):451–473.
9. Roberts LN, Helzer JE, Pryzbeck TR, et al. (1988). Alcohol disorders in the community: A report from the epidemiologic catchment area. In *Alcoholism: Origins and Outcome*, Rose RM, Barrett J, eds. New York: Raven Press.
10. Helzer JE, Pryzbeck TR (1988). The co-occurrence of alcoholism with other psychiatric disorders in the general population and its impact on treatment. *J Stud Alcohol* 49(3):000–000.
11. Sokolow L, Welte J, Hynes G, et al. (1981). Multiple substance abuse by alcoholics. *Br J Addict* 76:147–158.
12. Miller NS, Gold MS (1990). The diagnosis of alcohol dependence and cannabis dependence among cocaine addicts. *Adv Alcohol Subst Abuse* 8(3–4):33–42.
13. Miller NS, Millman RB, Keskinen S (1988). The prevalence of alcohol dependence among cocaine addicts in an inpatient population. *J Subst Abuse Treat* 6:37–40.
14. American Psychiatric Association (1987). Psychoactive substance use disorders. In *Diagnostic and Statistical Manual of Mental Disorders*, 4th Ed., pp. 165–185. Washington, DC: American Psychiatric Association.
15. Kosten TR, Rounsaville BJ, Babor TF, et al. (1987). The dependence syndrome across different psychoactive substances: Revised DSM-III. *Natl Inst Drug Abuse Res Monogr Ser* 76:255–258.
16. Miller NS, Gold MS, Cocores JA, et al. (1988). Alcohol dependence and its medical consequences. *NY State J Med* 88:476–481.
17. Miller NS, Gold MS (1988). Suggestions for changes in DSM-III-R criteria for substance use disorders. *Am J Drug Alcohol Abuse* 15(2):223–230.

CHAPTER 18

The Pharmacology of Narcotics: Natural, Semisynthetic, and Synthetic

History

Opioid addiction is a widespread phenomenon affecting our society. This chapter examines the evolution of addictive opioid use in this century. It also addresses issues of diagnosis, medical versus nonmedical use, pharmacological and nonpharmacological effects, and pharmacological and nonpharmacological treatment strategies.

Opium use has been known to have occurred throughout history, probably dating back to the time of the ancient Sumerians. The first undisputed reference to poppy juice is recorded in the writings of Theophrastus in the third century B.C. The term opium, derived from the Greek word for "juice," refers to juice from the poppy plant, *Papaver somniferum*. Arabian physicians knew the uses of opium, and Arabian traders introduced it to the Orient. By the middle of the sixteenth century, opium use was well established, carrying with it the well-known liabilities of addiction, tolerance, and dependence. In the eighteenth century opium smoking became popular in the Orient and Europe, although the addictive use of opium was more acceptable among the Orientals than the Europeans and remains so today (1).

Opium contains more than 20 distinct alkaloids. In 1806, morphine was isolated from opium by Serturner and named after Morpheus, the Greek god of dreams. In rapid succession, other derivatives of opium were isolated, including codeine by Rogiquet in 1832 and papaverine by Merck in 1848 (1).

Addictive use of opium in the United States came about as a result of its addictive properties as well as its unrestricted availability until the early twentieth century. The use of opium was common among immigrating Chinese laborers and also among wounded Civil War soldiers, contributing to its addictive use in the United States. Furthermore, because of the addictive potential of the opiates, their use in legitimate medical practice in itself produces a significant prevalence of addiction. Finally, the introduction of the hypodermic needle led to the particularly potent addictive and hazardous practice of intravenous administration of the opiates (2).

Discovery of the opioid agonist-antagonist as well as pure antagonists has led to interesting research findings and important clinical uses. Nalorphine, the first developed, is a mixed agonist-antagonist; it has the analgesic properties of morphine in addition to antagonistic actions. Studies of the properties of nalorphine led to the discovery of pure antagonists such as naloxone, and the use of these antagonists in conjunction with agonists made possible the discovery of opioid receptors as well as endogenous peptides that bind to these receptors (3–5).

The term opiate is used to designate drugs that are derived from opium, such as morphine, codeine, and heroin, a semisynthetic congener of morphine. The development of totally synthetic drugs led to the coining of the generic term opioid to refer to all these drugs, both naturally occurring opiates and the synthetic opiates with chemical structures and actions similar to morphine (Table 18.1).

"Narcotic" is a confusing term that, like many other terms in this area, has undergone changes in meaning with continued usage. Narcotic is a Greek word meaning stupor; it was and still is used to denote drugs that induce sleep. However, the term narcotic has acquired new meanings and now includes drugs that produce tolerance, dependence and addiction, such as opioids. It is therefore not a particularly useful pharmacological term (6,7).

Patterns of Use

Opioid addiction has been significantly prevalent for well over a hundred years. However, the patterns of use have changed considerably over the years. For example, at the turn of the century most of the opiate-addicted were Civil War veterans or users of patent medicines that contained a "tincture" of opium.

Many studies of opioid addiction classify as medical or nonmedical. However, this distinction between medical and nonmedical use is misleading because of the addictive potency of all opioids regardless of whether they are medically prescribed. Consequently, addiction, tolerance, and dependence rapidly occur in medical practice when opioids are used for more than a few weeks. Those at high risk for developing addiction to opioid analgesics in medical practice are individuals with chronic pain syndromes, such as those involving the back and joints, and professionals such as physicians, nurses, and pharmacists who have increased access to these drugs (8,9).

Medical opioid addicts typically present initially as individuals with an acute, or more frequently chronic, pain syndrome for which a less potent but still addicting opioid such propoxyphene (Darvon) or pentazocine (Talwin) is prescribed. As the pain persists and/or tolerance and dependence develop, the individual begins to rely on more potent opioids, such as oxyco-

TABLE 18.1. Classes of opioids.

Agonists
  Morphine
  Methadone
  Meperidine (Demerol)
  Oxycodone (Percodan)
  Propoxyphene (Darvon)
  Heroin
  Hydromorphone (Dilaudid)
  Fentanyl (Sublimaze)
  Codeine

Antagonists
  Naloxone (Narcan)
  Naltrexone (Trexan)

Mixed antagonists
  Pentazocine (Talwin)
  Nalbuphine (Nubain)
  Buprenorphine (Buprenex)
  Butorphanol (Stadol)

done (Percodan) and hydromorphone (Dilaudid). The typical pattern is for the addict to obtain the drugs from more than one physician source or from an illicit source, or through self-prescribing. The hallmark of the addicted patient is the unwillingness or inability to consider alternative methods of pain control or relief of symptoms despite adverse consequences of the opioid addiction (10,11).

Opioids that are used for recreational or nonmedical use, such as by the stereotypical "dope" addict, are usually obtained from illicit sources, although physicians may still be reliable sources. The prevalence of heroin addiction in the United States is less than 1%, considerably lower than the prevalence of alcoholism and cocaine addiction, which are approximately 20% and 5%, respectively. Most heroin addicts are intravenous users, although a minority use the drug intranasally. Before trying heroin, the typical addict uses other drugs, such as alcohol, marijuana, and tobacco, often addictively. The kind of people who become addicts may vary widely, but they tend to be males who live in the inner parts of large cities. An antisocial personality disorder may or may not predate the development of heroin addiction, but such a disorder frequently develops because of the pharmacological effects of heroin addiction combined with the high cost of obtaining it. Once addiction occurs, development in all areas of an individual's life, including educational, social, occupational, and psychosexual, is impaired and delayed as a result.

Once a heroin addiction develops, the prognosis is often very poor. At least 25% of opioid addicts will die within 10 to 20 years of active use, usually as a result of suicide, homicide, accidents, and infectious diseases such as tuberculosis or hepatitis (6,12).

As many as 50% to 75% of male and 25% to 50% of female opioid addicts have used and continue to use alcohol addictively, and can therefore be diagnosed as alcoholics. In addition, more than half of opioid addicts are also addicted to sedatives/hypnotics, usually benzodiazepines, regardless of whether their primary drug of choice is heroin, methadone, or neperidine (Demerol). Other drugs concurrently used addictively by heroin addicts include marijuana and cocaine. Monoaddiction to opioids alone is unusual. Again, among today's drug addicts, multiple drug addiction is the rule (13–15).

Street heroin available in the United States is diluted several times before it reaches the consumer. For example, a typical 100-mg bag bought on the street actually contains only 4 to 10 mg of heroin. In addition, the potency of the heroin depends on multiple variables, including the supply and factors that determine supply such as police activity and dealer interests. A more predictable source is the occasional unscrupulous physician who sells prescriptions of opioids to an addict. These so-called script doctors are sometimes difficult to prosecute because they use a front such as a pain or diet clinic to cover their true prescription practices. Finally, the opioid addicts may themselves have gotten hold of prescription pads and false Drug Enforcement Agency (DEA) numbers to procure drugs. Some heroin addicts prefer this prescription medication because of its superior quality control as well as the great reliability of the source. For example, experienced heroin addicts examined under controlled conditions cannot distinguish the effects of heroin from those of hydromorphone (Dilaudid), a potent opioid.

A common practice is to use heroin in combination with other drugs to produce certain effects. The additional drug may be an agonist-antagonist such as Talwin, an antihistamine, or a stimulant such as cocaine. The latter combination results in a "speed ball" that is administered intravenously. An additional combination is that of mixing the weak agonist, codeine, with the sedative glutethimide.

Diagnosis

The diagnosis of opioid addiction is made using the same criteria that are employed for the diagnosis of any drug addiction. These criteria include a preoccupation with the acquisition of the opioid, compulsive use in spite of adverse consequences, an inability to reduce the amount of use consistently to avoid adverse consequences, or a pattern of relapse to opioids after a period of abstinence. The persistent pursuit of the drug is particularly dramatic in opioid addicts who typically need to obtain financial resources illegally to purchase the illicit drugs, and who generally do this in a vigorous and aggressive manner.

The development of tolerance and dependence with repeated use of the drug is a characteristic feature of all the opioids. Tolerance is defined as the loss of an effect of a drug at a constant dose or the need to increase the dose of a drug to maintain the same effect. Dependence is the onset of predictable and stereotypic signs and symptoms that result from cessation of a drug and which are suppressed by more of it (16).

Tolerance and dependence may develop independently of the addictive use of an opioid. For example, a patient receiving an opioid for analgesia may develop tolerance and dependence initially without becoming preoccupied with acquiring, using, and relapsing to the drug after cessation of its use for analgesia. However, an opioid addict who uses the drug repetitively will almost always develop tolerance and dependence (16).

Another interesting but poorly understood feature of opioid addiction is that at some point, usually after several weeks, the addict reaches a maximum level of tolerance after which no further increase in dose is observed. However, the level of tolerance reached is often high for the eventual opioid dose may be as much as 10 times that of the original dose.

Studies of animals and humans have shown that even when opiates are available in unlimited supply, they tend to be self-administered at a constant dose after a period of increase in dose. This steady rate of self-administration allows the user to avoid both withdrawal symptoms and toxicity. It stands in marked contrast to the typical pattern of cocaine use, as the latter tends to be selfadministered erratically and excessively, frequently producing toxicity and death after a period of continuous use (16).

Tolerance and Dependence

The onset of an opioid withdrawal syndrome as well as its intensity and duration are determined by the drug's half-life, its dose, and the chronicity of use. The shorter the half-life, the more rapid the development of tolerance and dependence — and addiction. Drugs such as heroin or morphine that have a short half-life (2 to 3 hours) are characterized by the onset of withdrawal symptoms within 8 to 16 hours after the last dose. The peak withdrawal effect occurs between 36 and 72 hours after the last dose, with resolution of the acute effects of the withdrawal by 5 to 8 days. However, there is usually a protracted withdrawal caused by abstinence which consists of milder, persistent symptoms of anxiety and depression, including sleep and appetite disturbances, and which lasts weeks to months. A longer acting drug such as methadone with a prolonged half-life (24 hours) typically shows an onset of withdrawal symptoms within 2 to 3 days after last use, a peak effect at around 1 to 2 weeks, and persistent effects for months before resolution occurs (17).

The opioid withdrawal symptoms include nausea, diarrhea, coughing, lacrimation and rhinorrhea, profuse sweating, twitching muscles, and piloerection or "goose bumps," as well as mild elevations in body temperature, respiratory rate, and blood pressure. Yawning, insomnia, and sensations of diffuse body pain may also occur. Finally, and perhaps most dramatically, there is an intense drive or craving for more opioids that can be distinguished from the other withdrawal symptoms. The drug-seeking behavior resulting from this drive to use opioids will persist far beyond the acute pharmacological withdrawal period; further medication will only prolong it, making the goal of abstinence more difficult to attain (17).

An acute opioid overdose occurs when a user intentionally or inadvertently injects a much higher dose than usual that is above his threshold of tolerance. This may occur when tolerance has been lost after a period of abstinence or when a purer supply of heroin has been used. Furthermore, some overdoses may result from toxic and allergic reactions that occur in response to adulterants used to dilute the heroin. These acute toxic heroin reactions are characterized by a rapid development of pulmonary edema, respiratory distress, cyanosis, and an altered level of consciousness and coma. Fever and leukocytosis may develop as well as increased intracranial pressure and seizures.

Deaths from overdose of opioids result from direct effects on the brain that cause acute changes in the respiratory and cardiovascular systems. The opioids depress the brainstem response to carbon dioxide to the point of respiratory arrest and cardiovascular collapse. This depressant effect on brain function is synergistic with effects of other drugs such as alcohol and sedatives/hypnotics, which also depress the respiratory and cardiovascular systems in the brainstem (21,22).

Intoxication

Opioids as a class produce similar pharmacological effects. They cause an intoxication that is characterized by euphoria and a sense of well-being, analgesia, sedation, and somnolence. Other general effects, particularly with chronic use, include lethargy and apathy, anorexia, and depression and anxiety. More specific effects are pupillary constriction, constipation, decreased respirations, hypotension, nausea and vomiting, and depression of the immune system. Tolerance develops at different rates to all the pharmacological effects.

Opium and morphine occur naturally, and are the principal constituents of the poppy plant. The semisynthetic opioids, in contrast, are produced from the basic morphine molecule. These include diacetylmorphine (heroin), hydromorphone (Dilaudid), codeine, and oxycodone (Percodan). Finally, the purely synthetic opioids, which are similar in action to opium and morphine, include meperidine (Demerol), propoxyphene (Darvon), diphenoxylate, methadone, and pentazocine (Talwin). All these drugs produce euphoria, addiction, tolerance, and dependence, but it is the magnitude of the dose as well as the chronicity of use which determine how rapidly and severely these effects develop.

The opioids interact with opioid receptors throughout the brain and body. Endogenous opioid peptides, namely the enkephalins, endorphins, and dynorphins, are natural ligands that also interact with opioid receptors and have pharmacological properties similar to the exogenously administered drugs. Agonists are opioids that produce pharmacological effects similar to those produced by opium, whereas antagonists are opioids that block the opioid receptors by binding to them but producing no intrinsic effects. The mixed agonist-antagonists have both pharmacological properties similar to opium and blocking capacities at the opioid-receptor sites. For example, pentazocine, a mixed agonist-antagonist, has opioid effects and may displace morphine at the opioid-receptor sites, thereby precipitating withdrawal in a morphine-dependent individual. All opioid agonists, antagonists, and mixed agonist-antagonists interact with the same opioid receptors (20).

The mechanisms responsible for the development of tolerance and dependence are not precisely known. There is no consistent evidence to support the notion of changes in the opioid receptors or in the levels of endogenous opioid peptides that would result in these events. However, other biochemical systems that may contribute to the development of tolerance and dependence include alterations in intracellular modulators such as adenyl nucleotides, calcium and related substances, and neurotransmitters (20).

Opioids inhibit the gastrointestinal (GI) system, resulting in decreased GI motility with constipation and anorexia. In addition, liver function may be significantly impaired as a consequence of viral hepatitis contracted when the addict engages in needle sharing. Liver damage may also be caused by alcohol, malnutrition, and allergic and toxic reactions to adulterants. Finally, the intravenous injections themselves may produce local arterial occlusion, phlebitis, mycotic aneurysms, necrotizing angiitis, and angiothrombotic pulmonary hypertension (13,21,22).

The direct effects of opioids on the central nervous system include sedation by suppressing the reticular activating system in the brainstem, nausea and vomiting by activating the chemotrigger zone in the medulla, reduced pain perception by suppressing the spinal cord, thalamus, and periaqueductal grey region in the midbrain, and euphoria by stimulating the limbic system. In addition, acute and chronic administration of opioids produce decreases in luteinizing hormone (LH), testosterone, and cortisol, resulting in diminished libido, amenorrhea, impotency, inorgasmia, and reduced sperm count (18,19).

Some of the major adverse effects of opioid use are consequences of the adulterants in the drugs as well as of the nonsterile practices of intravenous use. For example, skin abscesses, cellulitis, and thrombophlebitis are frequent complications. Right-sided endocarditis is often caused by *Staphylococcus aures*.

Reported neurological complications of heroin use include transverse myelitis, acute inflammatory polyneuropathy, peripheral nerve lesions, toxic amblyopia secondary to quinine, rhabdomyolysis with myoglobinuria, fibrosing chronic myopathy, bacterial meningitis, subdural and epidural abscesses, and tetanus.

Acquired immune deficiency syndrome (AIDS) is probably the most dire consequence of the practice of sharing needles during intravenous drug use. Currently, more than half of all intravenous drug users, many of whom are opioid addicts, are positive for HIV antibodies and will at some point develop AIDS. The rate of death from AIDS in intravenous drug users is high, and this group is a major reservoir for the transmission of the AIDS virus to the general population as well.

Intervention and Treatment

The treatment of opioid overdose includes the intravenous administration of naloxone 0.4 mg. If the diagnosis of overdose is correct, naloxone should produce an increase in pupillary size and respiratory rate as well as increased alertness within several minutes. Repeated doses every 3 to 10 minutes may be necessary. If no response to naloxone occurs, the diagnosis of opioid overdose should be excluded (23).

Opioid withdrawal may be treated with either clonidine or methadone. It is important to remember that while the withdrawal may at times be very uncomfortable for the patient, it is medically benign. Morbidity and mortality from opioid withdrawal almost never occur. Clonidine has several advantages over morphine in that it is not an opioid, which means that completing the detoxification to an abstinent state is simpler and more likely to engender patient compliance. In addition, because clonidine does not have opioid toxicity, it can be given as needed to titrate the severity of withdrawal symptoms. Finally, the addiction liability to clonidine is low. The major disadvantages of clonidine are sedation and hypotension, which are usually dose related (24–26).

Clonidine can be used on an as-needed basis with the dose ranging from 0.1 to 0.3 mg. This can be given as often as every 4 hours for a total daily dose of 1.0 mg to 1.5 mg. The dose should be increased during the peak withdrawal period. For heroin, this peak occurs at 1 to 3 days; the dose should then be gradually tapered over the next 4 days. In contrast, for methadone the peak occurs at 1 to 2 weeks, and the dose of clonidine should then be tapered over the ensuing 2 weeks. This tapering is done to ensure that the withdrawal period is not covered by a dose of clonidine so high that toxicity occurs (Table 18.2).

Clonidine is an alpha$_2$ adrenergic agonist. It acts centrally in the locus ceruleus on the alpha$_2$ receptors located on the presynaptic neurons that contain norepinephrine. During withdrawal, the opioids release their suppression of the opioid receptors in the locus ceruleus. As a result, the locus

TABLE 18.2. Opiate withdrawal and detoxification.

Objective opiate withdrawal signs

1. Pulse 10 beats per minute or more over baseline or over 90 is no history of tachycardia and baseline unknown (baseline: vital sign values 1 hour after receiving 10 mg of methadone).
2. Systolic blood pressure 10 mm Hg or more above baseline or over 160/95 in nonhypertensive patients.
3. Dilated pupils.
4. Gooseflesh, sweating, rhinorrhea, or lacrimation.

Opiate detoxification

Heroin/morphine withdrawal (Clonidine)
Clonidine 20 μg/kg/day in three divided doses or 0.1–2 mg po tid for 4–5 days and taper over 4–6 days, or;
Clonidine 0.1 mg or 0.2 mg po every 4 hours prn for signs and symptoms of withdrawal. (Peak doses are between 2 to 4 days.)
Check blood pressure before each dose; do not give if hypotensive (for that individual, i.e., 90/60).

Methadone withdrawal (Clonidine)
Clonidine 20 μg/kg/day in three divided doses, or;
0.1–0.2 mg po tid × 14 days;
0.1–0.2 mg po bid × 3 days;
0.1–0.2 mg po every day × 3 days, or;
Clonidine 0.1–0.2 mg po every 4 hours po prn for signs and symptoms of withdrawal (18–20 days).
Check blood pressure before each dose; do not give if hypotensive (for that individual, i.e., 90/60).

Heroin/morphine withdrawal (Methadone)
Methadone test dose of 10 mg po in liquid or crushed tablet.
Additional 10 -mg doses are given for signs and symptoms of withdrawal every 4 hours.
Average dose is 30 mg in 24 hours.
Next day, repeat total first day dose in two divided doses (stabilization dose), then reduce by 3–5 mg per day until completely withdrawn.

---

ceruleus fires a sympathetic discharge. This discharge is inhibited by clonidine, which acts on the alpha$_2$ adrenergic receptors to suppress the release of the norepinephrine-containing neurons during withdrawal (27).

Methadone may also be used to treat opioid withdrawal. However, its use has several drawbacks; namely, it is an opioid with a high addictive and dependence-producing potential, making it difficult to wean during the tapering process. As the dose is lowered, the addict finds it increasingly difficult to comply with detoxification because of his slowly decreasing blood levels of methadone and the continuing protracted effects of withdrawal. The advantage of methadone is that it may be more effective in relieving the discomfort of the acute withdrawal because it is an opioid (28,29).

In practice, a test dose of methadone 10 mg is given for the onset of withdrawal signs and symptoms. This dose is repeated when the withdrawal reappears. The total dose for 24 hours is calculated (typically 30 mg for heroin withdrawal) and then given as a standing dose for 2 to 3 days. Subsequently, the dose is decreased by 5% to 10% during the next several days. The usual period of methadone administration for heroin withdrawal is 1 to 2 weeks; for methadone withdrawal it is 2 to 3 weeks (see Table 18.2).

The long-term approach to treatment of the opioid addict may take two basic forms, pharmacological and nonpharmacological. The former emphasizes methadone maintenance in conjunction with counseling and group and individual therapy. The overriding aim is to provide a legal opioid substitute that can be administered orally and monitored closely. The hope is to reduce criminal activity, providing an opportunity for the addicts to return to their family and employment. Methadone also provides an alternative to the high-risk practice of intravenous drug administration with all its attendant medical complications (30).

Methadone is a long-acting opioid that possesses almost all the properties of heroin. The maintenance dose may be as low as 30 mg to 40 mg per day, but usually higher doses (for example, 80 to 90 mg or more) are required. Methadone is administered orally in a liquid form. It is given once a day at a program center that is licensed to dispense methadone. Theoretically, the methadone not only decreases the addict's desire to use heroin but blocks the pharmacological effects of heroin if the latter is used. The major disadvantage of methadone maintenance is that the user remains in a drugged state and is consequently subject to sedation and other adverse effects on cognition and mood. Furthermore, because the addict continues to use an opioid, he tends to continue the practice of using multiple drugs such as alcohol, benzodiazepines, and marijuana. In this way, the methadone addict often continues to be an active polydrug addict. Thus, the effects and consequences of multiple drug addictions continue in the opioid addict who is maintained on methadone, and the original goals of the methadone maintenance are often not reached (31–33).

Another oral opioid antagonist, naltrexone, has not been shown to be of significant value in the treatment of opioid addiction. Naltrexone provides a deterrent to using opioids and, in this respect, is similar to Antabuse, which is used in the treatment of alcoholism. Naltrexone blocks the effects of opioids at the receptor site so that the euphoria and other effects of opioids are not experienced. The major problem with this method is the naltrexone must be taken every day to block the opioid effect. If the addict stops using the naltrexone, he can resume the other opioid use and overcome the naltrexone block in about 24 hours. He can even overcome the block at the same time if the other opioids are taken in sufficiently enough doses (34–36).

The nonpharmacological treatment of opioid addiction is based on abstinence and is similar to the treatment of alcohol addiction. For these patients who are motivated, the main goal is for the addict to develop a drug-free lifestyle. An inpatient or outpatient program emphasizing an abstinence approach and based on the principles of Narcotics Anonymous (NA) or Alcoholics Anonymous (AA) may be effective. Further, long-term follow-up in an aftercare program using group and individual therapies enhances the probability of continued abstinence. It is important to emphasize that the recovering addict must remain free from all drugs of addiction. If not, he faces a high risk of relapsing to opioids and is almost certain to become addicted to other drugs, if he is not already (37–40).

Continued regular attendance at NA or AA greatly enhances the probability that the addict will be able to maintain abstinence from drugs. Because of the relapsing nature of addiction, the long-term recovery from a drug addiction depends on an ongoing awareness of the nature of addiction, which is provided by the 12-step programs. In addition, the constant association with other addicts who are living a drug-free lifestyle using the 12 steps provides a supportive milieu as well as role models for identifying both the difficulties and successes in achieving and maintaining recovery.

For those addicts who use opioids ostensibly to treat pain, successful treatment of the addiction often results in a disappearance of the pain as well. This is because one of the major ways that an addiction is perpetuated is by the manifestation of the addiction, serving as a justification for the opioid use. When the addiction is adequately treated, the "need" for opioids to relieve pain frequently disappears.

References

1. Jaffe JH, Martin WR (1985). Opiate analgesics and antagonists. In *The Pharmacological Basis of Therapeutics*, 7th Ed., Gilman AG, Goodman LD, Rall TW, Murad F, eds., pp. 491–531. New York: Macmillan.
2. Oliverio A, Castellano C, Puglisi-Allegra S (1984). Psychobiology of opioids. *Int Rev Neurobiol* 25:277–337.
3. Croughan JL, Miller JP, Whitman BY, Schober JG (1981). Alcoholism and alcohol dependence in narcotic addicts: A prospective study with a five-year followup. *Am J Drug Alcohol Abuse* 8:85–94
4. Simon EJ, Hiller JM (1978). The opiate receptors. *Annu Rev Pharmacol Toxicol* 18:371–394.
5. Chang KJ, Cuatrecasas P (1981). Heterogeneity and properties of opiate receptors. *Fed Proc* 40:2729–2734.
6. Schuckit MA (1984). *Drug and Alcohol Abuse: A Clinical Guide to Diagnosis and Treatment*, 2d Ed. New York: Plenum Press.
7. Redmond DE Jr, Krystal JH (1981). Multiple mechanisms of withdrawal from opioid drugs. *Annu Rev Neurosci* 7:443.
8. Bonica JJ, ed. (1980). *Pain*. New York: Raven Press.
9. Wallot H, Lambert J (1984). Characteristics of physician addicts. *Am J Drug Alcohol Abuse* 10:53.
10. Simpson DD, Joe GW, Bracy SA (1982). Six-year follow-up of opioid addicts after admission to treatment. *Arch Gen Psychiatry* 39(11):1318–1323.
11. Vaillant GE (1973). A 20-year follow-up of New York narcotic addicts. *Arch Gen Psychiatry* 29:237.
12. O'Brien CP, Woody GE (1981). Long-term consequences of opiate dependence. *N Engl J Med* 304:1098.

13. Hartman N, Kreek MJ, Ross A, Khuri E, Millman RB, Rodriguez R (1983). Alcohol use in youthful methadone-maintained former heroin addicts: Liver impairment and treatment outcome. *Alcohol Clin Exp Res* 7(3):316–320.

14. Freed EX (1973). Drug abuse by alcoholics: A review. *Int J Addict* 8:451–437.

15. Carroll JF, Malloy MA, Kendrick BA (1977). Drug abuse by alcoholics: A literature review and evaluation. *Am J Drug Alcohol Abuse* 4:317–341.

16. Jaffe JH (1985). Drug addiction and drug abuse. In *The Pharmacological Basis of Therapeutics*, 7th Ed., Gilman AG, Goodman LD, Rall TW, Murad F, eds., pp. 532–581. New York: Macmillan.

17. Koob GF (1987). Neural substrates of opioid tolerance and dependence. *Natl Inst Drug Abuse Res Mongr Ser* 76:46–52.

18. Duggan AW, North RA (1983). Electrophysiology of opioids. *Pharmacol Rev* 35:219–282.

19. Basbaum AI, Fields HL (1979). Endogenous pain control systems: Brain stem spinal pathways and endorphin circuitry. *Annu Rev Pharmacol Toxicol* 19:245–267.

20. Akil H, Watson SJ, Young E, Lewis ME, Khachaturian H, Walker JM (1984). Endogenous opioids: Biology and function. *Annu Rev Neurosci* 7:223–225.

21. Holaday JW (1983). Cardiovascular effects of endogenous opiate systems. *Annu Rev Pharmacol Toxicol* 23:541–594.

22. Eckenhoff JE, Oech SR (1960). The effects of narcotics and antagonists upon respiration and circulation in man. *Clin Pharmacol Ther* 1:483–524.

23. Kleber HK, Riordan CE (1982). The treatment of narcotic withdrawal: A historical review. *J Clin Psychiatry* 43:30.

24. Gold MS, Redmond DE Jr, Kleber HD (1978). Clonidine blocks opiate withdrawal symptoms. *Lancet* 2:599–602.

25. Gold MS, Pottash AC, Sweeney DR, et al. (1980). Opiate withdrawal using clonidine. *JAMA* 243(4):343–346.

26. Rounsaville BJ, Kosten T, Kleber H (1985). Success and failure at outpatient opioid detoxification: Evaluation of the process of clonidine- and methadone-assisted withdrawal. *J Nerv Ment Dis* 173(2):103–110.

27. Gold MS, Redmond DE Jr., Kleber HD (1979). Noradrenergic hyperactivity in opiate withdrawal supported by clonidine reversal of opiate withdrawal. *Am J Psychiatry* 136:100–102.

28. Kreek MJ (1979). Methadone in treatment: Physiological and pharmacological issues. In *Handbook on Drug Abuse*, Dupont RI, Goldstein A, O'Donnell J, eds., pp. 57–86. Washington, DC: U.S. Govt. Printing Office.

29. Preston KL, Bigelow GE (1985). Pharmacological advances in addiction treatment. *Int J Addict* 20(6/7):845–867.

30. Senay EC, Mieta C, Dorus W, Soberu K, Baumgardner M (1986). Comprehensive treatment for heroin addicts: A pilot study. *J Psychoact Drugs* 18(2):107–116.

31. Strug DL, Hunt DE, Goldsmith DS, Lipton DS, Spunt B (1985). Patterns of cocaine use among methadone clients. *Int J Addict* 20(8):1163–1175.

32. Jackson G, Cohen M, Hanbury R, Korts D, Sturiano V, Stimmel B (1983). Alcoholism among narcotic addicts and patients on methadone maintenance. *J Stud Alcohol* 44:499–504.

33. Winston A, Jackson G, Suljaga K, Kaswan M, Skovron ML (1986). Identification and treatment of alcoholics who use opiates. *Mt Sinai J Med* 53(2):90–93.

34. Kleber HD, Kosten TR (1984). Naltrexone induction: Psychologic and pharmacologic strategies. *J Clin Psychiatry* 45:9.
35. Gold MS, Dackis CA, Pottash ALC (1982). Naltrexone, opiate addiction and endorphins. *Med Res Rev* 2:211–246.
36. Gritz ER, Shiffman SM, Jarvik ME, Schlesinger J, Charuvastra VC (1976). Naltrexone: Physiological and psychological effects of single doses. *Clin Pharmacol Ther* 19:773–776.
37. Peyrot M (1985). Narcotics anonymous: Its history, structure and approach. *Int J Addict* 20(10):1509–1522.
38. Woody GE, Luborsky L, McClellan AT, O'Brien CP (1985). Psychotherapy for opiate dependence. *Natl Inst Drug Abuse Res Mongr Ser* 58:9–28.
39. Miller NS (1987). A primer of the treatment process for alcohol and drug addiction. *Psychiatry Lett* 5(7):30–37.
40. Miller NS, Gold MS, Cocores JA, Pottash ALC (1988). Alcohol dependence and its medical consequences. *NY State J Med* 88(19):476–481.

CHAPTER 19

The Pharmacology of Nicotine

History

Columbus brought tobacco from the New World. In the following centuries, the smoking of tobacco spread throughout the world, despite vigorous opposition. The tobacco plant was named *Nicotiana tabacum* after Jean Nicot, who promoted his belief that the plant had medicinal value (1).

Nicotine is the basic addicting drug contained in cigarettes (2–4). Nicotine may also be the deadliest drug known to man in terms of overall prevalence of morbidity and mortality (1). The morbidity and mortality from nicotine addiction is greater than that from World Wars I and II, the Vietnam War, AIDS, and heroin and cocaine addiction combined. Tobacco use is linked to more than 390,000 deaths per year in the United States alone (2). The powerful lobbying forces of the tobacco industry have managed to keep supplies of nicotine available to the public in spite of efforts from medical and legal bodies to reduce advertising and educate the public about the adverse consequences of nicotine use.

There has been debate as to whether cigarettes are addicting and whether nicotine is the active ingredient in generating and sustaining the addiction (3). The reasons for the resistance to considering if nicotine is addicting or not has origins in attitudes toward addiction. Cigarette smoking and nicotine are good examples of the difficulty many people have in accepting addiction as a real phenomenon. Freewill and personal choice have prevailed as explanations why a 20-cigarette-per-day smoker will receive more than 70,000 boluses of nicotine per year in spite of the high rate of morbidity and mortality (6). It is also remarkable that it took the U.S. Surgeon General's office until 1988 to take an official position that cigarette smoking can be addictive.

The practice of smokeless tobacco is also popular and growing rapidly among young adults and children. The number of smokeless tobacco users in the United State is estimated at about 12 million. More than 80% of smokeless tobacco users first experiment with the drug before the age of 15 years (7,8).

Prevalence

Cigarette use often begins in young people. The National Institute for Drug Abuse (NIDA) surveys show that 51% of 8th-graders and 63% of 10th-grade students report having tried cigarettes; 16% of 8th-grade and 26% of 10th-grade students report having smoked a cigarette during the past month (girls, 23%, and boys 20%); and 12% of boys and 1% of girls reported having chewed tobacco or used snuff during the past month. Of those students who have tried cigarettes, 72% of the 8th graders and 41% of the 10th graders reported first use by 6th grade or earlier (9).

The use of cigarettes by the general population has shown only a slight decrease from 60 million in 1985 to 57 million in 1988. The combination of cigarettes with alcohol is particularly common, such that 85% of alcoholics smoke cigarettes and the overall prevalence rate of alcoholism is 16% in the general population in the United States. Moreover, cancer is the third leading cause of death, and alcohol and cigarettes are associated with several of the major types of cancer, that is, lung, gastrointestinal, and oropharynx (9).

The number of smokeless tobacco users in the United States is estimated at about 12 million. The marked resurgence of smokeless tobacco use among young people is a direct result of marketing by tobacco companies that use prominent sports figures and entertainers to promote their products. The average consumer of smokeless tobacco is between 18 and 24 years old (10).

Patterns of Use

Cigarette smoking ingests nicotine by the inhalation route. Studies show that, with inhalation, the drug reaches the brain within 7 seconds, more than twice as rapidly as it takes for heroin to reach the brain from an injection site in the arm. Inhalation is a particularly addicting mode of administration for a drug. This is also seen with crack, which is inhaled as vapors (11).

There are two basic methods of smokeless tobacco use—dipping and chewing. Dipping involves placing moist or dry tobacco between the cheek and gum, and chewing requires mastication of a wad of tobacco leaves in the cheek area. The blood nicotine level achieved using smokeless tobacco can be comparable to or exceed that achieved by smoking cigarettes. However, because of the route of administration the blood levels remain high longer, although not at as high a level as with inhalation (12).

Other forms of nicotine use are inhalation by pipe, cigar smoking, and snuff. These forms have their own peculiar liabilities, such as oral cancers and dental staining. All the forms of nicotine use are considered risk factors in bronchitis, emphysema, coronary artery disease, peripheral vascular disease, and a variety of other cancers (5,13).

Smokeless tobacco increases the risk of oral and pharyngeal cancer. Gingival blood flow is reduced by smokeless tobacco, resulting in ischemia and necrosis, gingival recession, soft-tissue alterations, and leukoplakia (8).

Intoxication

The intoxicating effects of nicotine are difficult to measure under laboratory conditions in humans and animals and hard for smokers to report. The intoxicating effects of nicotine are alertness, muscle relaxation, facilitation of memory or attention, and a decrease in appetite and irritability. Nausea and vomiting are not uncommon acute effects in the nontolerant user (4,14).

Although nicotine may provide a mild-to-moderate euphoric response to acute administration, tolerance develops rapidly so that continued use of nicotine does not appear to depend on euphoria as a psychological driving force. The current theory is that the reward center in the hypothalamus, which contains dopamine neurons in the ventral tegmentum, underlies the "craving" or drive to use drugs. Drugs that stimulate the dopamine neurons are neurochemically reinforced by the reward center (15). Nicotine has not been clearly shown to affect these dopamine neurons.

A measure of the reinforcing ability of a drug is the ability for the drug to induce self-administration. Self-administration is when a drug is sought for the drug effects and not motivated by some other reason for use. Nicotine is not particularly strongly self-administered under controlled conditions in laboratory animals. In a typical experiment, an animal is given access to a lever that delivers an intravenous injection of nicotine. It is difficult to induce animals to self-administer nicotine under these conditions. However, alcohol, another drug that rivals nicotine as a clinically addicting drug, is not a particularly strongly or avidly reinforced drug under controlled conditions. The more strongly self-administered drugs are stimulants and opiates. Of interest is that in humans, under controlled and uncontrolled conditions, the use of amphetamines, heroin, and alcohol increase cigarette smoking (16).

In contrast to the intense feelings of pleasure that follow the administration of amphetamine or heroin, there are no sensations produced by nicotine or smoking which can be described as highly enjoyable similar to these other drugs. In fact, the number of smokers who claim to smoke for pleasure is rather rare, and even those state that the pleasure is coincidental with some other pleasurable activity such as following a meal (3).

With all these limitations, when studies are performed, nicotine is a self-administered drug that follows other addicting drugs and behaviors, although less than some addicting drugs. Results of studies provide direct evidence that in doses comparable to those delivered by cigarette smoking, nicotine is a reinforcing drug and addicting. Nicotine meets the criteria required by other drugs that are considered addicting, such as barbiturates, amphetamines, and morphine (16–19).

Diagnosis

The diagnosis of nicotine addiction is straightforward and requires the application of the criteria of addiction. The diagnosis is somewhat easier in smokers because typically there is less denial regarding the loss of control over cigarette smoking. The preoccupation with acquiring nicotine is very dramatic in that addicted smokers are rarely without cigarettes, and will go to great lengths to obtain an adequate supply of nicotine. The compulsive use of cigarettes in spite of adverse consequences is dramatic and frightening. Clinical examples show continued smoking in spite of clear warnings on cigarette packages that smoking is dangerous to one's health. Physicians can recall unfortunate accounts of chronic lung patients who turn off the oxygen on which they are dependent to survive so that they can light up a cigarette. Moreover, the relapse or return to cigarette smoking after periods of abstinence is a common occurrence in nicotine addicts. Studies have confirmed a relapse rate of as high as 70% within the first 12 months (4,20).

The daily and repetitive use of nicotine in the form of inhalation or oral absorption is striking and easy to diagnosis clinically. The clinician is not met with the typical denial and rationalizations that are presented in addiction to other drugs. In fact, the nicotine addict may express a strong desire to quit smoking, but also admit the inability to do so. It is the one addiction that can be examined with the cooperation of the addict; however, the treatment of the addiction is no less difficult and challenging.

The diagnosis of nicotine addiction is easy to determine using the diagnostic criteria (32,33) or administering tests. Unlike most other drug addicts, nicotine-dependent patients can be reliable historians.

The Fagerstrom Tolerance Questionnaire (FTQ) is an easy-to-administer paper-and-pencil test consisting of eight questions that measure nicotine addiction, such as carbon monoxide and cotinine (35). The questionnaire is commonly used in research and clinical settings. Another self-report test is the Horn's Reason for Smoking Test, which measures individual differences in smoking patterns (36).

Tolerance and Dependence

The course of nicotine tolerance and dependence is predictable and variable as with other forms of drug addiction. Tolerance develops to many of, but not completely to all of, the effects of nicotine stimulation. Tolerance may develop incompletely to the increase in heart rate and blood pressure, arousal and hand tremor, and increase in plasma concentrations of certain hormones. However, tolerance develops readily to the nausea, vomiting, and depression. The development of tolerance, as with other drugs of addiction, results from pharmacodynamic changes rather than drug disposition (4).

The essential feature of nicotine withdrawal is that it occurs abruptly on the cessation of nicotine use. It occurs with all forms and routes of administration of nicotine. Changes in mood and performance from withdrawal can be detected within 2 hours of the last nicotine use, peak within 24 hours, and gradually subside within a few days to several weeks (4,21).

Associated correlates of withdrawal are slow waves on the electroencephalogram (EEG), decreased catecholamine, decreased metabolic rate, tremor, increased coughing, rapid-eye-movement sleep (REM) change, gastrointestinal disturbance, headache, insomnia, and impairment of tasks requiring vigilance (4,20).

The signs and symptoms of withdrawal are a drive or strong desire to use nicotine, irritability, frustration, anger, anxiety, depression, difficulty in concentrating, restlessness, decreased heart rate, and increased appetite or weight gain. The withdrawal is suppressed by the resumption of nicotine use as with other drugs that produce pharmacological dependence (4,22).

Pharmacokinetics

Tobacco contains 4000 compounds; the major constituents are nicotine, tar, and carbon monoxide. The actual nicotine content may vary from 0.2% to 5%, but is between 1% to 2% for smoking tobacco. The content of tar averages 1.0 mg, but varies from 0.5 to 35 mg (4,23).

Nicotine is readily absorbed from the respiratory tract, buccal membranes, and skin. As a strong base, it is absorbed better in an alkaline environment so that the small intestine is a better site for absorption than the stomach (4,23).

Approximately 80% to 90% is metabolized by the liver, lungs, and kidney. The major metabolites of nicotine are cotinine and nicotine-1'-N-oxide, which are formed by oxidation. The half-life of nicotine is approximately 2 hours. Both nicotine and its metabolites are rapidly eliminated by the kidneys. Nicotine is excreted in the milk of lactating women who smoke. The milk of lactating mothers may contain 0.5 mg per liter (4,23).

Neurochemistry

Nicotine has very specific properties that involve stereospecific receptors for nicotine and dopaminergic pathways. These receptors can be blocked with mecamylamine but not with muscarinic cholinergic or adrenergic blocking agents. Nicotine causes an increase in hand tremor, an arousal EEG (low voltage, fast activity), decreased muscle tone, and decreased deep tendon reflexes. Nicotine causes the release of norepinephrine and dopamine from brain tissue and, depending on the dose, increases or inhibits the release of acetylcholine (24–26).

Other Drug Use

As mentioned, a high percentage, more than 85%, of alcoholics are also addicted to nicotine whereas only 29% of Americans are thus addicted (5,7). Preliminary evidence suggests that cocaine and marijuana addicts reduce their cigarette consumption during the active use of these other drugs. They tend to return to higher levels of nicotine use when not using the other drugs.

Intervention and Treatment

There is growing evidence that traditional 12-step approaches work for nicotine addiction as with other drugs of addiction. Smokers Anonymous (SA) is a growing organization that has patterned itself after Alcoholics Anonymous and Narcotics Anonymous. The first step, requiring abstinence, is readily applicable to nicotine addiction as are the other steps. The peer support is powerful in assisting the nicotine addict into recovery and maintaining a sustained and continuous abstinence from nicotine (27,28).

Nicotine replacement with nicotine gum or nicotine polacrilex is used. The amount of nicotine absorbed depends on numerous variables, and must be carefully monitored by the physician and user to achieve success. For instance, swallowed nicotine is not absorbed well while gentle chewing that promotes absorption through the buccal mucosa produces the best results (29,30). Also, most of the nicotine absorbed is metabolized during the first pass through the liver by way of the portal system (32,33).

Clonidine is being used to treat nicotine withdrawal, and has been showing some preliminary results. Clonidine is a alpha$_1$-agonist that inhibits the release of norepinephrine from presynaptic neurons in the locus ceruleus. Clonidine appears to reduce the desire for more nicotine, irritability, anxiety, restlessness, and depression. Some serious side effects are sedation and hypotension. Transcutaneous clonidine is available (31–34).

Scopolamine is a belladonna alkaloid that is used to treat motion sickness. The anticholinergic action of scopolamine, as with mecamylamine, is thought to be the mechanism of action. Studies have shown that these agents reduce the craving and withdrawal symptoms from nicotine (36,38, 39).

All these pharmacological agents have specific indications and are to be used for a limited duration, during the withdrawal period only. They do not have efficacy to prevent relapse during extended abstinence. These agents should also be used in conjunction with other modalities of treatment as mentioned, as with other drug addictions, to reduce the risk for relapse (40,41).

References

1. Penn WA (1902). *The Soverance Herbe: A History of Tobacco*. p. 56. New York: Grant Richards.
2. Johnson LM (1942) Tobacco smoking and nicotine. *Lancet* 2:742.
3. Warburton DW (1988). The puzzle of nicotine use. In *The Psychopharmacology of Addiction*, Chap. 3. New York: Oxford University Press.
4. Taylor P (1985). Ganglinic stimulating and blocking agents. In *The Pharmacological Basis of Therapeutics*, 7th Ed., Gilman AG, Goodman LA, Rall TW, Murad F, eds., Chap. 10. New York: Macmillan.
5. U.S. Department of Health & Human Services (1988). *The Health Consequences of Smoking: Nicotine Addiction. A Report of the Surgeon General*. Washington, DC: U.S. Gov. Printing Office.
6. Jarvik ME (1967). Tobacco smoking in monkeys. *Ann NY Acad Sci* 142:280–294.
7. U.S. Public Health Service (1986). *The Consequences of Using Smokeless Tobacco. A Report of the Advisory Committee of the Surgeon General*. DHEW Publications No. (PHS) 86-2874. Washington, DC: U.S. Gov. Printing Office.
8. Glover ED, Schroeder KL, Henningfield JE, et al. (1988). An interpretive review of smokeless tobacco research in the United States: Part I. *J Drug Educ* 18(4):285.
9. National Institutes of Drug Abuse (1989). *National High School Survey*. National Institute of Drug Abuse. Washington, DC: US Gov. Printing Office.
10. Maxwell JC (1980). Maxwell manufactured products report: Chewing snuff is growth segment. *Tob Rep* 107:32.
11. Siegal RK (1982). Cocaine smoking. *J Psychoact Drugs* 14:272–341.
12. Gritz ER, Baer-Weiss V, Benowitz NL (1981). Plasma nicotine and cotinine concentration in habitual smokeless tobacco users. *Clin Pharmacol Ther* 30:201.
13. Hoffman D, Hecht SS (1985). Nicotine-derived *N*-nitrosamines and tobacco related cancer. *Cancer Res* 45:2285.
14. Wesnes K, Warburton DM (1983). Smoking, nicotine and human performance. *Pharmacol Ther* 21:189–208.
15. Wise RA (1982). Neuroleptics and operant behavior: The anhedonia hypothesis. *Behav Brain Sci* 5:39–53.
16. Henningfield JE (1984). Pharmacological basis and treatment of cigarette smoking. *J Clin Psychiatry* 45:24–34.
17. Russell MAH (1971). Cigarette smoking: Natural history of a dependence disorder. *Br J Med Psychol* 44:1–16.
18. Schuster CR, Thompson T (1969). Self-administration of and behavioral dependence on drugs. *Ann Rev Pharmacol* 9:483–502.
19. Mello NK, Mendelson JH, Sellers ML, et al. (1980). Effects of heroin self-administration on cigarette smoking. *Psychopharmacology* 67:45–52.
20. American Psychiatric Association (1987). *Diagnostic and Statistical Manual of Mental Disorders*, 3d Ed. (Revised). Washington, DC: American Psychiatric Association.

21. Pomerleau OF, Rosecrans J (1989). Neuroregulatory effects of nicotine. *Psychoneuroendocrinology* 14(6):407–423.
22. Shiffman SM (1979). The tobacco withdrawal syndrome. In *Cigarette Smoking as a Dependence Process*, Krasnegor NA, ed. Washington, DC: National Institute for Drug Abuse.
23. Warburton DM (1987). The functions of smoking. In *Tobacco Smoke and Nicotine: A Neurobiological Approach*, p. 178–199. New York: Plenum Press.
24. Warburton DM (1975). *Brain, Behaviour and Drugs*. London: Wiley.
25. Jarvik ME, Henningfield JE (1988). Pharmacological treatment of tobacco dependence. *Pharmacol Biochem Behav* 30:279.
26. Cocores JA, Sinaikin P, Gold MS (1989). Scopolamine as treatment for nicotine polacrilex dependence. *Ann Clin Psychiatry* (1):203–204.
27. Alcoholics Anonymous World Services, Inc. (1976). *Alcoholics Anonymous*, 3d Ed., p. 58. New York: Alcoholics Anonymous World Services.
28. Jeanne E (1984). *The Twelve Steps for Smokers*, p. 3. Center City, MN: Hazeldon Foundation.
29. Schneider N (1988). *How to Use Nicotine Gum & Other Strategies to Quit Smoking*. New York: Pocket Books.
30. Bobo JK (1989). Nicotine dependence and alcohol epidemiology and treatment. *J Psychoact Drugs* 21(3):323.
31. Benowitz NL (1983). The use of biologic fluid samples in assessing tobacco smoke consumption. *Natl Inst Drug Abuse Res Monogr Ser* 48:6.
32. Noland MP, Kryscio RJ, Riggs RS, et al. (1988). Saliva cotinine and thiocyanate: Chemical indicators of smokeless tobacco and cigarette use in adolescents. *J Behav Med* 11(5):423.
33. Nanji AA, Lawrence AH (1988). Skin surface sampling for nicotine: A rapid, noninvasive method for identifying smokers. *Int J Addict* 23(11):1207.
34. Glassman AH, Jackson WK, Walsh BT, et al. (1984). Cigarette craving, smoking withdrawal, and clonidine. *Science* 226:864.
35. Glassman AH, Stetner MS, Walsh BT, et al. (1988). Heavy smokers, smoking cessation, and clonidine. *JAMA* 259(19):2863.
36. Bachynsky N (1986). The use of anticholinergic drugs for smoking cessation: A pilot study. *Int J Addict* 789.
37. Sees KL, Stalcup SA (1989). Combining clonidine and nicotine replacement for treatment of nicotine withdrawal. *J Psychoact Drugs* 21(3):355.
38. Cocores JA, Gold MS (1989). Transdermal scopolamine for nicotine dependence: Use in non-addicts versus recovering addicts. In *Proceedings of the American Society of Addiction Medicine*, 20th Annual Conference, Atlanta, Georgia, p. 22.
39. Cocores JA, Gold MS (1991). Nicotine dependent psychiatric patients. In *The Clinical Management of Nicotine Dependents*, Cocores JA, ed., p. 420. New York: Springer-Verlag.
40. Cocores JA, Goias PR, Gold MS (1990). The medical management of nicotine dependence in the workplace. *Ann Clin Psychiatry* (1):237–240.
41. Cocores JA, Pottash AC (1991). Outpatient management of nicotine dependence. In *The Clinical Management of Nicotine Dependence*, Cocores JA, ed., p. 331. New York: Springer-Verlag.

CHAPTER 20

The Pharmacology of Nonprescription Medications

History

Over-the-counter medications (OTC) are defined as proprietary medications or drugs sold "over the counter" in stores, such as pharmacies, grocery stores, etc. These drugs do not require prescriptions for purchase and are often not used as a result of a recommendation of a physician. The motivation for use is often self-determined for common ailments that may or may not require the attention of a physician.

The most commonly used OTC medications are analgesics, cough and cold remedies, vitamins, and antacids (Table 20.1). There are estimated to be between 100,000 and 500,000 different kinds of OTCs. The Food and Drug Administration (FDA) does not maintain accurate records of all brand names. One type of generic drug may be packaged under several brand names in a variety of preparations. Possibly 300,000 over-the-counter medicines contain 500 significant active ingredients (1–3).

Pattern of Use

A study performed in the 1970s by the National Academy of Science–National Resource Council determined the efficacy of OTC medications. The findings indicated that 15% were effective, 27% were probably effective, 46% were possibly effective, and 11% were ineffective. Thus, more than half of the OTCs tested did not show convincing effectiveness (4).

The problems most likely to be treated with a nonprescription medicine are included in Table 20.2. As expected, minor ailments, particularly those which are chronic, recurring, and without a known etiology to treat are common. Of interest are those ailments or conditions which are not likely to be treated with OTCs. These conditions have more specifically known etiologies, for example, heredity, food intake, and aging (5).

TABLE 20.1. Usage of OTCs.[a]

	Annual dollar volume
Internal analgesics	1,015,060,000
Cough and cold	946,260,000
Vitamins	559,090,000
Antacids	492,060,000
Laxatives	287,530,000
External analgesics	156,480,000
Acne/medicinal soap	117,750,000
Antidiarrheals	108,620,000

[a]From Ref. 7.

Intoxication

The adverse reactions are common and predictable from the drug class and actions. The analgesics (e.g., aspirin), laxatives, antihistamines, sympatho-mimetics, and alcohol-based OTCs, caffeine, and nicotine produce expected untoward effects based on their pharmacological toxicities (6).

It is important to recognize that the diagnostic clues to the existence of an OTC misuse/abuse are clinical conditions that have many etiologies, both drug and nondrug related. The practice to have a differential diagnosis that includes OTC medication is clear. Because they are commonly used for disorders that are chronic and common, OTC use and toxicity should be

TABLE 20.2. OTC treatment usage.[a]

	Percent who treat with OTCs
Adult problems most likely to be treated with a nonprescription medicine	
Headache	71
Lip problems	70
Athlete's foot	66
Chronic dandruff	61
Common cold	60
Migraine headache	59
Painful, dry skin	58
Adult problems not likely to be treated with an OTC	
Bruises	6
Baldness/hair loss	5
Overweight	5
Underweight	4
Age spots	4

[a]From Ref. 5.

considered often (Table 20.3). Patients may not offer that they are taking OTCs, or may even omit their use on questioning because nonprescription drugs are not always considered "real" medications (Table 20.3).

The adverse reactions may also occur because (1) most OTCs contain several ingredients; (2) many OTCs can be used for multiple symptoms; (3) instructions on labels are often unclear; (4) many customers consider them safe because they can be bought without a prescription; and (5) future sales of agents depend on whether the patient feels an effect, thus manufacturers may add unnecessary ingredients to provide stimulation (7).

Toxicity

The toxicities of OTC indications are frequent and sometimes severe. The vitamins have many mechanisms by which toxicity may develop. Their metabolites may have direct toxic effects; megadoses of water-soluble vitamins may lead to dependence states, and if they are abruptly discontinued withdrawal symptoms may develop that may mask the symptoms or signs of a concurrent disease. Vitamins may interact with drugs or with other vitamins, and the use of megadoses of water-soluble vitamins may be associated

TABLE 20.3. Diagnosing misuse or abuse of OTC drugs.[a]

Drug class	Diagnostic clues
OTC analgesics	Gastritis Heme-positive stools Nephropathy Elevated alkaline phosphatase
Laxatives	Continuing diarrhea Metabolic abnormalities (hypokalemia, hypocalcemia) Nonspecific inflammatory changes at rectal biopsy
Antihistamines and anticholinergics	Mental status abnormalities Unusual reactions to prescription psychotropic medications
Sympathomimetics	Arrhythmias Hypertension Chronic sinus or nasal congestion
Alcohol-based OTCs	Elevated liver enzymes Worsening of preexisting chronic conditions History of alcohol abuse
Caffeine	Anxiety Insomnia Tachyarrhythmias
Nicotine	Stigmata of smoking or oral tobacco use (stained teeth, fingers) and presence of tobacco products History of alcohol abuse

[a]From Ref. 14.

with concurrent intake of high doses of fat-soluble vitamins. See Table 20.4. Disorders that are aggravated by megadoses of water-soluble vitamins are presented in Table 20.4 (8,9).

The OTC stimulants may lead to familiar toxicity of stimulants such as hypertension, anxiety, depression, paranoid delusions, suspiciousness, supraventricular and ventricular arrhythmias, myocardial injury, or seizures. Treatments of these disorders are presented in Table 20.5 (10,11).

Prevalence

The elderly, aged 65 years or over, spend half as much money on OTCs as on prescription medications. The American public spends 4 to 8 billion dollars per year on self-prescribed and self-administered drugs for self-diagnosed illnesses. A survey performed in 1979 in 16 states and Washington, D.C. interviewed 30,000 individuals. The findings were that 68% had used analgesics within the previous 6 months, 17% had used a sedative, and 37% had used a vitamin. By the age of 2 years, about 79% of the children studied had received some type of medication (12).

The use of prescription drugs appears to be declining and the practice of self-medication to be increasing. It has been estimated that two-thirds to three-fourths of all ailments are self-managed by the individual of the family without seeking professional medical advice (13).

A simple way of comprehending that magnitude of the use of OTC medication is to assume approximately 100,000 million individuals buy at least 1 OTC per year. Simple multiplication reveals that the number of purchases range in the millions of such medications per year.

Tolerance and Dependence

Tolerance and dependence do develop to a variety of the OTC drugs. The tolerance develops to many effects for a given drug and only to a limited extent, so that toxicity cannot be always avoided. Only certain drugs show well-defined withdrawal syndromes, although many more may also do so depending on the definition of the dependence syndrome (14,15).

TABLE 20.4. Mechanisms of vitamin toxicity.[a]

Vitamins or their metabolites may have direct toxic effects.
Megadoses of water-soluble vitamins may lead to dependency states, and withdrawal symptoms may develop if they are abruptly discontinued.
Vitamins may mask the symptoms or signs of a concurrent disease.
Vitamins may interact with drugs or with other vitamins.
The use of megadoses of water-soluble vitamins may be associated with concurrent intake of high doses of fat-soluble vitamins.

[a]From Ref. 9.

TABLE 20.5. Disorders that are aggravated by megadoses of water-soluble vitamins.[a]

Disorder	Vitamin	Mechanism effect
Asthma	Nicotinic acid	Histamine release
Diabetes mellitus	Nicotinic acid	Hyperglycemia
	Vitamin C	False positives for glucosuria
Peptic ulcer disease	Nicotinic acid	Histamine release and increased acidity
Liver disease	Nicotinic acid	Leakage of liver enzymes
		Cholestatic jaundice
		Massive necrosis
Gout	Nicotinic acid	Elevated serum urate
		Acute gouty arthritis
Nephrolithiasis	Vitamin C	Uricosuric agent
	Vitamin C	Oxaluria
G-6-PD deficiency	Vitamin C	Increased RBC lysis
Megaloblastic anemia	Folate	Masks B_{12} deficiency
	Vitamin C	Decreased B_{12} absorption
Sideroblastic anemia	Vitamin C	Increased iron absorption
Diarrhea	Vitamin C	
	Pantothenic acid	} Promote diarrhea
	Nicotinic acid	
Cardiac disease	Nicotinic acid	Promotes arrhythmias
Skin disease	Nicotinic acid	Causes acanthosis nigricans
CNS disorders	Vitamin B_6	Causes convulsions
	Vitamin B_1	Causes irritability
	Folate	Causes insomnia
Scurvy	Vitamin C	Rebound deficiency
Parkinson's disease	Vitamin B_6	Antagonizes L-dopa
Sensory neuropathy	Vitamin B_6	Destroys dorsal roots

[a]From Ref. 9.

Common effects of OTCs to which tolerance develops include sedation, hypnosis, stimulation, insomnia, hypertension, hypotension, and tachycardia. The withdrawal syndrome for anticholinergics is general somatic distress, anxiety or agitation, sleep disturbance characterized by excessive vivid dreaming and insomnia, and movement disorder and excitement. The alcohol-based OTCs may reveal an abstinence alcohol withdrawal syndrome with headache, anxiety, depression, tremors, elevation in blood pressure. Caffeine- and other stimulant-containing preparations may show a withdrawal syndrome consisting of depression, anxiety, hypersomnia, somatization, and hyperphagia.

Neurochemistry

The action of anxiety of the OTCs are predictable on the basis of their neurochemistry. Only a brief discussion of the major classes of OTCs will be presented in this chapter, and not exhaustively.

The analgesics, particularly aspirin, have a principal effect on the platelets to inhibit their aggregation to prevent hemostases. This action makes aspirin an attractive agent to use in prophylaxis for thromboembolic events in cardiac and cerebrovascular disease. Aspirin also exerts its antipyretic effect by resetting the thermostat in the hypothalamus at a lower level to inhibit fever production. Aspirin exhibits its analgesic effect by stabilizing neuronal membranes to lower excitation of sensory nerve injuries (6,7).

Laxatives have a variety of mechanisms from simply providing bulk for stool formation to stimulating the bowel by acting as an irritant. Antihistamines, both H-1- and H-2-receptor blockers, act as histamine receptors to block histamine action. Anticholinergic medications act at cholinergic receptors in the parasympathetic nervous system by blocking the action of acetylcholine receptors in the cardiovascular and central nervous systems (15).

Sympathomimetics act by stimulating the sympathetic nervous system. Phenylpropanolamine acts as a direct agonist on norepinephrine alpha$_2$ receptors and by releasing norepinephrine to produce vasoconstriction. Ephedrine and pseudoephedrine are both alpha- and beta-adrenergic agonists and produce effects on the norepinephrine alpha$_2$ receptors. However, by acting on beta receptors, they may produce vasodilatation. Caffeine is a potent releaser of epinephrine, and to a lesser extent norepinephrine, from the adrenal medulla (Table 20.6) (11).

Intervention and Treatment

Intervention may begin by knowing first the ways in which people learn about OTC indications. The informational sources for introducing and describing the indications for which the OTC medications are used include: advertising, 30%; friends/relatives, 23%; pharmacists, 20%; physicians, 14%; and product labels, 13%. Curiously, professionals are the sources of information only 34% of the time (16).

Advertising is by far the most common method for the users to become acquainted with these drugs and to learn their uses. Inherent in advertising are obvious biases to promote the product, encourage its use, and claim efficacy. The motive to objectively inform and educate the potential consumer is questionable (17).

Friends and relatives are perhaps a reliable source of information but again may not provide an unbiased report, and are not qualified diagnosticians. In spite of their genuine intent to help, their recommendation may be misleading. Pharmacists and physicians are the knowledgeable informed sources in most cases. However, the pharmacist who sells the OTC drugs does have some profit motive behind his recommendations. The physician, on the other hand, is more likely to prescribe for his credibility and not endorse OTC medications routinely.

The consumer may use product labels to choose an OTC, but these sources of information are not well-regulated by the FDA. The same problems associated with advertising are also inherent in product labels. The ethanol

TABLE 20.6. Treatment of toxic reactions to OTC stimulants.[a]

Drug	Sign or symptom	Treatment	Comment
Phenylpropanolamine	Hypertension	Rapidly acting antihypertensive agent (nitroprusside of phentolamine) Sitting position may be helpful if hypertension is postural Maintain adequate urine output; acidific action of urine may be useful if urine pH is >7.0	Duration of toxic reaction is generally less than 6 hr · · · Acidification of urine may promote myoglobinuric renal failure
	CNS toxic effect	Supportive	· · ·
	Other (arrhythmias, myocardial injury)	Not established	Control of hypertension is most important because of risk of intracerebral hemorrhage; contribution of other cardiac toxic effects of drug to morbidity and mortality is not established
Ephedrine, pseudoephedrine	Hypertension	Same as for phenylpropanolamine	· · ·
	Tachyarrhythmias	β-Blocker	This therapy could cause hypertension by antagonizing β_2-mediated vasodilation and unmasking α-mediated vasoconstriction
Caffeine	Hypertension plus tachyarrhythmia	May require both β-blocker and antihypertensive agent	· · ·
	Supraventricular tachyarrhythmias	β-blocker	· · ·
	Ventricular tachyarrhythmias	· · ·	· · ·
	Seizures	A benzodiazepine	
	Other CNS toxic effects	Supportive	· · ·
	Hypotension	Not established	Hypotension may be due to peripheral vasodilation, secondary to a tachyarrhythmia, or possibly due to a direct myocardial toxic effect

[a]From Ref. 11.

TABLE 20.7. Ethanol content of some pharmaceuticals available in the rsa.[a]

Product name	Manufacturer/ supplier	Schedule category[b]	Alcohol content % v/v[c]	Maximum daily alcohol intake (ml)[d]
Actifed Syrup	Calmic	S2	4.0	1.2
Aktivanad Tonic	Noristan	NS	11.0	5.0
Alertonic	Mer-National	S5	15.0	6.8
Balsem vita (all colours)	Lennon	NS	±86.4	4.3
Benylin Expectorant	Parke-Davis	S2	5.0	3.0
Beracal Lotion	SCS Pharmalab	S1	0.8	—
Betapyn Syrup	Restan	S2	14.5	13.1
Borstol Cough Mixture	Group Labs	NS	16.4	19.7
Chamberlain's Diarrhoea Mixture	Chamberlain	NS	56.0	16.8
Chief Cough Mixture	Williamson	NS	±30.0	9.0
Clearasil Skin Cleanser	Richardson	NS	19.0	—
Daenite Cold and Flu Mixture	Restan	S2	35.0	31.5
Darosed Syrup	SCS Pharmalab	S2	1.23	0.75
Day Nurse Cough Syrup	Beechams	S2	15.5	18.6
Demazin Expectorant	Scherag	S2	7.0	4.2
Dilinct Syrup	Restan	S2	10.0	9.0
Emprazil-A Syrup	Wellcome	S1	9.4	2.8
Eskamel Ointment	SKF	NS	12.0	—
Expigen Syrup	Adcock-Ingram	NS	7.1	4.3
Ferlixir Syrup	Nattermann	NS	12.5	3.8
Gripe Water	Lennon	NS	2.93	1.3
Grippon Syrup	Alex Lipworth	S2	10.0	3.0
Ipradol Syrup	Petersen	S2	6.72	2.0
Lewensessens	Lennon	NS	45.0	4.5
Listerine Mouth Wash	Warner	NS	26.7	—
Liviton Tonic	Vesta	NS	14.3	2.9
Melisana Herbal Tonic	Noristan	NS	82.2	49.3
Meprogesic Syrup	Alex Lipworth	S2	5.0	4.5
Nethaprin Expectorant	Mer-National	S2	8.5	6.8
Nite Nurse	Beechams	S2	14.8	3.0
Nitepax Syrup	MPS	S1	0.8	0.3
Panado Syrup	Winthrop	NS	8.5	7.7
Periactin Syrup and Periactin B-C Syrup	MSD	S1/S2	5.0	4.0
Phensedyl Linctus	Maybaker	S2	7.0	2.1
Physeptone Linctus	Wellcome	S7	12.3	3.7
Pynstop Syrup	Rio Ethicals	S2	10.0	3.0
Retin-A Gel	Janssen	S3	97.0	—
Sentinel Ulcer Mixture	Martyn	S2	56.0	8.4
Silgastrin-Gel	Ethimed	S1	1.0	0.4
Silomat Composit Syrup	Boehringer	S1	1.6	0.5
Sloan's Liniment	Chamberlain	NS	50.0	—
Stopayne Paediatric Syrup	Adcock-Ingram	S2	10.0	3.0
Syndol Niteduty	Mer-National	S2	19.2	5.8

TABLE 20.7. *Continued*

Product name	Manufacturer/supplier	Schedule category[b]	Alcohol content % v/v[c]	Maximum daily alcohol intake (ml)[d]
Tai Ginseng Tonic	Peppina	NS	21.0	9.5
Tixylix Linctus	Maybaker	S2	3.8	1.1
Tylenol Elixir	Pharmedica	NS	7.0	6.3
Versterkdruppels	Lennon	NS	40.0	6.0
Vicks Acta Plus	Richardson	NS	10.0	2.5
Waterbury Tonic	Chamberlain	NS	11.0	9.9
Woods Peppermint Cure	Lennon	NS	11.27	9.0
Zaditen Syrup	Wander	S3	2.39	0.25

[a]From Ref. 18.
[b]NS = Non-scheduled and freely available.
[c]The alcohol content was supplied by the manufacturer/supplier, when not listed on the product label or package insert.
[d]Based on the recommended daily intake of product.

content of medications is frequently not clearly or not at all indicated on the product (See Table 20.7).

Thus, the consumer of OTC medications is left with no clearly objective and unbiased source of information, and must self-diagnose and self-medicate almost by trial and error. The method for deciding on an OTC combined with their toxicity make it important for the user to weigh carefully the risk of benefits before using the OTC medications. In spite of these questions about consumer-informed choices, surveys regarding consumer attitudes toward OTC do not reveal a problem (16,17,18).

References

1. Pepper GA (1986). Rational use of OTCs. *Nurse Pract* 2:00–00.
2. Esmay JB, Wertheimer AI (1979). A review of over-the-counter drug therapy. *J Community Health* 5(1):00–00.
3. Tolbert RB (1987). Health professionals should monitor workers' over-the-counter drug use. *Occup Health & Saf* 56:52–54.
4. Shands VP, Goff LD, Goff DH (1983). Rx for OTC users: Improved health education *J Occup Saf Health* 53(7):423–426.
5. Anon (1984). What patients know about OTC limits. *RN* 47:75–82.
6. Rodman MJ (1981). The drug interactions we overlook. *RN* 44:37–41.
7. Lamy PP (1982). Over-the-counter medication: The drug interactions we overlook. *J Am Geriatr Soc* 30(11; Suppl.):569–575.
8. Ovesen L (1984). Vitamin therapy in the absence of obvious deficiency: What is the evidence. *Drugs* 27:148–170.
9. Alhadeff L, Gualtieri CT, Lipton M (1984). Toxic effects of water-soluble vitamins. *Nutr Rev* 42(2):34–40.

10. Bravo EL (1988). Phenylpropanolamine and other over-the-counter vasoaction compounds. *Hypertension* 2:II7–II10.
11. Pentel D (1984). Toxicity of over-the-counter stimulants. *JAMA* 252(14):1898–1903.
12. Vener AM, Krupka LR, Cluno JJ (1982). Drugs (prescription, over-the-counter, social) and the young addict: Use and attitudes. *Int J Addict* 17(3):399–415.
13. Spencer R, Alexander D (1986). Clients regarding over-the-counter drug use. *J Community Health Nurs* 3(1):3–9.
14. Kofoed LL (1985). OTC drug overuse on the elderly: What to watch for. *Geriatrics* 40(10):55–60.
15. Disauer SC, Greden JF, Snider RM (1987). Antidepressant withdrawal syndromes: Phenomenology and pathophysiology. *Int J Clin Psychopharmacol* 2:1–19.
16. Grahn JL (1983). Relationship of consumers' perceptions of drugs to drug use. *Public Health Rep* 98(1):85–90.
17. Vener AM, Krupka LR (1986). Over-the-counter drug advertising in gender-oriented popular magazines. *J Drug Educ* 16(4):367–381.
18. Dangor CM, Veltman (1985). Ethanol content of some pharmaceuticals available in the RSA. *S Am Med J* 68:172–173.

CHAPTER 21

The Pharmacology of Phencyclidine

History

Phencyclidine (PCP, angel dust, peace pill, cadillac, crystal joints, DOA) was synthesized in the 1960s by Parke-Davis Laboratories. The drug was originally intended for use as a surgical anesthetic, but it was found to produce violent postoperative psychosis (1,2). Because of its side effects, which included muscular rigidity as well as nightmares and frank delirium with frightening hallucinations and delusions, PCP was removed from the market for human use a few years after its introduction. It is still used as a tranquilizer in veterinary surgery.

Prevalence

PCP was a popular street drug in the mid-1970s but then declined in use. In recent years, the drug has again become popular in the United States (3-6). Classified as a Schedule II drug, along with morphine, amphetamines, and other highly addictive drugs, PCP is considered both an "upper" and a "downer" because it has both stimulant and depressant effects. The drug has hallucinogenic properties similar to those of lysergic acid diethylamide (LSD) and marijuana (7), as well as dangerous medical, psychiatric and pathological effects (8,9).

PCP is thought to be one of the most widely available psychoactive drugs in the United States (6). A high use of PCP is reported in Los Angeles, Washington, D.C., and New York City, and increasing use is being reported throughout the country. Unfortunately, the drug is most popular among young people, particularly those aged 6 to 20 years.

Patterns of Use

PCP is usually smoked in a manner similar to marijuana. The drug is mixed with dried leaf materials, such as marijuana, tobacco, or parsley. Like cocaine, it is also snorted or sniffed through the nose. Oral administration, in

pill or liquid form, is also prevalent. Less often, the drug is injected intravenously (10).

Because PCP is inexpensive and easy to manufacture, it is often sold
deceptively in place of drugs that are scarce or costly. Drug dealers frequently use PCP to adulterate or enhance other drugs with similar effects, such as
LSD, cocaine, and marijuana.

Intoxication

Nystagmus and hypertension are hallmarks of PCP intoxication. The nystagmus is irregular, with jerky eye movement in any direction. Blood pressure may increase to 160/105 mm Hg or higher. Stroke and cerebral hemorrhage have occurred after PCP use. Sinus tachycardia may occur, along with
shortness of breath and increased respiratory rates. Respiratory and cardiac
arrest are possible sequelae of high doses of PCP. Hyperthermia, with body
temperatures as high as 108°F (42°C), has been reported (11).

Muscular rigidity and immobility of body movement are commonly associated with low to moderate doses of PCP. Bizarre posturing and movement
disorders, such as tremors, writhing, and jerky movements, are not uncommon. Generalized tonic-clonic seizures and status epilepticus may occur
with higher doses. Deep tendon reflexes are often increased.

The autonomic nervous system is commonly stimulated by PCP, resulting
in diaphoresis, increased salivation, increased bronchial secretions, and
urinary retention. Wheezing and severe bronchial spasms may compromise
breathing. The pupils may be any size. Death from PCP is caused by respiratory depression, seizures, or cardiovascular collapse (11,12).

The psychological effects of PCP are unpredictable. With low doses, PCP
users may have a clear sensorium, or they may be disoriented and confused.
The subjective effects of the drug include euphoria, sedation, drunkenness,
and slow or speeding thoughts.

Objective signs of PCP use include slurred or pressured speech, rapid and
varied use of words, echolalia, and illogical, uncoordinated thinking. Psychotic reactions, including auditory and visual hallucinations, delusions,
and paranoid thinking, can occur at any dose but are more common with
higher doses (13).

Under the influence of PCP, the user may be subdued and mute, staring
off into space. Less commonly, the individual may become agitated, fearful,
and violent (14). PCP can distort perceptions to the point that the user
commits a violent crime or commits suicide out of fear and confusion or in
response to paranoid delusions and auditory commands. (In this regard,
PCP is a drug dangerous to nonusers who come into contact with those who
are under its influence.) Psychotic reactions, with hallucinations, delusions,
catatonia, and stupor, can last weeks or months after PCP use. With large
doses, the user may become comatose and unresponsive to verbal or physi-

cal stimuli. The question of permanent brain damage resulting from PCP use has not been settled (14).

The most significant observable change is in the personality of the user. Mood fluctuations, distortions in thinking, deterioration in attitudes, lack of personal responsibility, and impairment in judgment regularly accompany PCP use.

Tolerance and Dependence

Addiction to PCP may be defined as preoccupation with the use of PCP and compulsive use of PCP despite adverse consequences. The confirmatory criterion of addiction is a return to PCP use despite previous adverse consequences. Depression, school problems, and family difficulties are often given as reasons for drug use, but it is more likely that the drug use caused the other problems. In treatment, it is important to detect the denials and rationalizations that promote and sustain drug use.

PCP users develop tolerance to the effects of the drug; increasingly higher doses are required to induce euphoria and hyperactive behavior. Physical dependence on the drug is signified by withdrawal symptoms of nervousness, anxiety, and depression. The depression may be deep and severe, and the individual may become suicidal.

Chronic users of PCP may experience anxiety, depression, and loss of memory, particularly recent memory, for months or years. Many of these symptoms and signs subside only after prolonged abstinence (15).

Pharmacokinetics

PCP is almost completely metabolized by the liver, with very little excreted unchanged in the urine. However, PCP, like marijuana, has a very long half-life and can remain in the body for days, weeks, and perhaps months. This may explain some of the drug's long-term psychological and physical effects.

Other Drugs

PCP users commonly use other drugs as well. More than 60% drink alcohol, and least 40% use opiates or marijuana. Therefore, any history of PCP use should include questions about other drugs (15,16).

The use of illicit drugs impedes the maturation process in adolescence. The prolonged effects of PCP on mood and memory may be dangerous to the adolescent user. PCP and other drugs also affect relationships between the adolescent and family members, teachers, and others, especially the police. Drug use impairs judgment and affects emotional responses.

Adolescence is difficult enough in the sober state; drugs accentuate and exaggerate the normal challenges of this period. Adolescents need to develop a healthy self-awareness and a sense of identity. When young people live on the border of reality, with drug-induced hallucinations, delusions, or false alterations of emotions, they have little chance of achieving self-fulfillment (17).

Intervention and Treatment

Pharmacological Management

The two major states that often require pharmacological intervention are PCP intoxication and psychosis. The intoxicated state is usually transient and is treated supportively by keeping the patient calm and safe. A quiet place with reassuring staff is indicated for the protection of both the user and others. Patients with PCP intoxication frequently are anxious, depressed, agitated, and paranoid; their perceptions are often distorted, hallucinatory, and unpredictable.

Chlordiazepoxide (Librium) 25 to 200 mg, or diazepam (Valium) 10 to 30 mg or more, may be necessary to calm and sedate the patient. Dosage should be titrated to cover the acute period of intoxication. Vital signs should be monitored frequently, because hypertension may occur. Calming and sedating the patient will often suffice to lower the blood pressure (7,11).

PCP-induced psychosis is similar to the intoxicated state but usually lasts longer. The usual symptoms of anxiety, paranoia, delusions, hyperactivity, assaultiveness, and exaggerated muscular strength may persist for days or even several weeks before they gradually resolve. Again, the treatment goal is to restrain the patient in a quiet, safe place. Talking the patient down is not recommended, because this technique may only increase the patient's agitation and paranoia (9,10).

High-potency neuroleptics with low anticholinergic effects are useful in control of the symptoms of PCP psychosis. Haloperidol (Haldol) may be given intramuscularly or orally in doses similar to those used in acute idiopathic psychosis. Low-potency neuroleptics such as chlorpromazine (Thorazine) and thioridazine (Mellaril) have undesirable anticholinergic effects that worsen the delirium and psychosis. Acidification of the urine enhances excretion of the drug. The urine should be maintained below pH 5 (12).

Nonpharmacological Treatment

Because many PCP users are addicted to both PCP and other drugs, such as alcohol or marijuana, a thorough history and medical evaluation are indicated to determine the duration, extent, and consequences of drug use. If the user denies other drug use, the physician should seek corroborative information from family members, teachers, or employers. Not infrequently, persistent inquiry uncovers a relatively long history of drug use (possibly years of use in adolescents). Cooperation from those who are responsible for the addict is essential in persuading the addict to accept help.

Effective and early treatment for drug addiction is available. Individual psychotherapy is not useful in treating drug addiction. Group therapy, facilitated by physicians, psychologists, and counselors, is the principal means of treatment (15,18). Successful treatment for drug addiction includes total abstinence from all nonmedical drugs and an inpatient or outpatient program specific for drug addiction. These treatment programs often are based on a "12-step" abstinence approach.

The follow-up period is critical to continued abstinence and recovery. Aftercare sessions that meet weekly for a period of months ensure monitoring and support. Frequent attendance at regular meetings of Alcoholic Anonymous or Narcotics Anonymous is the single best predictor of a successful recovery from PCP drug use (19).

References

1. Cohen S (1977). Angel dust. *JAMA* 238:515-516.
2. Cohen S (1981). *The Substance Abuse Problems*. New York: Haworth.
3. Nicholi AM, Jr. (1984). Phencyclidine hydrochloride (PCP) use among college students: Subjective and clinical effects, toxicity, diagnosis and treatment. *J Am Coll Health* 32:197-200.
4. Senay EC, Becker CE, Schnoll SH (1977). *Emergency Treatment of the Drug-Abusing Patient: For Treatment Staff Physicians*. Rosslyn, VA: National Drug Abuse Center.
5. Drug Enforcement Administration (1981). *Drug Abuse Warning Network (DAWN) 1980 Annual Report*, p. 130. Washington, DC: Drug Enforcement Administration.
6. Hinkely S, Greenwood J (1984). *Emergency Room Visits in DAWN Projected to the Nation*. Washington, DC: Drug Enforcement Administration.
7. Showalter CV, Thornton WE (1977). Clinical pharmacology of phencyclidine toxicity. *Am J Psychiatry* 134:1234-1238.
8. Allen RM, Young SJ (1978). Phencyclidine-induced psychosis. *Am J Psychiatry* 135:1081-1084.
9. Fauman MA, Fauman BJ (1978). The psychiatric aspects of chronic phencyclidine (PCP) use: A study of phencyclidine users. In *Phencyclidine (PCP) Abuse: An Appraisal*, Petersen RC, Stillman, RC, eds., pp. 183-200. Rockville, MD: National Institute on Drug Abuse.
10. McAdams MT, ed. (1980). *Phencyclidine Abuse Manual*. Los Angeles: University of California Extension.
11. Kline NS, Lindenmayer JP (1981). *Psychotropic Drugs: A Manual for Emergency Management of Overdosage*, 2d Ed. Oradell, NJ: Medical Economics.
12. Done AK, Aronow R, Miceli JN (1978). The pharmacokinetics of phencyclidine in overdose and its treatment. In *Phencyclidine (PCP) Abuse: An Appraisal*, Petersen RC, Stillman RC, eds., pp. 210-217. Rockville, MD: National Institute on Drug Abuse.
13. Linder RL, Lerner SE, Burns RS (1981). *PCP, the Devil's Dust: Recogni-*

tion, Management and Prevention of Phencyclidine Abuse. Belmont, CA: Wadsworth.

14. Fauman MA, Fauman BJ (1979). Violence associated with phencyclidine abuse. *Am J Psychiatry* 136:1584–1586.
15. Smith DE, Wesson DR, Buston ME, et al. (1978). The diagnosis and treatment of the PCP abuse syndrome. In *Phencyclidine (PCP) Abuse: An Appraisal,* Petersen RC, Stillman, RC, eds., pp. 218–228. Rockville, MD: National Institute on Drug Abuse.
16. Schuckit MA, Morrissey ER (1978). Propoxyphene and phencyclidine (PCP) use in adolescents. *J Clin Psychiatry* 39:7–13.
17. DeAngelis GG, Goldstein E (1978). Long-term treatment of adolescent PCP abusers. In *Phencyclidine (PCP) Abuse: An Appraisal,* Petersen RC, Stillman, RC, eds., pp. 254–271. Rockville, MD: National Institute on Drug Abuse.
18. Miller NS, Gold MS (1987). The medical diagnosis and treatment of alcohol dependence. *Med Times* 115(9):109–126.
19. Miller NS (1987). A primer of the treatment process for alcoholism and drug addiction. *Psychiatry Lett* 5(7):30–37.

CHAPTER 22

The Pharmacology of Sedatives/Hypnotics

History

The classification for the sedatives/hypnotics is a source of confusion for even dedicated pharmacologists. The method of classification probably arose as primarily an attempt to describe the subjective and behavioral effects produced by these drugs, that is, sedation and hypnosis (1,2).

The members of the class are remarkably similar in their pharmacological properties but significantly differ in their chemical structure. The barbiturates are the prototype drug and constitute the principal member of the sedative/hypnotic class if the benzodiazepines are not included. The benzodiazepines belong in the class of sedative/hypnotic drugs if actual pharmacological properties are used for classification. The benzodiazepines are classified as tranquilizers because of ingenious marketing techniques.

The term tranquilizer was derived to emphasize a particular characteristic of all sedative/hypnotic drugs, which is to tranquilize or to produce tranquility. The distinguishing characteristic of a tranquilizer is to induce calmness without sedation. Barbiturates were referred to as tranquilizers before the introduction of the benzodiazepines. The claim that benzodiazepines do not produce sedation has not withstood clinical experience. Furthermore, many of the benzodiazepines are used interchangeably for sedation and hypnosis (3,4).

The use of barbiturates and other sedative/hypnotic drugs has declined (with a few exceptions) with the advent of the benzodiazepines in 1960. The reasons for this trend are the similarity of the benzodiazepines to barbiturates in sedative/hypnotic effects; less lethal acute toxicity with benzodiazepines; addiction, tolerance, and dependence with sedatives/hypnotics, although the benzodiazepines may be equal to the sedative/hypnotic drugs in these respects (5,6).

Other members of the sedative/hypnotic class are chloral hydrate (Notec), ethchlorvynol (Placidyl), glutethimide (Doriden), meprobamate (Miltown), methyprylon (nodular), paraldehyde (parol), and triclofos (triclos). The pharmacological properties are more alike than distinct. Abuse, addiction, tolerance, and dependence develop readily to all members of the class.

Prevalence

The historical development of the sedatives/hypnotics is also marked by similarities. The introduction of one sedative/hypnotic drug for another has been heralded by unguarded optimism and misguided claims. History has repeated itself with each new drug. The toxicities, abuse, addiction, and development of tolerance and dependence remained in force for each subsequent drug that appeared on the market. Only a variation on the same theme distinguished one drug from the other with some minor improvements in untoward effects. The essential features of the drugs remained the same.

The bromides were the first sedatives, after alcohol, to be marketed specifically for their sedative/hypnotic effects in 1826. Barbituric acid was the next to be introduced, in 1903, followed by chloral hydrate (Mickey Finn) in 1932, meprobamate in 1955, and the benzodiazepines in 1961. The reasons for the failure of each class of drugs was that it was not possible to treat only the target symptoms, that is, anxiety, depression and insomnia, without the development of abuse and addiction to the drugs. The neurochemical location of action in the limbic system of the drugs may also suggest vulnerability to abuse and addiction. Finally, it may be illogical to suppose that a drug will sedate and induce sleep without producing sedation and hypnosis as side effects. Tolerance and dependence are regular accompaniments to frequent drug use, and are natural adaptations of the nervous system to the presence of a foreign chemical. The absence of the drug requires suppression of these adaptations of tolerance and dependence (6,7).

The prevalence of use is difficult to obtain because of a variety of reasons. The user frequently minimizes the amount of use and denies the consequences of the use so that he can continue to use the drug. Physicians who prescribe these drugs do not appreciate their potential for abuse and addiction. The pharmaceutical houses have a large financial investment to promote and sell the sedative/hypnotic drugs that continue to be among the most frequently used drugs in the United States and throughout the world. Finally, public institutions and legal bodies do not respond to the magnitude of the problem in any constructive or lasting way. The typical measure is to either excuse the use or to advocate punishment and intimidation without clearly and fully addressing the salient problems (8,9).

Only estimates through surveys are available for the prevalence rates of use of the sedatives/hypnotics. One survey that has been conducted annually since 1975 has provided nonmedical use of the sedative/hypnotic drugs among high-school seniors. Another survey performed nationally in the United States six times during a 13-year period (1972–1984) has provided additional information about the nonmedical use of drugs among persons living in households. In 1984, the two surveys showed that 14% to 19% of high-school seniors and young adults (18–25 years old) reported past non-medical use of sedatives/hypnotics. In both surveys, these lifetime prevalence rates were generally below those for other major drug classes except heroin and opioid analgesics: alcohol (93%–95%), tobacco cigarettes (70%–77%), marijuana 59%–64%), stimulants (18%–28%), cocaine (16%–28%), and hallucinogens (15%–21%). The high-school survey did not show the decrease (5,6).

The major problem with these surveys is that they do not assess the medical use of the sedatives/hypnotics. Abuse and addiction can occur readily in the medical populations of sedative/hypnotic users for the reasons already stated. The distinction between medical and nonmedical use is not always sharp, and frequently the two overlap considerably. Any survey or assessment would need clear definitions for medical and nonmedical use, abuse, addiction, tolerance, and dependence. Unfortunately, those definitions are rarely applied in studies of prevalence rates.

Further, certain populations are at higher risk than others for sedative/ hypnotic use. These include the chronically ill, the elderly, those already using or addicted to other drugs such as alcohol, stimulants (cocaine), and virtually any drug of abuse and addiction, and those who suffer from the target symptoms for which the sedative/hypnotic drugs are intended (10–13).

Patterns of Use

Drug self-administration studies in laboratory animals have examined a variety of sedative/hypnotic drugs for pattern of use. A high level of self-administration is maintained in the barbiturates by self-injection of the drugs. The development of observable addiction, tolerance, and dependence occurs readily to many of the barbiturates, particularly the short-acting compounds.

The best-validated human experimental approach for providing information about the abuse liability of drugs is to use placebo-controlled, double-blind methodologies to characterize subjective effects and/or behavior-reinforcing properties in human subjects. The abuse and addiction potential of a drug may be inferred from the ability of the drug to serve as a reinforcer, that is, to increase the probability of behavior that results in its administration, and the ability of the drug to produce pleasant subjective effects. The results of these studies are similar to those from the animal data for self-administration. The sedatives/hypnotics, particularly the barbiturates and methaqualone, are self-administered in a pattern of use consistent with abuse and addiction occurring frequently and distinctly (13,14).

Opioid users often take sedatives/hypnotics, as do alcoholics and cocaine addicts. The shortacting barbiturates such as pentobarbital ("yellow jackets") or secobarbital ("red devils") are preferred to longacting agents such as phenobarbital. Other commonly used sedatives/hypnotics are meprobamate, glutethimide, methyprylon, methaqualone, and the benzodiazepines. Paraldehyde and chloral hydrate are still around but have been replaced by the other drugs that have less noxious side effects (15,16).

The patterns of use are many and varied in instances, but adhere to the general principles of use, abuse, and addiction of sedatives/hypnotics overall. They range from regular use for anxiety and insomnia to episodes of gross intoxication and to prolonged compulsive daily use of large quantities of drug. A preoccupation with acquisition and maintaining adequate supplies, compulsive use in spite of adverse consequences, and a recurrent pattern of relapse develop. Some users develop tolerance and may not show obvious intoxication in spite of frequent and heavy doses. The original contact with the drug is often through a physician or the "street" vendor.

In the medical patient, the problem may develop gradually over, time whereas use of the drug may accelerate rapidly when prescribing to the addict. The medical patient begins using the drug for insomnia or anxiety and progresses through increasing doses while the addict required high doses initially. Eventually, the drug is a major priority of the user's life. Neither the patient nor the physician may recognize the existence of abuse and addiction that frequently has occurred. Both assume that the anxiety, tremulousness, and insomnia that emerge when the drug is discontinued are a return of the symptoms for which the drug was initially prescribed. More likely these symptoms represent withdrawal from the drug that may be protracted over weeks and months (17–20).

The most common route of administration by far is oral, although a few inject the drug intravenously, as in mainlining, and others inject the drug subcutaneously, as in skin popping. The sedatives/hypnotics are administered intravenously for anesthesia and to treat seizures acutely. Otherwise, the oral route is by far the choice for the treatment of anxiety, insomnia, and seizures.

Intoxication

The members of the sedative/hypnotic class depress the activity of all excitable tissue, particularly nerve cells, in reversible and transient action on acute administration. The central nervous system (CNS) is exquisitely sensitive to doses of sedatives/hypnotics that produce little effect on skeletal, cardiac, or smooth muscle. In larger doses, as in acute intoxication, the drugs can suppress cardiovascular function and activity in other peripheral organs.

The effects of acute administrations of the sedatives/hypnotics are related to the dose in a positive incremental gradation. In low doses, the drugs are sedating, and as the dose is increased, the magnitude of the sedation is increased until hypnosis is reached. The level of hypnosis is deepened through the stages of coma until depression of all CNS function occurs. All degrees of sedation, hypnosis, and coma are correlated with the blood level of the drug. The CNS concentration for the drug is proportional to the unbound or free concentration in the blood (21).

The subjective effects are predictable and stereotypic in the nontolerant individual for a given member of the sedative/hypnotic class. Early drug effects are diminished attention and concentration, impaired recent or short-term memory, euphoria, decreased abstraction, reduced cognitive abilities, and a sensation of intoxication. As the blood level increases, the alertness is significantly compromised, mood is depressed, and intellectual function is decreased at blood levels considerably lower than those observed in tolerant individuals.

The objective effects are visible and measurable. Incoordination of motor movements occurs in gait, hand–eye tasks, saccadic eye pursuit, and truncal equilibrium with relatively low doses of drug such that skilled maneuvers as driving an automobile or motor performance under dangerous circumstances are risky. On examination, nystagmus, finger-to-nose and heel-to-shin ataxia, uncoordinated rapid alternating movements of the hands, and tandem walking are evident. Respiration are decreased in number and in depth, and blood pressure and pulse may be lowered, especially in higher doses. The tonus of the gastrointestinal musculature and its amplitude and rhythmic contractions are decreased (22).

The effects from even a single dose, such as 200 mg of secobarbital, has been showed to interfere with performance of driving or flying for as long as 10 to 22 hours. These aftereffects may be prolonged considerably, as for days following several successive doses. Many of the drugs will accumulate after repeated administrations with increasing effects even after the development of tolerance in chronic use (23,24). In some individuals, particularly the extremes of age — the young and old — a paradoxical excitement occurs in response to single low doses. This is especially true in pain states (25,26).

The effects on the electroencephalogram (EEG) are striking. In small doses, the drug decreases low-frequency electrical activity and increases the low-voltage, fast activity (15–35 Hz). The fast activity is predominant in the frontal regions and spreads to the parietal and occipital regions. As the dose is increased, the appearance of low-frequency activity alternates with occasional brief periods of electrical silence, until in high doses, the periods of electrical silence predominate in a pattern of burst suppression. Electrocerebral silence may occur in sufficiently high doses, as in the barbiturate-induced coma that mimics the EEG pattern seen in brain death (27).

Hypnotic doses of the drugs always alter sleep in a dose-dependent fashion. The drugs decrease sleep latency, increase delta bursts and fast activity, decrease the number or stage shifts to stages 0 and 1 (number of awakenings), and decrease body movements. Stages 3 and 4 sleep (slow-wave sleep, SWS) are significantly shortened. The latent period before rapid-eye-movement (REM) sleep is prolonged, and the number of REM cycles and REM activity are diminished. Some tolerance occurs to the effects on sleep with days of repeated use. The total effect of tolerance to the hypnotic drugs may be as much or more than 50% of the original effect on sleep. A rebound effect on discontinuation during withdrawal from the drugs constitutes an excessive increase above baseline of stage 2 and REM sleep that may persist for weeks. These rebound phenomena are accompanied by sleep disturbances over the period of demonstrable EEG effects and longer (28–32).

The effects from the chronic use of the sedatives/hypnotics are similar for all members of the class. The primary organ affected by the drugs is the CNS. Numerous studies have documented persistent symptoms and syndromes that accompany and follow chronic sedative/hypnotic use. The major brain functions altered by the drugs are mood, cognition, attention and concentration, insight and judgment, memory, affect, and emotional rapport in interpersonal relationships. Changes in personality that resemble significant personality disorders may develop in regular users of sedatives/hypnotics. Characteristics of antisocial, histrionic, paranoid, and other personality traits can occur in chronic use of the drugs (33).

Tolerance and Dependence

Two major forms of tolerance develop in response to the acute and chronic administration of barbiturates. Pharmacokinetic and pharmacodynamic tolerance are means to reduce the effect of a particular does or doses of sedative/hypnotic drugs. Pharmacokinetic tolerance refers to the absorption, metabolism, and elimination for disposition of the drug. The sedative/hypnotic drugs are quite lipid soluble, having a high lipid-to-water ratio. The nonionized form favors lipid solubility. In usual doses, the sedatives/hypnotics are readily absorbed through the gastrointestinal tract into the systemic circulation. A redistribution stage occurs, particularly with the more lipid-soluble, short-acting sedatives/hypnotics that favors the rapid uptake by fat depot and muscle. In this redistribution the drug disappears from the bloodstream but is not transformed or eliminated from the body. When the equilibrium is in the direction of the blood compartment, the drug is slowly released back to the blood from tissue storage. This phenomenon of redistribution accounts in the body for a long-lasting subjective and behavioral effect (34,35).

The barbiturates compete with other substrates that are metabolized by the cytochrome P-450. The barbiturates and other sedative/hypnotics combine with the cytochrome P-450 system to inhibit the biotransformation of those drugs that also combine with that system. More often, however, the barbiturates cause a marked increase in the microsomal enzyme system to accelerate the metabolism of other drugs including the sedatives/hypnotics themselves. This drug-induced biotransformation of itself and other drugs is another source of tolerance and cross-tolerance. Various anesthetics, ethanol, and the sedative/hypnotic drugs are metabolized by and induce the microsomal enzymes to produce multidirectional cross-tolerance. Of concern is that excessive activation of these enzymes can cause dangerous exacerbations of porphyria in persons with intermittent porphyria (3).

Pharmacodynamic tolerance is an adaptation that occurs at the receptor level. For barbiturates, this is usually a cellular change at the membrane level. The cellular membrane becomes more ordered as tolerance develops. Pharmacodynamic tolerance develops both acutely and chronically in response to the single or repetitive administration of the sedative/hypnotic drugs. Acute tolerance appears to occur significantly earlier than does the induction of microsomal enzymes in response to a single dose of barbiturate. The acute tolerance develops without a change in blood level of drug. Chronic administration of the drug over time will result in a gradual increase in pharmacodynamic tolerance only if the dose is increased. Otherwise the degree of pharmacodynamic tolerance remains unchanged after reaching a peak in only a few days of drug administration. Tolerance to the effects on mood, sedation, and hypnosis occurs more readily, and is greater than that to the anticonvulsant and lethal effects so that the therapeutic index decreases with an increase in tolerance. The dose of barbiturate or other sedative/hypnotic may be increased sixfold as tolerance develops. Pharmacokinetic tolerance through stimulation of microsomal enzymes accounts for only a two- to threefold increase in the dose, whereas pharmacodynamic tolerance accounts for the remainder (36).

The concept of dependence is not well understood. Pharmacological dependence does not constitute addiction. Addiction is preoccupation with acquisition, compulsive use, and relapse to drugs. Dependence is marked by the onset of predictable signs and symptoms of withdrawal from a drug on the cessation of use of the drug. Furthermore, the administration of the drug during withdrawal will abort the appearance of signs and symptoms of that drug. Continued use of the drug may be to offset the discomfort of withdrawal in some instances, particularly if the withdrawal is severe. Withdrawal from sedatives/hypnotics is marked by anxiety and depression that can be especially severe. However, the cycle of increasing tolerance followed by a more severe dependence that allows further increases in drug use is often ended by the escalation of the anxiety and depression.

The withdrawal syndrome is a spectrum that contains a wide array of signs and symptoms occurring in a temporal sequence. Anxiety and depression are rather constant symptoms while others occur less frequently. These symptoms are clinically significant when they appear, and some are potentially dangerous. Tremors, seizures of a partial and generalized type, and a delirium with hallucinations, often visual, and delusions, often paranoid, are less common in appearance in the spectrum. The withdrawal syndrome from the sedatives/hypnotics is similar for all members of the class and differ only in severity and temporal onset in the signs and symptoms. The shorter acting drugs typically have a more severe, earlier, and abrupt onset of withdrawal. Conversely, the longer acting drugs have a milder, later, and more gradual onset of withdrawal. As a useful rule of thumb, the withdrawal syndrome for sedatives/hypnotics is similar to alcohol withdrawal, which can be used as the prototype for the sedative/hypnotic class of drugs (35,37,38).

The presence of tolerance and dependence does not necessarily mean that addiction has occurred. Drug-seeking behavior is the hallmark of addiction. Tolerance and dependence are frequently developed in addiction because use is often regular and in increasing doses. Tolerance and dependence are expected adaptations of the body to the persistent presence of the drug, but do not signal addictive use because tolerance and dependence follow regular use of many drugs that are not used addictively. Tolerance and dependence are guides to the frequent use of a drug but addiction may or may not be present (36,39).

Other Drug Use

Various drugs act synergistically with sedatives/hypnotics todproduce dangerous and lethal depression of respirations and cardiovascular function. Frank hypotension and shock can result from sublethal doses in combination with other drugs. Any combination of the sedatives/hypnotics, ethanol, antihistamines, isoniazid, methylphenidate, and monoamine oxidase inhibitors can increase the CNS depressant action beyond that which would be expected from the sum of the effects of the drugs.

Because the sedatives/hypnotics — particularly the barbiturates — induce the microsomal enzymes, a significant acceleration of the disappearance of many drugs occur. Some examples are corticosteroids, oral anticoagulants, digoxin, beta-adrenergic antagonists, doxycline, oral contraceptives, griseofulvin, quinine, phenytoin, sulfadimethoxine, testerone, tricyclic antidepressants, and zoxazolamine. The metabolism of vitamin D and K may be accelerated to produce deficiencies in the coagulation factors II and VIII. Neonates have coagulation defects when the mothers have been taking pentobarbital. Elderly patients may have already low levels of calcium in the plasma, which is responsible, in part, for the high number of bone fractures that occur in that population. Barbiturates competitively inhibit the metabolism of the cyclic antidepressants as well as other drugs.

Neurochemistry

Not all the members of the sedative/hypnotic class have been as well studied as the barbiturates and benzodiazepines, in particular. The barbiturates act throughout the CNS by directly inhibiting neuronal function at polysynaptic and gamma-aminobutyric acid- (GABA-) ergic sites. GABA, an inhibitory neurotransmitter in the CNS, is ubiquitous and is found at both presynaptic and postsynaptic inhibitory neurons (40).

At low doses, barbiturates inhibit the CNS preferentially at various sites, particularly the mesencephalic region where the reticular activating system (RAS) is located. The RAS is responsible for wakefulness, and is the area that is inhibited by the sedatives/hypnotics to product sedation and hypnosis (15,41).

The barbiturates, in addition to their inhibitory effect on the polysynaptic neurons, also potentiate the GABA-ergic neurons. The barbiturates act by potentiating GABA-induced increases in chloride ion conductance and reducing glutamate-induced depolarization at about the same concentrations. At high concentrations, the barbiturates depress calcium-dependent action potentials, reduce the calcium-dependent release of neurotransmitters, and enhance chloride ion conductance in the absence of GABA. Although the barbiturates resemble the benzodiazepines in facilitating the GABA-ergic inhibition, barbiturates do not displace the benzodiazepines from the binding sites. Instead, the barbiturates enhance the binding affinity for benzodiazepines. These findings suggest that the entire macromolecular complex, composed of GABA-ergic receptors, chloride ionophores, and binding sites for benzodiazepines, is important for the depressant actions of the barbiturates (42).

The barbiturates also affect the membrane order of the cells. The neuronal membranes are composed of bilipid layers. These bilipid layers are composed of phospholipids arranged with the polar heads toward the outside of the membrane and the nonpolar long-chain fatty acids towards the inside. The order of the membrane is determined by this alignment of the phospholipids. The more tightly packed are the fatty acids, the more ordered is the membrane.

The barbiturates act to disorder the membranes on acute administration. The degree of membrane order is measured by fluorescence polarization and electron spin resonance. Important proteins such as receptor complexes and ionophores are embedded in a noncovalent fashion in the membrane. The membrane becomes increasingly ordered with chronic administration of the drug. Behavioral tolerance correlates with the increased order of the membrane.

The lethal dose of sedative-hypnotic drugs varies with several factors. The short-acting drugs are more lethal than the long-acting drugs because of rapid onset of action, high uptake into the lipid-rich brain, and potent suppression of nervous function. The usual fatal dose of secobarbital is 2 to 3 g, whereas that for phenobarbital is 6 to 10 g.

The signs and symptoms of barbiturate poisoning are judged by the effect on the CNS and the cardiovascular system. Moderate intoxication resembles alcohol intoxication, and with increasing doses, CNS depression and cardiovascular suppression occur. The loss of consciousness is followed by signs of coma. The deep tendon reflexes are diminished, as are the responses to noxious stimuli, and the Babinski sign appears. The EEG initially shows slowing, then burst suppression, and finally an isoelectric or flat reading that is indistinguishable from brain death. If respirations are adequately supported, the state of the EEG is reversible as the blood level of drugs drops. For this reason, brain death cannot be confirmed in the presence of alcohol and drugs, because the clinical examination and the EEG may revert to normal as the drug effect disappears. Other organ systems need to be adequately supported during the period of drug-induced suppression. The cardiovascular system as well as the renal system may require pharmacological support if the patient is to survive fatal doses of depressant drugs. It is essential to maintain an open airway, perhaps by mechanical ventilation, and hydration, vasopressors, and hemoperfusion dialysis may be required (43,44).

Intervention and Treatment

The treatment of withdrawal is necessary to avoid morbidity and even mortality from the adverse consequences. The sedative/hypnotic drugs, including alcohol and benzodiazepines, have cross-tolerance and dependence to one another so that any may be substituted for the other. A common approach is to calculate the dose equivalency for drug with one particular sedative/hypnotic that is frequently used, such as librium, valium, or phenobarbital. A long-acting sedative/hypnotic is selected because it does not need to be covered for its own withdrawal. The time course for administration is determined by the drug for which the withdrawal is being treated. For short-acting drugs, a week to 10 days is usually sufficient, whereas for intermediate or long-acting drugs, 2 weeks may be necessary (Table 22.1) (45–47).

It is important for the clinician and patient to agree on a set schedule at the outset to avoid misattribution of drug-seeking behavior to true withdrawal signs and symptoms. Precise calculations of dose equivalency may be a futile exercise because of the difficulty and unreliability of the drug-taking histories in many users. An adequate approach is to categorize the drug use into mild, moderate, and heavy, from which the substitute drug can be approximated. Caution is always urged in interpreting the differences between the signs and symptoms of withdrawal and drug-seeking behavior. The redistribution is less for drugs of lower lipid solubility. Barbiturates and many other sedatives/hypnotics distribute to fetal blood, and concentrations approach those in maternal plasma (3).

Depression of the CNS with apathy, decreased concentration, clouding of consciousness, drowsiness, lethargy, and sleepiness are common sequelae from repetitive use of the sedatives/hypnotics. Tolerance develops only partially to these aftereffects. Subtle distortions of mood and impairment of judgment and motor skills may be demonstrable, and the period between doses of drug may be excitatory with anxiety, mild tremors or shakiness. Nightmares or night terrors may be caused by the deprivation of REM sleep and/or stage 4 sleep (48,49).

Paradoxical excitement occurs in the very young and old. This is an unusual reaction in which the drug causes excitement rather than the expected

TABLE 22.1. Dose conversions[a] for sedative/hypnotic drugs equivalent to secobarbital 600 mg and diazepam 60 mg.

Drug	Dose (mg)
Benzodiazepines	
Alprazolam	6
Chlordiazepoxide	150
Clonazepam	24
Clorazepate	90
Flurazepam	90
Halazepam	240
Lorazepam	12
Oxaxepam	60
Prazepam	60
Temazepam	90
Barbiturates	
Amobarbital	600
Butabarbital	600
Butalbital (in Fiorianal)	600
Pentobarbital	600
Secobarbital	600
Phenobarbital	180
Glycerol	
Meprobamate	2400
Piperidinedione	
Glutethimide	1500
Quinazolines	
Methaqualone	1800

[a]For patients receiving multiple drugs (e.g., flurazepam 30 mg/day, diazepam 30 mg/day, phenobarbital 150 mg/day), each drug should be converted to its diazepam or secobarbital equivalent. In the preceding example, patient is receiving equivalent dose of diazepam 100 mg/day or secobarbital 1000 mg/day. Adapted from Perry PJ, Alexander B. Sedative/hypnotic dependence: patient stabilization, tolerance testing, and withdrawal. *Drug Intell Clin Pharm* 1986:20: 532-537.

sedation or hypnosis. The idiosyncratic reaction most frequently is associated with phenobarbital and *N*-methylbarbiturates.

Hypersensitivity reactions occur most often in those individuals who have a history of allergic reactions such as asthma, urticaria, angioedema, and similar conditions. The hypersensitivity reactions to sedative/hypnotic drugs are localized swellings, particularly of the eyelids, cheeks, or lips, and erythematous dermatitis. Rarely, exfoliative dermatitis may be associated with phenobarbital; the condition includes skin eruptions, fever, delirium, and marked degenerative changes in the liver and other organs with a fatal outcome (3).

Barbiturates enhance porphyrin synthesis, so that they are absolutely contraindicated in patients with acute intermittent porphyria or porphyria variegate. In unusual doses, sedatives/hypnotics may compromise respirations where respiratory insufficiency already exists. Fatal respiratory depression may result from oral, or particularly intravenous, administration (3).

References

1. Gary NE, Tresnewsky O (1983). Clinical aspects of drug intoxication: Barbiturates and a potpourri of other sedatives, hypnotics and tranquilizers. *Heart Lung* 12:122–127.
2. Mendelson WB (1977). *The Use and Misuse of Sleeping Pills: A Clinical Guide.* New York: Plenum Press.
3. Breimer DD (1977). Clinical pharmacokinetics of hypnotics. *Clin Pharmacokinet* 2:93–109.
4. Nicoll RA (1979). Differential postsynaptic effects of barbiturates on chemical transmission. In *Neurobiology of Chemical Transmission*, Otsuka M, Hall ZW, eds., pp. 267–278. New York: Wiley.
5. Johnston LD, O'Malley PM, Backman JG (1975–1984). *Drugs and American High-School Students.* DHHS Publication No. (ADM) 85-1394. Washington, DC: U.S. Govt. Printing Office.
6. Miller TD, Cisin IH, Gardner-Keaton H, et al. (1982). *National Survey on Drug Abuse: Main Findings.* DHHS Publication No. (ADM) 83-1263. Washington, DC: U.S. Govt. Printing Office.
7. Fejer D, Smart R (1973). The use of psychoactive drugs by adults. *Can Psychiatr Assoc J* 18:313–320.
8. Williams P, Murray J, Clare AA (1982). Longitudinal study of psychotropic drug prescription. *Psychol Med* 12:201–206.
9. Fink RD, Knott DH, Beard JD (1974). Sedative-hypnotic dependence. *Am Fam Physician* 10:116–122.
10. Allgulander C (1978). Dependence on sedative and hypnotic drugs. *Acta Psychiatr Scand (Suppl.)* 27C:1–120.
11. Borkovec TD (1982). Insomnia. *J Consult Clin Psychol* 50:880–895.
12. Lader M (1986). The use of hypnotics and anxiolytics in the elderly. *Int Clin Psychopharmacol* 1(4):273–283.
13. Ator NA, Griffiths RR (1987). Self-administration of barbiturates and benzodiazepines. A review. *Pharmacol Biochem Behav* 27(2):391–398.
14. Allgulander C (1986). History and current states of sedation — Hypnotic drug use and abuse. *Acta Psychiatr Scand* 73(5):465–478.
15. Richter JA, Holman JR (1982). Barbiturates; Their in vivo effects and potential biochemical mechanisms. *Prog Neurobiol* 18:273–319.
16. Sampson I (1983). Barbiturates. *Mt Sinai J Med* 50(4):283–288.
17. APA (1978). *Diagnostic and Statistical Manual of Mental Disorders*, 1987 3d Ed. Revised. Washington, DC: *American Psychiatric Association*.
18. Sellers EM (1978). Addictive drugs: Disposition, tolerance and dependence interrelationships. *Drug Metab Rev* 8:5–11.
19. Hawthorne JW, Zabora JR, D'Lugolf BC (1982). Outpatient detoxification of patients addicted to sedative-hypnotics and anxiolytics. *Drug Alcohol Depend* 9:143–151.

20. Wikler A (1976). Review of research on sedative drug dependence at the addiction research center and University of Kentucky. In: *Predicting Dependence Liability of Stimulant and Depressant Drugs*, Thompson T, Unna KR, eds., pp. 147–163. Baltimore: University Park Press.
21. Tang M, Kenny J, Falk JL (1984). Schedule-induced ethanol dependence and phenobarbital preference. *Alcohol* 1(1):55–58.
22. Idestrom CM (1954). Flicker fusion in chronic barbiturate usage. *Acta Psychiatr Scand (Suppl.)* 91:1–93.
23. Fishman RH, Yanai J (1983). Long-lasting effects of early barbiturates on central nervous system and behavior. *Neurosci Biobehav Rev* 17(1):19–28.
24. Okamoto M, Rao S, Walewski JL (1986). Effects of dosing frequency on the development of physical dependence and tolerance to pentobarbital. *J Pharmacol Exp Ther* 238(3):1004–1008.
25. Svensmark O, Buchthal F (1963). Accumulation of phenobarbital in man. *Epilepsia* 4:199–206.
26. Hay D, Milne RM, Gilleard CT (1986). Hypnotic drugs, old people and their habits: A general practice study. *Health Bull (Edinb)* 44(4):218–222.
27. Michenfelder JD (1982). Barbiturates for brain resuscitation: Yes and no. *Anesthesiology* 57:74–75.
28. Hartmann E (1976). Long-term administration of psychotropic drugs: Effects on human sleep. In *Pharmacology of Sleep*, Williams RL, Karacan I, eds., pp. 211–223. New York: Wiley.
29. Feinberg I, Hihi S, Cavness C, March J (1974). Absence of REM rebound after barbiturate withdrawal. *Science* 185:534–535.
30. Kales A, Kales J (1983). Sleep laboratory studies of hypnotic drugs: Efficacy and withdrawal effects. *J Clin Psychopharmacol* 3:140–150.
31. Kales A, Kales J, Soldatos CR (1982). Insomnia and other sleep disorders. *Med Clin North Am* 66:971–991.
32. Kales A, Soldatos CR, Bixler EO, Kales JD (1983). Rebound insomnia and rebound anxiety: A review. *Pharmacology* 26:121–137.
33. Griffiths RR, Bigelow GE, Liehson I (1983). Differential effects of diazepam and pentobarbital on mood and behavior. *Arch Gen Psychiatry* 40(8):865–873.
34. Richter SA, Harris P, Handord P (1982). Similar development of tolerance to barbital-induced inhibition of avoidance behavior and loss of righting reflex in rats. *Pharmacol Biochem Behav* 16:467–471.
35. Fraser HF, Wilker A, Essia CF, Isbell H (1958). Degree of physical dependence, induced by secobarbital or pentobarbital. *JAMA* 166:126–129.
36. Miller NS, Dackis CA, Gold MS (1987). The relationship of tolerance, dependence and addiction: A neurochemical approach. *J Substance Abuse Treat* 4:197–207.
37. Wikler A (1968). Diagnosis and treatment of drug dependence of the barbiturate type. *Am J Psychiatry* 125:758–765.
38. Okamoto M (1984). Barbiturate tolerance and physical dependence: Contribution of pharmacological factors. *Natl Inst Drug Abuse Res Monogr Ser* 54:333–347.
39. Khanna JM, Mayer JM (1982). An analysis of cross tolerance among ethanol, other general depressants and opioids. *Subst Alcohol Actions-Misuse* 3(5):243–257.

40. Ho IK, Harris RA (1981). Mechanism of action of barbiturates. *Annu Rev Pharmacol Toxicol* 21:83–111.
41. Macdonald RL, McLean MJ (1982). Cellular bases of barbiturate and phenytoin anticonvulsant drug action. *Epilepsia* 23(1):517–518.
42. Study RE, Barker JL (1981). Diazepam and (−)-pentobarbital: Fluctuation analysis reveals different mechanism for potentiation of gamma-aminobutyric acid responses in cultured central neurons. *Proc Natl Acad Sci* 11:7180–7184.
43. Steer CR (1982). Barbiturate therapy in the management of central ischemia. *Dev Med Child Neurol* 24:219–231.
44. Martin PR, Kapur BM, Whiteside EA, Sellers EM (1979). Intravenous phenobarbital therapy in barbiturate and other hypnosedative withdrawal reactions: A kinetic approach. *Clin Pharmacol Ther* 26:256–264.
45. Perry DJ, Alexander B (1986). Sedative/hypnotic dependence: Patient stabilization, tolerance testing, and withdrawal. *Drug Intell Clin Pharm* 20:532–537.
46. Benzer D, Cushman P (1980). Alcohol and benzodiazepines withdrawal syndromes. *Alcohol Clin Exp Res* 4:243–247.
47. Reinberg A (1986). Circadian rhythms in effects of hypnotics and sleep inducers. *Int J Clin Pharmacol Res* 6(1):33–44.
48. Nicholson AN (1980). Hypnotics: Rebound insomnia and residual sequelae. *Br J Clin Pharmacol* 9:223–225.
49. Seidel WF, Dement WC (1982). Sleepiness in insomnia: Evaluation and treatment. *Sleep* 5(2):5182–5190.
50. NIDA (1977). *Sedative/Hypnotic Drugs: Risks and Benefits*. Rockville, MD: National Institute on Drug Abuse.

CHAPTER 23

The Pharmacology of Interactions Between Medical and Psychiatric Drugs

History

Drug interactions are clinical responses from a combination of two or more drugs that cannot be explained by only one drug. The clinical responses may be beneficial or harmful. A drug may facilitate the action of another drug in a clinically useful way, or may interact with another drug to produce an adverse reaction or simply reduce the clinical efficacy of one or both drugs. Some drug interactions are commonly encountered, whereas others are infrequent (1,2).

The clinician from any specialization needs to be aware of the potential interactions between drugs, many having wide therapeutic indications and uses. Morbidity, mortality, and compliance are directly attributable to interactions between psychiatric and medical drugs. Knowledge of specific drug interactions is particularly important for psychiatric patients, who may present with a variety of somatic and psychological complaints that are indistinguishable from drug effects (3,4).

When a new symptom appears as a manifestation of a clinical state that is treated with drugs, either the clinical state or the drugs may cause the symptoms and the physician is presented with a diagnostic dilemma. These clinical challenges are enhanced as the number of drugs is increased when medical and psychiatric illnesses occur together, making it likely that significant drug interactions will occur. An understanding of the disease states as well as the drug interactions, which produce symptoms that individual drugs would not, is imperative for definitive diagnosis and proper treatment.

Diagnosis

The ability of physicians to recognize drug interactions may be impaired by (i) lack of information of drug interactions and the tendency to view and report drug interactions as reactions to a single drug; (ii) the tendency of physicians to attribute new symptoms during treatment to the underlying disease; (iii) the tendency to ascribe a severe drug reaction to the patient's idiosyncratic response to a single drug, rather than to a drug interaction; (iv) lack of training in pharmacokinetics, resulting in use of therapeutic agents as "tonics" rather than as chemicals with known or predictable absorption, distribution, and excretion; and (v) the large number of potential drugs involved in drug interactions, which are difficult to recall. Even when the physician knows the drugs and dosages prescribed, multiple-drug therapy leads to mistakes in drug administration (5,6).

Epidemiological studies have demonstrated that the rate of adverse reactions to drugs increases from 4.2%, when 5 or fewer drugs are used, to 45% when 20 or more drugs are prescribed. The rationale for drug choice and the therapeutic goals and guidelines for toxicity must be firmly established on both clinical and pharmacological grounds before the use of multiple drugs can be justified. When polypharmacy is unavoidable, knowledge of the frequency and mechanisms of drug interaction is essential. An informed physician can detect drug interactions early and avoid serious toxicity, or intentionally allow a drug interaction to occur if it is beneficial (5,6).

Other Drugs

Drug reactions have increased in number and severity because of (i) the increased number and availability and use of prescription drugs; (ii) introduction of industrial drugs into the public environment; (iii) the increased number and availability of nonprescription drugs; (iv) the increased number and availability of illicit or street drugs; (v) the practice of the concept that if one drug works, then more than one is better; (vi) the practice of using drugs, singly or in combination, empirically or on a trial-and-error basis, to "see" if the drugs work; (vii) the practice of "covering" oneself by using drugs in questionable clinical settings; (viii) the notion that the use of drugs is better than not using drugs even when the indications for the drugs are not clear; (ix) the pressure from reimbursement agencies to approve on a basis of objective criteria for treatment such as drugs given rather than clinical judgement based on observation; and (x) the advertisement and promotion of pharmaceutical agents that overstate the efficacy and understate the toxicity of drugs.

Drugs are used excessively either singly or in combination. Polypharmacy has become a way of life for the American public. Physicians frequently prescribe multiple therapeutic agents simultaneously; even when a single drug is prescribed, the ingestion pattern of other drugs by a patient may vary. Over-the-counter preparations contain agents that influence the metabolism, absorption, and elimination of many drugs. Antihistamines and anticholinergic drugs are commonly used without prescription and knowledge by physician in combination with prescribed drugs. These agents produce a variety of central nervous system effects such as confusion, sedation, and delirium and of peripheral nervous system effects such as hypotension, constipation, urinary retention, and sweating (7–10).

A physician is naturally reluctant to think that his treatment contributes to a patient's disability, and thus adverse drug reactions are denied or minimized. There is a tendency to attribute new symptoms to the underlying disease rather than to occult drug toxicity. All too frequently, laboratory data or new symptoms that do not "fit" into the anticipated course of a disease are ignored. Life-threatening clinical situations often lead to the irrational use of drugs, and the urgency and hopelessness mask the effects of drug reactions.

Sound clinical and pharmacological knowledge are requisite to safe therapeutics. Knowledge of the pharmacology of the drug combined with its biochemistry is absolutely necessary to use drugs efficaciously and safely.

Unfortunately, drug treatment of any kind is often compromised by lack of full compliance by the patient. Common errors of compliance to a regimen by a patient may be of omission, purpose (taking drugs for the wrong reasons), dosage, timing or sequence, adding drugs not prescribed, or premature termination of drug therapy. Multiple drugs, frequent-dose regimens, and the physical features of the medication itself often foster poor compliance. Patients taking three or more drugs are less likely to use them as directed. Further, the more frequently a drug is directed to be taken, the less likely it will be taken as prescribed. Omission rates doubled when the number of drugs prescribed was increased from one to four, and doubled when the administration was increased from once daily to four times daily. Considerable confusion may also develop when multiple drugs of similar appearance are prescribed for the same patient.

Patients frequently discontinue drugs at the emergence of minor untoward effects. Because drug interactions increase as a function of the number of drugs prescribed, the compliance decreases with the addition of more drugs, even if the drugs are given to counteract other side effects from other drugs, such as anticholinergic drugs given for extrapyramidal effects. The consequences of noncompliance are often not fully appreciated by the physician. Overutilization of the prescribed drugs accounts for 65% of problems with compliance. Poor compliance leads to underutilization of the prescribed drug that deprives the patient of the intended therapeutic benefits. Thus, 75% of patients referred for evaluation of "refractoriness" of seizure control to phenytoin were found not to taking the drug as prescribed.

The pattern of drug use among alcoholics and drug addicts has paralleled the practice of polypharmacy among physicians. Eighty percent of alcoholics less than 30 years old are addicted to another drug in addition to alcohol. The drugs in order of decreasing frequency of use are marijuana, cocaine, sedatives/hypnotics (benzodiazepines, barbiturates), hallucinogens, and opiates. The practice by drug addicts of using more than two drugs concurrently is strikingly common and consistent. "Polypharmacy" by alcoholics and drug addicts is the rule rather than the exception. Because many of these patients come to the attention of various types of physicians, knowledge of drug interactions between drugs of addiction and prescribed

drugs is critical in understanding clinical responses to pharmacologic therapeutics.

Classifications of Drug Interactions: Pharmacokinetics and Pharmacodynamic Actions

The number of drugs presently known to be involved in drug interactions is
too large to hold in memory. Classification of interactions by pharmacological type, chemical nature of drugs, and the pharmacokinetics mechanism of
interaction provides a guide for application to the clinical setting. The pharmacological effect of a drug or its active metabolite is related to the free
concentration of the active drug at its receptor site. The receptor may be
intracellular or extracellular. The free concentration of drug or active metabolite is increased or decreased as a result of a variety of pharmacokinetics
and pharmacodynamic actions (2,3).

1. Direct chemical or physical interactions
2. Interactions in gastrointestinal absorption
3. Interactions from protein binding
4. Interactions at the receptor site
5. Interactions from accelerated metabolism
6. Drug interactions from inhibition of metabolism
7. Interactions from alteration in renal excretion
8. Interactions from alterations in pH or electrolyte concentrations (2,3)

Common Interactions Between Medical and Psychiatric Drugs

Psychiatric patients that receive psychotropic medications are relatively
evenly represented in all age groups. The various medical drugs are prescribed as indicated by medical conditions. Psychiatric patients tend to
be maintained acutely and chronically on combinations of psychiatric
drugs. The combinations of phenothiazine and anticholinergic drugs as well
as antidepressants and tranquilizer/sedative/hypnotic drugs are common.
Therefore, the interaction between psychiatric drugs is important to consider in addition to the interaction between medical and psychiatric drugs. The
emphasis of the following discussion is on the more common medical and
psychiatric drug interactions (11,12).

Antidepressants

The tricyclic antidepressants are involved in many clinically important drug
interactions. The tricyclic antidepressants bind to plasma albumin competitively with phenytoin, phenylbutazone, aspirin, aminopyrine, scopolamine,

and phenothiazine. When these drugs are given in combination, the blood level of the tricyclic antidepressants is increased to enhance the effects clinically, and especially the toxicity (13).

The cardiac effects of the antidepressants resemble those of quinidine and the phenothiazine; in intoxicated patients, sudden death from arrhythmias and congestive heart failure is frequent. Myocardial depression may be severe in patients with overdoses of tricyclic antidepressants; complete heart block may occur. The tricyclics have both direct and indirect effects on cardiovascular physiology. Because the adrenergic neuronal uptake of norepinephrine is impaired by the tricyclics, the sensitivity to adrenergic agents is increased. They are also alpha-blocking agents, and frequently cause postural hypotension in those individuals who have peripheral adrenergic dysfunction, such as the presence of another antiadrenergic drug or a drug that has similar actions.

The metabolic breakdown of the tricyclic drugs is impaired by neuroleptics, methylphenidate, and certain steroids, including hydrocortisone and oral contraceptives, resulting in an increase in the blood levels. The metabolic degradation is enhanced by barbiturates, other sedatives, and cigarettes, which induce the microsomal enzymes to lower the blood levels thereby reducing the clinical effects of the tricyclic antidepressants (11,12).

The sedative effects of the tricyclics potentiate other sedatives such as alcohol, barbiturates, and benzodiazepines. The anticholinergic activity of the tricyclics is additive with antiparkinsonism agents, other antimuscarinic compounds, antihistamines, and phenothiazine.

The tricyclic antidepressants act on mechanisms responsible for biogenic amines and other drugs that act via the biogenic amines. The tricyclics block the reuptake by the presynaptic neuron of norepinephrine, dopamine, and serotonin to enhance their effects at the postsynaptic site. The enhancing effects of tyramine are blocked because the tricyclics prevent its uptake into the presynaptic sites where the neurotransmitters are stored for release by tyramine into the synapse. Similarly, guanethidine is not taken up by the presynaptic neuron to inhibit the adrenergic effects. The tricyclic antidepressants inhibit the peripheral effects of amphetamines by the same mechanism. The central nervous system (CNS) effects of amphetamines are enhanced because the tricyclics do not interfere with the amphetamine-induced release of dopamine from the CNS neurons but inhibit the hepatic metabolism of the amphetamines (11,12).

The simultaneous administration of tricyclic antidepressants and monoamine oxidase (MAO) inhibitors is a particularly potentially dangerous practice that is to be avoided. The MAO inhibitors inhibit the enzyme monoamine oxidase, which degrades the biogenic amines in the presynaptic neuron. The result is an increase in the concentration of biogenic amines for release into the synapse. The action of the tricyclics to increase the level of biogenic amines at the postsynaptic site is potentiated by the greater available biogenic amines for release from MAO inhibition. The syndrome that results from the interaction of the two drugs is characterized by hyperpyrexia, convulsions, hypertension, and coma.

The MAO enzyme degrades the biogenic amines in the presynaptic neuron, and the MAO inhibitor prevents the degradation to increase the concentration of biogenic amines in the presynaptic neurons. Any drugs that promote the release of the biogenic amines from the presynaptic neuron will intensify the effects of the biogenic amines. Amphetamines and tyramine act to release the amines from storage sites in the nerve ending.

When the enzyme monoamine oxidase is inhibited, the biogenic amines are not being dominated for inactivation. The potential effects of the biogenic amines remain active although not clinically visible until provoked by another drug interaction. Administration of a precursor to a biogenic amine concurrently with MAO inhibitors may result in increased concentrations in the biogenic amines in the brain. Levodopa or 5-hydroxytryptamine increases levels of catecholamine to produce signs of CNS excitation in animals and man, with agitation and hypertension as common signs.

Hypertensive crisis is a most serious toxic effect of MAO inhibitors that results from interactions with other drugs. The amine tyramine acts to increase the release of catecholamine from the presynaptic storage sites. The combination of increased levels of catecholamine from MAO inhibition and their enhanced release through tyramine produces a marked rise in blood pressure and other cardiovascular changes. Headache, epistaxis, and cerebral hemorrhage have occurred during the hypertensive crisis. The same hypertensive reaction may occur with a combination of MAO inhibitors and sympathomimetic amines, such as methyldopa, dopamine, tricyclic antidepressants, reserpine, and guanethidine.

Tyramine is found in a variety of naturally occurring foods such as cheese, beer, wine, pickled herring, snails, chicken liver, coffee, citrus fruit, canned figs, broad beans, chocolate, and cream products. Patients should be given a list of foods to be avoided.

MAO inhibitors also interfere with detoxication mechanisms for other certain drugs. They prolong and intensify the effects of generalized depressants such as alcohol, anesthetics, sedatives, antihistamines, analgesics, anticholinergic agents, and antidepressants.

Lithium

Lithium is eliminated by the body by renal excretion. Approximately 95% of lithium is eliminated in the urine following a single dose, and urinary excretion of lithium increases with chronic administration. Reabsorption of lithium by the proximal convoluted tubule can be increased by diuretics that deplete sodium to lead to lithium retention, for example, furosemide, ethycrynic acid, and thiazides, because less sodium is available to compete with lithium for reabsorption by the tubule and subsequent increased lithium levels with toxicity. Renal excretion of lithium can be increased by administration of osmotic diuretics, acetazolamide, triamterene, phenothiazines, or aminophylline. Thiazide diuretics may correct the nephrogenic diabetes insipidus syndrome caused by lithium (14,15).

Lithium produces sedation in clinical doses in some patients; the effect is intensified by other sedatives and depressants such as alcohol, barbiturates, and benzodiazepines (16,17).

Neuroleptics

The phenothiazines, thioxanthenes, butyrophenones, and others, especially those of low potency, interact with a number of drugs to produce clinically important signs and symptoms (18,19).

The neuroleptics potentiate other CNS depressants, an effect that has been utilized in anesthesiology. Sedatives, hypnotics, antihistamines, anticholinergics, alcohol, and analgesics are among drugs that interact with the neuroleptics, particularly the low-potency and high-anticholinergic agents, to produce sedation and hypnosis. Respiratory depression from other drugs may be enhanced additively or synergistically by the neuroleptics; the phenothiazines, particularly, potentiate the CNS effects of barbiturates, alcohol, and narcotics (20).

The phenothiazines block the antihypertensive effect of guanethidine. Phenothiazines promote hypotension so that interaction with antihypertensive drugs is remarkable, although the effects of the combination are unpredictable (21).

Thioridazine may partially nullify the inotropic effect of digitalis by a quinidine-like action that itself may cause myocardial depression, decreased efficiency of repolarization, and increased risk of tachycardia and tachyrhythmia. The electrophysiological effects and the changes in cardiac electrolyte composition induced by phenothiazine resemble those produced by quinidine. The antimuscarinic effects of the phenothiazine produce a tachycardia that may oppose actions of beta blockers on the chronotropic action of the heart. The arrhythmia tends to be paroxysmal, resembling the arrhythmias induced by quinidine; in the periods of normal sinus rhythm intervening between runs of ventricular tachycardia, a prolonged Q-T interval be seen.

Drugs such as phenobarbital and other sedatives and anticonvulsants induce microsomal drug-metabolizing enzymes that increase the metabolism of the neuroleptic drugs in a clinically significant fashion that results in lowered blood levels for phenothiazines. Phenothiazine blood levels are increased when tricyclic antidepressants are given because of inhibition of their metabolism by the tricyclics. Conversely, the metabolic breakdown of tricyclic antidepressants is slowed to increase tricyclic blood levels when neuroleptics are given. Phenothiazine also enhance the clearance of phenobarbital. Phenothiazine blood levels are increased if given with estrogens. Phenothiazines may potentiate the effects of other neuroleptics, alpha-methyldopa, or thyroxine through their dopamine-blocking, L-adrenergic

antagonism and displacement of thyroxine from binding with thyroid globulin.

The anticholinergic effects of the low-potency neuroleptic drugs may interact additively with drugs that posses similar anticholinergic properties as
well as antagonistically with cholinergic agents such as physostigmine and
pilocarpine.

The extrapyramidal effects of phenothiazines and other classes of neuroleptics are antagonized by drugs that possess anticholinergic or dopaminergic actions. The dopaminergic blockade at dopamine receptors by the
neuroleptics is reversed by several dopamine agonists such as L-dopamine,
bromocriptine, and apomorphine. Anticholinergic drugs and dopamine
agonists are used to counteract the extrapyramidal effects of tremor, rigidity,
and dystonia more easily than others such as bradykinesia, akathisia, and
tardive dyskinesia. Severe extrapyramidal reactions and hypertensive crises
may be seen if phenothiazines are used in combination with MAO inhibitors.

Antiparkinsonian agents are often given during phenothiazine administration to prevent the appearance of the extrapyramidal signs. These combinations of anticholinergic and antihistamines with phenothiazines, thiothix-
enes, butyrophenones, and others may cause hyperpyrexia, the masking of
the appearance of tardive dyskinesia, and reduction in the effectiveness of
the phenothiazine. The combination of a phenothiazine with a tricyclic
antidepressant may not only cause but also mask tardive dyskinesia.

The seizure threshold is reduced by the neuroleptics so that the anticonvulsant effect of many of the anticonvulsants is antagonized. Caution is
suggested in the use of neuroleptic drugs in the presence of anticonvulsants
as the effect is relatively constant and consistent. These drugs are relatively
contraindicated in individuals with a seizure disorder or a tendency to have
seizures.

Benzodiazepines

The benzodiazepines, although classified as tranquilizers, are basically seda-
tive/hypnotic drugs that interact with other drugs similarly to those interactions with sedative/hypnotic drugs such as the barbiturates. The CNS depression produced by benzodiazepines is diffuse and additive, perhaps
synergistic when combined with other CNS depressants. Respiratory depression that is lethal can result from the interaction of benzodiazepines with
other depressants such as alcohol and barbiturates.

The ability of the benzodiazepines to induce hepatic metabolism does not
appear to be significant clinically. Most benzodiazepines raise the seizure
threshold in acute administration but lower it during the period of withdrawal after chronic use in any interval when the blood level declines significantly. This is a particular problem with the short-acting benzodiazepines
such as alprazolam.

Confusional states can occur because of the interaction between benzodiazepines and other drugs that adversely affect concentration and memory. Benzodiazepines reduce the attention span and recent memory in therapeutic doses when given alone so that the addition of any agent that also has these effects, augmenting the impairments in brain function (21–23).

Common Interactions Between Alcohol and Drugs

The sedative and depressant effects of alcohol on the CNS are additive and synergistic with other drugs. Those drugs, in particular, are sedatives/hypnotics, anticonvulsants, antidepressants, antianxiety drugs, and analgesic agents. The depressant effect of these drugs with alcohol produces impairment in mental and motor functions ranging from inattention, poor memory, mood disturbances, incoordination, ataxia, and lethargy to stupor and coma.

Some interesting and distressing effects of chronic alcohol use are the production of antagonism between hypertension and antihypertensive therapy. Regular alcohol use causes a sustained elevation in blood pressure in virtually anyone. The basis for the alcohol-induced hypertension is the discharge of the sympathetic nervous system during alcohol withdrawal. Alcohol withdrawal follows a declining blood alcohol level so that the blood pressure is elevated as often as alcohol is ingested. The result is that the need for antihypertensive medication is greater and the compliance is less in the setting of active and frequent alcohol consumption.

Gastrointestinal symptoms are quite common in regular alcohol use. Alcohol is irritating to the gastrointestinal mucosa, producing a chemical inflammation and ulceration, particularly after chronic use. Alcohol effects on the gastrointestinal tract are counter to therapies that are aimed at relieving the effects on inflamed and ulcerated mucosa from any cause (24).

Unusual side effects are unpleasant reactions to the combination of alcohol and oral hypoglycemic agents, metronidazole, or cephalosporins that are similar to a disulfiram reaction. A disulfiram reaction includes nausea, vomiting, headache, lightheadedness, hypotension, and malaise. The combination of oral hypoglycemics and insulin with alcohol is to intensify the hypoglycemic effect because alcohol produces hypoglycemia by itself. Alcohol can also interfere with the therapeutic actions of a wide variety of drugs by altering their metabolism, usually increasing the metabolic rate.

Cannabis is an hallucinogen that has properties that are similar to alcohol and cocaine as well as psychiatric symptoms for which psychotropic drugs are given. Cannabis produces sedation, depression of mental and motor function, hypotension, illusions of space and time, and intense anxiety as in generalized anxiety and panic attacks, paranoid thinking, and depression of mood. These effects mimic psychiatric signs and symptoms, and may either aggravate underlying psychiatric illness or produce new psychiatric symptoms that neutralize the therapeutic effects of psychotropic medications.

Furthermore, other untoward effects of therapeutic drugs are intensified by the effects of cannabis listed previously and by interactions with cannabis (25).

Cocaine potentiates the responses of sympathetically innervated organs that are stimulated by norepinephrine and epinephrine. Cocaine blocks the reuptake of catecholamines at adrenergic nerve endings that enhance nerve transmission in the synapse by intensifying the catecholamine effect. Through this mechanism as well as its local anesthetic action on nerve transmission, cocaine produces a variety of signs and symptoms that are similar to psychiatric illness and untoward effects from other drugs. There are many drug interactions of cocaine and psychotropic and medical drugs. Cocaine produces euphoria, anxiety, hyperactive behavior, hallucinations and delusions, hypertension, tachycardia, anorexia during intoxication, and depression, hyperphagia, somnolence, and anxiety during withdrawal. These effects worsen similar symptoms already present or counter therapeutic agents such as antidepressants, antipsychotics, and antihypertensives that are intended to treat these symptoms (26).

Phencyclidine (PCP) produces many effects that are similar to those of alcohol, cannabis, and cocaine. The sedation, anxiety, depression, euphoria, hallucinations, delusions, hypertension, increased motor strength and activity, violent and irrational, even suicidal, behavior are indistinguishable from the psychiatric syndromes. Any psychotropic or medical drug given must take into account the wide and dramatic effects and potential interactions with PCP.

Opiate effects may be exaggerated and prolonged by phenothiazines, MAO inhibitors, and tricyclic antidepressants. The respiratory depressant, sedative, hypotensive, and analgesic effects of the opiates are enhanced by the phenothiazines and tricyclics.

References

1. Karch FE, Lasagna L (1975). Adverse Drug Reactions: A critical review. *JAMA* 234:1236–1241.
2. Mangini RJ, ed. (1985). *Drug Interactions: Facts and Comparisons* St. Louis: Lippincott.
3. Murad F, Gilman AG (1985). Drug interactions (Appendix III). In *The Pharmacological Basis of Therapeutics*, 7th Ed., Gilman AG, Goodman LS, Rail TW, Murad F, eds., pp. 1734–1750. New York: Macmillan.
4. Venning GR (1983). Identification of adverse reactions to new drugs. *Br Med J* 286:199–547.
5. Gram LF, Christiansen J, Overo KF (1973). Pharmacokinetic interaction between tricyclic antidepressants and other pharmaca. *Acta Psychiatr Scand (Suppl.)* 243:52–53.
6. Morselli PL (1977). Psychotropic drugs. In *Drug Disposition During Development*, Morselli PL, ed., pp. 431–474. New York: Spectrum Publications.
7. Linnoila JF, George L, Guthrie S (1982). Interaction between antidepressants and prephanazine in psychiatric patients. *Am J Psychiatry* 139:132–1331.

8. Sepala T, Linnoila M, Elonen E, Mattila MJ, Maci M (1975). Effect of tricyclic antidepressants and alcohol on psychomotor skills related to driving *Clin Pharmacol Ther* 17:515–522.
9. Sulser F, Robinson SE (1978). Clinical implications of pharmacological differences among antipsychotic drugs. In *Psychopharmacology: A Generation of Progress*, Lipton MA, DiMascio A, Killarm KD, eds., pp. 943–954. New York: Raven Press.
10. White K, Simpson G (1981). Combined MAO-tricyclic antidepressant treatment: A reevaluation. *J Clin Psychopharmacol* I:264–282.
11. Kaufman JS (1976). Drug interactions involving psychotherapeutic agents. In *Drug Treatment of Mental Disorders*, Simpson LL, ed., pp. 289–309. New York: Raven Press.
12. Ayd FJ, Jr., Bacwell B, eds., (1970). *Discoveries in Biological Psychiatry*. Philadelphia: Lippincott.
13. Folks DG (1983). Monoamine oxidase inhibitors: Reappraisal of dietary considerations *J Clin Psychopharmacol* 3:249–252.
14. Himmelhock JM, Poust RI, Mallinger AG (1977). Adjustment of lithium dose during lithium—chlorothiazide therapy. *Clin Psychopharmacol Ther* 22:225–227.
15. Depaulo JR, Jr., Correa EI, Sapir DG (1981). Renal toxicity of lithium and its implications. *John Hopkins Med J* 149:15–21.
16. Tupin JP, Schuller AB (1978). Lithium and haloperidol incompatibility reviewed. *Psychiatr J Univ Ottawa* 3:245–231.
17. Johnson FN, Johnson S (1978). *Lithium in Medical Practice*. Baltimore: University Park Press.
18. Shader RI, DiMascio A (1970). *Psychotropic Drug Side Effects: Chemical and Theoretical Perspectives*. Baltimore: Williams & Wilkins.
19. Sakalis G, Curry SH, Mould GP, Lader MH (1972). Physiologic and clinical effects of chlorpromazine and their relationship to plasma level. *Clin Pharmacol Ther* 13:931–946.
20. Loga S, Curry S, Lader M (1975). Interactions of orphenadrine and phenobarbitone with chlorpromazine: Plasma concentrations and effects in main. *Br J Clin Pharmacol* 2:197–208.
21. Marden CD, Tarsy D, Baldessarini RJ (1975). Spontaneous and drug-induced movement disorders in psychiatric patients. In *Psychiatric Aspects of Neurologic Disease*, Benson DF, Blumer D, eds., pp. 219–265. New York: Grune and Stratton.
22. Greenblatt DJ, Divoll M, Abernathy DR, Ochs HR, Shader RI (1983). Clinical pharmacokinetics of the newer benzodiazepines. *Clin Pharmacokinet* 8:233–252.
23. Greenblatt DJ, Sader RI, Abernathy DR (1983). Current status of benzodiazepines. *N Engl J Med* 309:354–358, 410–416.
24. Miller NS, Gold MS, Cocores JA, Pottash AC (1988). Alcohol dependence and its medical consequences. *NY State J Med* 88(9):476–481.
25. Miller NS, Gold MS, Millman RB (1989). Cocaine. *Am Fam Physician* 39(2):115–120.
26. Miller NS, Gold MS (1989) The diagnosis of marijuana (cannabis) dependence. *J Subst Abuse Treat* 6:183–192.

CHAPTER 24

The Pharmacology of Drug Testing: Indications and Methodology

History

The use of drug testing in the interest of health care has its roots in the occupational medicine movement. As early as 1916, medical departments began to be established in U.S. industry, leading to the formation of the American Association of Industrial Physicians and Surgeons. More recently, there has been an Employee Assistance Programs (EAP) movement among employees in U.S. industry (now known as AOMA—American Occupational Medication Association). This movement has led to the development of programs designed to assist the employee with a drug problem before more punitive action, such as termination, is considered.

Several factors have fueled the increasing interest in drug testing in this country. Of primary importance are well-documented epidemics of drug use, which are creating crises of a national and international magnitude. In addition, drug testing has been recognized as playing an important role in forensic techniques as well as in the Occupational Safety and Health Act of 1970 (OSHA). Finally, economic pressures stemming from increased competition to U.S. industry from foreign countries have increased interest in attacking drug use in the workplace in an effort to improve the quality and productivity of U.S. workers (1).

Today, government agencies, private corporations, amateur and professional bodies, and other organizations responsible for safety and performance are employing drug testing. Opponents of the practice are defending the rights and civil liberties of the individual, and it is likely that ongoing debates and controversy will continue regarding protection of the legal rights of those who use drugs, the safety and health needs of the individual, and the legalities of assuring the rights of those who are adversely affected by the user of drugs.

Drug testing is legal when both parties involved in the drug testing agree that it is within the constitutional rights of the individual. In practice, drug testing can be performed any time there is a contract between the tester and the person being tested. Legal contention may result when such agreement does not exist and drug testing is either required or imposed. Meanwhile, with all its attendant risks and benefits, drug testing is likely to remain and almost certainly increase in use as an effective tool in health and industry.

Curiously, medicine as a profession has been slow to capitalize on the assets of drug testing despite the fact that laboratory testing is already an indispensable part of clinical practice. In other areas of medicine, physicians tend to favor and readily adopt testing procedures designed to improve diagnosis and monitor response to treatment. One reason drug testing has not "caught on" in medicine is linked to the nature of drug and alcohol abuse and addiction. When there is a need to diagnose a drug problem, efforts to obtain history and documentation often do not include the efficacious use of drug testing. In general, physicians rely on patient cooperation and compliance for the testing procedures they order for diagnosis and treatment. Unfortunately, however, drug use, abuse, and addiction are conditions that possess inherent denial and resistance to their detection and modification in a clinical setting (2).

Unfortunately, drug use, abuse, and dependence do not fit the medical model. Drug dependence, particularly, is viewed as a personal preference or lifestyle that is under the control of the individual and not as an illness to be treated by medical practice. Physicians are powerful forces in the lives of those who are afflicted with drug and alcohol problems and, consequently, have a dramatic impact on the course of a drug problem. Most drug users and dependents are seen by a physician at some point in their drug use for drug-related or coincidental health problems. A thorough history and examination for drug and alcohol use would yield enormous benefits for the patients and ultimately satisfaction for the physician. Drug testing may be an integral part of that evaluation just as a complete blood count (CBC), chest x ray, or electrocardiogram (EKG) is for other conditions (3).

Diagnosis

The principal indications for drug testing in current practice are (i) evaluation of a new patient, especially when the clinical picture suggests drug use; (ii) evaluation of all adolescents, especially those with behavioral problems; (iii) evaluation of all high-risk patients (e.g., those with relatively greater exposure and access to drugs; (iv) evaluation of all new patients with acute and chronic syndromes, especially when the presentation is atypical or there is a failure to respond to treatment; (v) evaluation of an unexpected or unexplained mental state or performance change; (vi) monitoring response to inpatient and outpatient treatment for drug and alcohol addiction and other psychiatric illness; and (vii) employment monitoring when an agreement exists between employers and employees (Table 24.1).

The need for drug testing is underscored by statistics that indicate that drug use, particularly illicit use, is widespread. In a large drug screening in the U.S. government, one in six members of the federal work force were

TABLE 24.1. Spectrum of possible psychiatric presentations resulting from certain drugs of abuse.

Drug	Anorexia nervosa	Schizophrenia	Acute psychosis	Major depression	Manic depression	Personality changes	Organic brain syndrome	Panic anxiety disorder	Other
Alcohol	+	+	+	+	+	+	+	+	+
PCP[a]	+	+	+	+	+	+	+	+	+
Toluene	+			+		+		+	
Marijuana		+	+	+		+		+	
Amphetamine	+	+	+	+	+	+		+	
Cocaine	+		+	+	+	+		+	
Sedatives/hypnotics			+	+		+	+	+	
Heroin				+		+	+	+	
Methadone				+		+		+	

[a]PCP, Phencyclidine.

found to use illicit drugs regularly, and 44% of all new employees screened had used drugs such as marijuana and cocaine within the previous year. In another large-scale drug screening, one-third of applicants to the New York Transit Authority had positive tests for drugs in their urine during preemployment evaluation. A spot check of U.S. Navy personnel in San Diego, California, and Portsmouth, New Hampshire, in 1983 revealed 47% were smoking marijuana. This figure is now down to 2% after widespread adoption of drug-screening programs (1).

In most instances, the five major drugs of interest in drug testing are marijuana, cocaine, amphetamines, opiates, and phencyclidine (PCP), although screening for other drugs may be indicated. Polydrug use, abuse, and addiction are the rule. For example, as many as 80% of alcoholics under the age of 30 use another drug in addition to alcohol, most commonly marijuana, followed by cocaine and PCP. A little known fact is that 98% of all cocaine addicts have used marijuana, and from 50% to 75% of opiate users have used or are using marijuana, benzodiazepines, and cocaine. Furthermore, 90% of Americans have at least tried alcohol, and from 10% to 20% or more have a problem with alcohol. Twenty-five million people have at least tried cocaine, 5 to 6 million use it regularly, and 12 to 13 million use it once a year (4,5). The need for drug screening extends beyond illicit drugs to legal prescription medications, as 81 million prescriptions were filled in 1985 for benzodiazepines. According to the 1985 Drug Abuse Warning Network (DAWN) reports, benzodiazepines were "mentioned" in 18,492 emergency room (ER) visits, morphine and heroin in 14,696 ER visits, and cocaine in 13,501 ER visits (6). These ER visits were for a variety of reasons pertaining to medical and psychiatric problems directly or indirectly related to the drug use.

In the national household study done by the National Institute for Drug Abuse (NIDA) in 1985, the lifetime prevalence of use by individuals 18 to 25 years old was 60% for marijuana, 11.5% for hallucinogens, 17.3% for stimulants, 11.0% for sedatives, 12.2% for tranquilizers, 11.4% for analgesics, and 1.2% for heroin (6). This prevalence rate indicates that nearly half the U.S. population has used marijuana and substantial numbers have used other drugs. From these statistics alone, it is evident that drug use is no longer the providence of the less fortunate or "the other guy." Convenient cliches and stereotypes cannot be used to explain drug use, as drugs are used by many individuals in all walks of life (7). It is a pervasive practice with adverse consequences affecting almost everyone.

Intoxication

Drug and alcohol use can induce virtually any psychiatric symptom or syndrome as well as many medical symptoms and syndromes that are indistinguishable from the idiopathic form. The severity of the alcohol- and drug-induced psychopathology may range from mild anxiety and sadness to frank mania and delirium, and there are many variations between these two extremes. Because the symptoms and syndromes caused by drugs and alcohol are frequently indistinguishable from those with other etiologies, it is important to identify drugs and alcohol in the history or confirm their presence by drug testing.

Some of the major psychiatric syndromes induced by drugs and alcohol are mania, depression, anxiety disorders, personality disorders, schizophrenia, eating disorders, and delirium and dementia (organic mental disorders). Some of the major medical syndromes are gastrointestinal, cardiovascular, endocrinological, traumatic, rheumatological, and dermatological in origin. These conditions may be induced either during the period of drug intoxication and/or withdrawal, depending on the particular drug action (8–15).

Cocaine, for instance, causes mania, personality disturbances, hypertension, cardiac arrhythmias, anorexia, and self-inflicted excoriating lesions of the skin during intoxication. During withdrawal, it induces severe depression with suicidal thinking, hyperphagia, and hypersomnia. PCP intoxication produces mania, personality disturbances with violent outbursts, hypertension, cardiac arrhythmias, and vivid visual and auditory hallucinations, whereas the withdrawal is characterized by impulsivity, poor judgment, and depression with suicidal thoughts. Heroin use may be associated with endocarditis, arthritis, acquired immune deficiency syndrome (AIDS), and other consequences of intravenous drug use. The practice of inhalation of organic solvents, such as glues, aerosols, and gasoline, produces organic brain syndromes, such as delirium and dementia, cardiac arrhythmias, and hepatocellular damage (5,16–19) all of which may or may not be reversible (see Table 24.1). Marijuana has many effects on brain and behavior that typically include anxiety, depression, poor concentration and memory loss, hallucinations, paranoid ideation and delusions, poor motivation, and a general deterioration in personality.

The diagnosis of a drug or alcohol problem is greatly enhanced by drug testing, especially when the clinical picture suggests the presence of abuse, addiction, tolerance, and dependence. Furthermore, it is important that the physician know the definitions of these terms to adequately diagnosis and describe drug problems as well as to use drug testing effectively and efficiently (3).

For example, recreational use of drugs is for relationships or to complement a social or recreational event. In contrast, drug or alcohol "abuse" is defined as use outside of an accepted norm or standard of use for a particular society. This can include transient impairments from abnormal use of a drug or alcohol. However, when the drug becomes the center of attention or priority for the user, the term that applies is addiction rather than abuse. Addiction is defined as preoccupation with the acquisition of drugs, compulsive use in spite of adverse consequences, recurrent use, and inability to control or reduce the use effectively, resulting in a pattern of recurrent use or relapse after abstinence. The behaviors of addiction are universal; they transcend norms or standards of use and are not dependent on the characteristics of a particular drug (20).

The development of tolerance is the need to increase a dose of a drug to maintain the same effect or the loss of a drug to maintain the same effect or the loss of an effect at a constant dose of a drug. Pharmacological dependence occurs when stopping the drug results in predictable signs and symptoms, depending on the particular drug. Characteristically, the signs and symptoms or withdrawal are suppressed by the drug (20) when it is given in sufficient doses at an appropriate time during withdrawal.

Contrary to popular notion, tolerance and dependence are not specific for addiction. While dependence (addiction) is frequently accompanied by tolerance and dependence, these may and frequently do occur without the development of dependence (addiction). For instance, opiate analgesics are used in the treatment of acute pain with subsequent rapid development of tolerance and the onset of a predictable withdrawal syndrome on cessation of use, but frequently without preoccupation, compulsive use, and relapse to opiate use. Predictably, tolerance and dependence are necessary adaptations of the brain to regular use of drug in response to the presence of the drug. Because dependent use is frequently repetitive, pharmacological tolerance and dependence readily occur in the dependence (addiction) syndrome (21). Also, the detection of tolerance may be impeded by denial of use (common in addiction) and by subtle, insidious onset of tolerance, such as is true of alcohol (Table 24.2).

To successfully diagnose drug addiction, it is important to recognize and circumvent these obstacles to the clinical diagnosis. Denial, rationalization, and minimization by users and others, lack of skill and knowledge in diagnosis elements of abuse/addiction/tolerance/dependence, lack of awareness that effective treatments for drug and alcohol addiction do exist and are available, and an increasing lack of reimbursement for drug and alcohol

TABLE 24.2. Definitions of diagnostic terms for abnormal alcohol and drug use.

Abuse
Use outside the accepted norm
Abnormal use
Not addiction
Dependence (addiction)
Preoccupation with acquisition of alcohol/drugs
Compulsive use in spite of adverse consequences
Recurrent pattern of use/relapse
Tolerance
Need to increase dose of drug to achieve same effect
Loss of effect from drug at a particular dose
Pharmacological dependence
Stereotypic set of signs and symptoms of cessation of use of drug
Drug will abort its withdrawal symptoms

problems are some of the reasons for low diagnosis of drug addiction. Drug testing is an aid to reduce these obstacles by providing documentation and confirmation of drug use and addiction (22–24) in spite of odds against identification.

Pharmacokinetics

Sensitivity and Specificity

The sensitivity and specificity of the method for drug testing determine greatly the utility of the test. Sensitivity is the ability to detect the presence of the drug at low levels, while specificity is the degree of accuracy in detecting only the drug desired. It is important to note that the test methods used for drug testing vary greatly in their sensitivity and specificity. Unfortunately, many physicians who use and interpret drug testing are unaware that some of the laboratory tests used most frequently tend to be low in both sensitivity and specificity. Thin-layer chromatography (TLC) has both low sensitivity and specificity; enzyme immunoassay (EIA) has high sensitivity but less specificity. Moreover, some tests yield only qualitative information detecting the presence of the drug without reliably measuring the quantity of the drug. Quantitative tests, in contrast, give information on the amount of the drug that is present in body fluids, which is important in differentiating low levels of drugs that persist for prolonged periods from higher levels in recent use (2,8,22). For instance, a steadily declining urine level of cannabinoid metabolites followed by an abrupt significant rise in the metabolites indicates recent use of marijuana (Table 24.3).

Source of Specimen

The target of the methodology in drug testing is measuring either the parent drug or its metabolite or both. Although urine and blood may both be assayed, it is important to know that urine contains 1000 times more drug

TABLE 24.3. Sensitivities of urine drug testing methodologies (ng/ml).

	TLC[a]	EMIT	GC/MS
Amphetamines	2000	300	25
Barbiturates	2000	300	50
Benzodiazepines	–	1000	50
(Cocaine) BE	2000	75–300	20
Marijuana/THC	20-SP	20–100	20
(Opiates)(morphine)	2000	300	20
PCP	–	75	20

[a]Abbreviations: TLC, thin-layer chromatography; EMIT, Enzyme Multiplied Immunoassay Technique; GC/MS, gas chromatography/mass spectrometry; BE, benzoylecognine; PCP, phencyclidine; SP, special procedure, not detected by routine TLC.

than blood, and therefore is preferable as the source to examine in most instances. However, examination of blood is useful in identifying recent use, as detection indicates that the drug has been ingested close in time to sampling so that biotransformation and elimination from the blood have not yet occurred. For example, cocaine is detectable in blood for only a number of hours, but by certain methods it can be detected for days in the metabolite form. In addition, the drug screens for various laboratories vary in the number and types of drugs that are assayed and the methodologies of tests employed. Usually, a clinician must specify the drugs of interest or at least be aware of the type of tests performed by the laboratory. Otherwise, only those drugs deemed routine by the laboratory will be done (2,8,22) and only according to their selected methodologies.

Elimination Time

Elimination time is an important factor in clinical interpretation of results of drug testing. For any given test, it is important to know how long a result is likely to be positive in relation to the time of last use of the drug. Some drugs have a relatively long elimination time, especially if the metabolite is also identifiable; that is, marijuana itself is detectable for days while its metabolites, δ-9-THC (tetrahydrocannabinol) and 11-*nor*-δ-THC-9-carboxylic acid (THCA), are detectable for weeks by certain methods. Even short-acting drugs like cocaine can be identified by the presence of their metabolites for prolonged periods after the parent drug has been cleared; that is, cocaine is 98% eliminated from the blood in 5 hours, while its metabolite, benzoylecognine (BE), is detectable for 2 to 4 days. It is critical that the test for a drug be ordered sufficiently close in time to the drug ingestion so as to be able to detect it by any method (2,8). A commonly used drug, alcohol, is metabolized rapidly so that blood and urine are positive for only hours after last use. Alcohol's metabolites are too common to the body and efficiently utilized in endogenous biochemical pathways to be reliably measured, for example, acetic acid (Table 24.4).

Cutoff Levels

The cutoff value reflects the level of the sensitivity of the drug test. It determines whether a test is reported as positive or negative by the laboratory, and depends on the capability of the methodology as well as the needs of the clinician. The cutoff value is ordinarily selected by the laboratory but can be specified by the physician, according to the clinical indications for drug testing. Frequently the level is set high to avoid false-positives and litigation. This is sometimes overly defensive, however, as valid and reliable results are obtainable if a lower or more sensitive cutoff value is use. It is important to emphasize that the physician can order whatever cutoff value is needed or desired, but the value may need to be specified by the laboratory. For instance, a cutoff value for cannabinoids of 100 ng/ml will miss many

TABLE 24.4. Temporal profile of drugs identified by drug testing.

Alcohol — hours
Cocaine — hours, days
Marijuana — weeks, months
Benzodiazepines — weeks, months
Opiates — days, weeks
Barbiturates — weeks, months
PCP[a] — weeks, months
Obstacles to clinical diagnosis
   Denial, rationalization, and minimization by users and others
   Lack of skill and knowledge in diagnosing elements of abuse/addiction/tolerance/depen-
   dence
   Lack of knowledge of effective treatments available for drug and alcohol addiction
   Lack of reimbursement for drug and alcohol problems

[a]PCP, phencyclidine.

significantly positive samples that would be detected by a cutoff value of 20 ng/ml (2,8) (Table 24.5).

False-Positives and -Negatives

The meaning of false-positive or false-negative results is important to understand for proper interpretation of the report. A "false-negative" result is a negative result from the method when the drug is actually present but not

TABLE 24.5. Testing parameters for individual drugs.

Drug	Half-life (hr)	EMIT cutoff (mg/ml)[a]	GC/MS cutoff (ng/ml)	Detectability range (days)
Amphetamines	10–15	300	100	1–2
Barbiturates				
SH	20–30	300	100	3–5
L	48–96	–	–	10–14
Diazepam	20–35	300	–	2–4
Benzodiazepines–Nordiaz	50–90	300	100	7–9
Cocaine				
C	0.8–1.5	–	–	0.2–0.5
BE[a]	–	300[a]	50	2–4
Methaqualone	20–60	300	50	7–14
Opiates–codeine–morphine	2–4	300	100	1–2
Phencyclidine (PCP)	7–16	75	10	2–8
Cannabinoids	10–402	20–100	10	2–8 (acute) 14–42 (chronic)

[a]Abbreviations: EMIT, Enzyme Multiplied Immunoassay Technique; GC/MS, gas chromatography/mass spectrometry.

detected in the sample. A "false-positive" result is the positive result from the method when the drug is not actually present but detected in the sample. Contrary to popular belief, false-negative results are far more common than false-positive results in clinical practice. A study done by the Centers for Disease Control (CDC) found that 75% of the participating labs reported false-negatives on a urine specimen containing 4000 ng/mL of the cocaine metabolite BE, a value far above concentrations that are evident clinically in usual states of use at the time of detection by most laboratories by usual methods. Another survey by the CDC confirmed that high rate of false-negative results by finding that 91% of the labs had unacceptable false-negative rates for cocaine and BE. Also, most clinicians are not aware that marijuana, PCP, LSD, and other commonly used or abused illicit drugs are not identified at all in most TLC systems, which are still used by many laboratories. False-positive results are very unusual but should be confirmed routinely by laboratories with a more sensitive and specific test such as gas chromatography/mass spectrometry (GC/MS) (25,26) (Table 24.6).

The confusion rising from the use of drug testing may arise in part from such variables. These variables in drug testing are frequently not sufficiently appreciated by most clinicians who rely on laboratory testing in clinical practice in addition to the myriad of clinical variables. Further, detectability of a drug depends on the type of drug, size of the dose, frequency of use, the route of administration, and individual variation in drug metabolism. In turn, these variables are dependent on the time of the last dose, the sample collection method, and the sensitivity and specificity of the analytical method used for drug testing.

TABLE 24.6. Limits of sensitivity for tests used in drug testing.

Detection	Sensitivity	
	Ranges (ng/ml)	Cost/sample range ($)
Chromatographic		
TLC[a]	1000–2000	3–10
GLC	10–300	20–40
HPLC	20–300	40–60
GC/MS	5–100	40–100
Immunological		
EIA	300–1000	2–6
RIA	2–20	2–10

[a]Abbreviations: TLC, thin-layer chromatography; GLC, gas–liquid chromatography; HPLC, high-pressure liquid chromatography; GC/MS, gas chromatography/mass spectrometry; EIA, enzyme immunoassay; RIA, radioimmunoassay.

Methodologies

Methods

The analytical methods available for drug testing are of two basic types, chromatographic and competitive binding/immunoreactive. Chromatographic techniques include thin-layer chromatography (TLC), gas-liquid chromatography (GLC), high-pressure liquid chromatography (HPLC), and combined gas chromatography/mass spectrometry (GC/MS); competitive binding/immunoreactive techniques are radioimmunoassay (RIA) and enzyme immunoassay (EIA) (2,8,22).

TLC

TLC is reserved mainly for detecting toxic ranges of only a few selected drugs in drug screening. Although it is relatively fast and inexpensive, an experienced technician is required to process and interpret the TLC plates. Further, TLC is a qualitative test; it yields only a positive or negative result without a quantitative measurement of the amount of drug present. Its main drawbacks, however, are its low sensitivity and low specificity. The minimum amount of drug or metabolite necessary to yield a positive result is 1000 to 2000 ng/mL, which is very large in comparison to other methods (see Table 24.3).

TLC relies on a reproducible migration pattern by the drug on a thin layer of absorbent (e.g., a silica-coated glass plate). Characterization of a particular drug is achieved by color reactions produced by spraying the plate with color-complexing reagents. The method was originally designed to detect very high-dose, recent drug use or toxic blood levels from a number of drugs used simultaneously. It is a reasonable test in an emergency room, where the drugs taken are unknown and there is a need for quick determination of toxic levels (2,8).

TLC should be ordered with extreme caution and interpreted with suspicion, as lower levels of drugs are not detected by this method, nor are TLC screens generally admissible as forensic evidence. Negative results for cocaine and other drugs are meaningless by the TLC method, and positive results should be confirmed by a second, more specific method because of the low specificity and sensitivity of TLC (2,8) (see Table 24.6).

GLC

GLC is an analytical method that separates molecules by use of a glass or metal tube that is packaged with material of a particular polarity. The sample of drug is vaporized at the injection site and carried through the column by a steady flow of gas. The column terminates at a detector that permits recording and quantification. The time to pass through a column is the retention time, and each drug has a particular retention time for a given column.

HPLC

HPLC is similar to GLC but uses a liquid rather than a gas to propel the sample through the column. Some drug classes are better chromatographed on HPLC (i.e., tricyclic antidepressants and benzodiazepines), while other drugs are better detected with GLC, so that the two methods are complementary in a given laboratory. It is important to know that GLC and HPLC are significantly more specific and sensitive than TLC. However, these methods require extraction, derivation, column separation, and detection, all of which increase the time for testing (2,8) (see Table 24.6).

GC/MS

GC/MS is the ultimate laboratory method of detection. It analyzes a given drug according to a fragmentation pattern that is specific for that particular drug. The fragmentation pattern is produced by the breaking of weaker bonds of the drug molecules under stress. A perfect match with a fragmentation pattern in a computer library is considered an absolute confirmation of the drug, and is referred to as "fingerprinting" of the molecules. The range of sensitivity of the method is less than 50 ng/ml, or 100 to 1000 times more sensitive and far more specific than the TLC system. Common drugs of abuse and addiction are readily identified in small amounts (i.e., marijuana, cocaine, heroin). The expenses of the technique make GC/MS impractical for screening but vital for confirmation of drug presence and identity (2,8) (see Table 24.6).

RIA and EIA

RIA and EIA are immunological methods that employ antibodies against the specific drugs or competing drug molecules or enzymes, which are labeled with a radioactive tracer. Because the antibody sites are limited, the number of radioactively tagged molecules displaced is used to calculate the amount of unlabeled drug in the mixture. The principal drawback of the immunological method is the cross-reactivity of parent drugs and metabolites with the antibodies, which in reality is low. Although the cross-reactivity may produce a false-positive reaction, the result can be and should be confirmed by the more specific method, GC/MS. Because the sensitivity is high and the specificity still reasonably high, the EIA and RIA are commonly employed as screening techniques. The Enzyme Multiplied Immunoassay Technique (EMIT, trademark of SYVA Co.) is the test most widely used for marijuana. In general, the EIA system is very popular because it does not require timely extraction and centrifugation procedures. It lends itself to automation and is considerably less expensive than most other methods.

GC/MS, GLC, HPLC, and some RIA methodologies may be applied to all bodily fluids, including serum. Because blood levels are better indicators of recent use, it is sometimes important to obtain a blood level in evaluating a clinical state of intoxication. In contrast, RIA, EIA, and TLC are not ordinarily designed to detect drug levels in the blood, but are used in analyzing urine (2,8,25) (see Table 24.6).

Intervention and Treatment

It cannot be overemphasized that it is essential that all urine specimens be collected under direct supervision, including witnessing micturition. An unsupervised urine sample is always suspect, as urine samples can be substituted, contaminated, and adulterated easily, even by novices. Testing supposedly recently voided urine for basal body temperature may obviate the need for supervision in the future, but for now, testing should be supervised. A first-void urine (ie., the first urination in the morning) has the highest concentration of drug with the highest specific gravity (to detect dilution of urine), and it will therefore have the greatest likelihood for detection. The drugs of interest and the type of methodology for drug testing need to be specified, and the cutoff value for the sensitivity selected or at least known. Urine and blood samples when indicated, should be ordered for the following conditions: (i) for diagnosis, particularly for a differential diagnosis in atypical cases; and (ii) to monitor treatment progress on an inpatient or outpatient basis. For example, urine screens may be done several times a week. Drug testing during treatment acts as a deterrent to drug use and helps to identify reasons for those who relapse (27–29) (see Table 24.4).

The "office" testing procedure with the fastest turnaround and adequate accuracy is the EIA. Many offices, clinics, and even employers have the equipment and personnel to rapidly test urine samples. "Dipstick" testing offers no advantages and many disadvantages with false-positives and false-negatives. Office testing is comprised by laboratory turnaround. A test that is delivered to a good lab in the early evening should be reported to the physician the next morning by EIA or RIA even if GC/MS confirmation is pending. Labs are certified by CDC or National Pathology organizations (CAP), or, more recently for drug testing, by the National Institute on Drug Abuse (NIDA). We recommend knowing the laboratory to which you send your patient (i.e., patient samples) — its certification, quality assurance programs, and proficiency testing. We also recommend a visit to the lab if at all possible.

An illustrative example of how clinical testing can be useful is seen in the treatment of cocaine addiction. Cocaine is a commonly used drug, and its use is often denied by the users. Relapse to cocaine is high even in treatment programs, and the physician can use drug testing rather than self-reports to monitor response to treatment. For example, cocaine and its metabolite BE are detectable by TLC in the urine for only about 12 to 20 hours after cocaine is last used; by EIA, to 48 hours; by RIA, to 3–4 days; and by GC/MS, to 7–8 days after last use. It is important to know the clinical history of last use in relation to the time of collection, as well as whether the collection of the sample was supervised. This information is used in conjunction with cutoff value in order to interpret the results of the drug testing (2,8,24) (see Table 24.4).

The treatment of the drug- or alcohol-using patient requires a certain level of mutual trust. Drug testing simplifies the physician–patient relationship by taking drug use and detective-like interrogation out of the therapy. Urine is routinely taken, and consequences of positives follow. Urine testing should be expected as a part of treatment and, ideally, as a condition of treatment.

In conclusion, laboratory testing can aid a clinician in making a differential diagnosis and eliminating drugs from active consideration as a cause of psychiatric symptoms. Testing of blood is useful in forensic and diagnostic questions when the clinician needs to know what drug or drugs the person was influenced by at the time (and hours before) relative to the mental status exam (change in behavior, accident, etc.). It is also useful in treatment planning and monitoring response to treatment in both in patient and outpatient settings. In occupational settings, drug testing can be used as an early indication that a problem exists and also as a successful prevention tool. It is important that the physician have an understanding of available test methodologies, including their advantages and limitations, to use drug testing effectively and efficiently in clinical practice.

References

1. Pottash ALC, Gold MS, Extein I (1982). The use of the clinical laboratory. In *Inpatient Psychiatry: Diagnosis and Treatment*, Sederer LI, ed. Baltimore: Williams & Wilkins.
2. Gold MS, Dackis CA (1986). Role of the laboratory in the evaluation of suspected drug abuse. *J Clin Psychiatry* 47(Suppl):17–23.
3. Miller NS, Gold MS (1987). The medical diagnosis and treatment of alcohol dependence. *Med Times* 115:109–126.
4. DeMilio L, Gold MS, Martin D (1986). Evaluation of substance abuse. In *Diagnostic and Laboratory Testing in Psychiatry*, Gold MS, Pottash ALC, eds. New York: Plenum Press.
5. Gold MS, Estroff TW (1985). The comprehensive evaluation of cocaine and opiate abusers. In *Handbook of Psychiatric Diagnostic Procedures*, Hall RCW, Beresford TP, eds. New York: Spectrum.
6. NIDA (1985). *National Household Survey on Drug Abuse*. National Institute on Drug Abuse. Washington, DC: U.S. Govt. Printing Office.
7. Wolfe SM (1987). Drug-induced tranquility. *Health Lett* 6–8.
8. Verebey K, Gold MS, Mule SJ (1986). Laboratory testing in the diagnosis of marijuana intoxication and withdrawal. *Psychiatr Ann* 16:235–241.
9. Estroff TW, Gold MS (1984). Medication and toxin-induced psychiatric disorder.

In *Medical Mimics of Psychiatric Disorders*, Extein I, Gold MS, eds. Washington DC: American Psychiatric Press.

10. Estroff TW, Gold MS (1986). Medical and psychiatric complications of cocaine abuse and possible points of pharmacologic intervention. *Adv Alcohol Subst Abuse* 5:61-76.

11. Estroff TW, Gold MS (1984). Psychiatric misdiagnosis. In *Advances in Psychopharmacology: Predicting and Improving Treatment Response*, Gold MS, Lydiard RB, Carman JS, eds., pp. 34-66. Boca Raton, FL: CRC Press.

12. Weissman MM, Pottenger M, Kleber H, et al. (1977). Symptom patterns in primary and secondary depression: A comparison of primary depressives with depressed opiate addicts, alcoholics and schizophrenics. *Arch Gen Psychiatry* 34:854-862.

13. Thacore VR, Shukla SRP (1976). Cannabis psychosis and paranoid schizophrenia. *Arch Gen Psychiatry* 33:383-386.

14. Beamish P, Kiloh LG (1960). Psychoses due to amphetamine consumption. *J Ment Sci* 106:337-343.

15. Extein I, Dackis CA, Gold MS, et al. (1986). Depression in drug addicts and alcoholics. In *Medical Mimics of Psychiatric Disorders*, Extein I, Gold MS, eds., pp. 133-162. Washington, DC: American Psychiatric Press.

16. Gold MS, Washton AM (1984). *Adverse Effects on Health and Functions of Cocaine Abuse; Data from 800 Cocaine Callers: Trends, Patterns and Issues in Drug Abuse*. Natl Inst Drug Abuse Res Monogr Ser 1, (2), Rockville, MD: National Institute for Drug Abuse.

17. Gold MS, Dackis CA, Pottash ALC, et al. (1986). Cocaine update: From bench to bedside. In *Advances in Alcohol & Substance Abuse*, Vol. 6, Stimmel B, ed., pp. 1-5. New York: Haworth Press.

18. Estroff TW, Gold MS (1987). Chronic medical complications of drug abuse. *Psychiatr Med* 3:267-286.

19. Yago KB, Pitts FN, Burgoyne RW, et al. (1981). The urban epidemic of phencyclidine (PCP) use: Clinical and laboratory evidence from a public psychiatric hospital emergency service. *J Clin Psychiatry* 42:193-196.

20. Jaffe JH (1985). Drug addiction and drug abuse. In *The Pharmacological Basis of Therapeutics*, 7th Ed., Gilman AG, Goodman LS, Rall TW, Murad F, eds., pp. 532-581. New York: Macmillan.

21. Miller, NS, Dackis CA, Gold MS (1987). The relationship of addiction, tolerance, dependence: A neurochemical approach. *J Subst Abuse Treat* 4:197-207.

22. Gold MS, Pottash ALC, Estroff TW, et al. (1984). Laboratory evaluation in treatment planning. In *The Psychiatric Therapies, Part 1: The Somatic Therapies*, Karusu TB, ed. Washington DC: APA Commission on Psychiatric Therapies.

23. Verebey K, Martin D, Gold MS (1986). Drug abuse: Interpretation of laboratory tests. In *Diagnostic and Laboratory Testing in Psychiatry*, Gold MS, Pottash ALC, eds., pp. 155-167. New York: Plenum Press.

24. Gold MS, Pottash AC, Extein I (1984). The psychiatric laboratory. In *Clinical Psychopharmacology*, Bernstein JG, ed., pp. 29-58. United Kingdom: John Wright.

25. CDC (1974). *Toxicology and Drug Abuse Survey III: Proficiency Testing*. Atlanta, GA: Centers for Disease Control.

26. Hansen JH, Caudill SP, Boone DJ (1985). Crisis in drug testing—Results of CDC blind study. *JAMA* 25:2382-2387.

27. Washton AM, Gold MS, Pottash AC (1985). Cocaine abuse treatment outcome. In *Abstracts of New Research*, APA 138th Annual Meeting. Washington DC: American Psychiatric Association.
28. Washton AM, Gold MS, Pottash AC (1987). Naltrexone in addicted physicians and business executives. *Natl Inst Drug Abuse Res Monogr Ser* 55:135–190.
29. Miller NS (1987). A primer of the treatment process for alcoholism and drug addiction. *Psychiatry Lett* 5:30–37.

CHAPTER 25

The Pharmacological Treatment of the Acute Intoxication and Detoxification of Alcohol and Drugs of Abuse and Addiction

History

The effects of drug and alcohol may be caused by the stimulation or inhibition of different neurotransmitters, chiefly gamma-aminobutyric acid, acetylcholine, norepinephrine, dopamine, serotonin, and beta-endorphin. The biopsychiatric model focuses on putative neurotransmitter activity to diagnose and treat overdose and addiction. This model explains how different drugs exert their effects and provides a rationale for specific pharmacological intervention in the drug-dependent patient.

Alcohol and drug addiction are often misdiagnosed because of the multiple signs and symptoms associated with each drug and the varying, complicated presentations that result from drug–drug interactions. Misdiagnosis can result in significant morbidity and even mortality.

The biopsychiatric model may assist physicians in the accurate diagnosis and efficient treatment of drug intoxication and withdrawal. The advantage of this model is that only a few principles must be mastered. These principles can then be applied to most drug-dependent situations (1).

The biopsychiatric model is based on the principle that drugs of abuse and addiction do not interact uniquely with the brain to produce highly specific symptoms. In fact, they increase or inhibit the rate of release of only a limited number of known neurotransmitters. A basic knowledge of neurotransmitter activity helps physicians recognize drug abuse and addiction. Once drug dependence is diagnosed, treatment follows the specific neurotransmitters that have been affected (2).

Neurotransmitters

Six neurotransmitters—gamma-aminobutyric acid (GABA), acetylcholine, norepinephrine, dopamine, serotonin, and beta-endorphin—account for most of the symptoms seen with the drugs most commonly abused in the United States (Figure 25.1) (1).

Neurotransmitter/ central action	Drugs of abuse that affect neurotransmitter action	Central location
γ-Aminobutyric acid (GABA) General inhibition of other neurotransmitters	Alcohol Barbiturates Benzodiazepines Chloral hydrate Ethchlorvynol Meprobamate Methaqualone (?) Phencyclidine	Throughout brain
Acetylcholine Counterbalances dopamine Maintains memory Initiates short-term memory	Phencyclidine	Caudate nucleus Lentiform nucleus Cerebral cortex Nucleus basalis of Meynert Nigrostriatal tract Reticular activating substance
Norepinephrine Modulates mood Maintains sleeping state	Amphetamines Cocaine Opiates Phencyclidine	Nucleus locus ceruleus Pontine and medullary cell groups

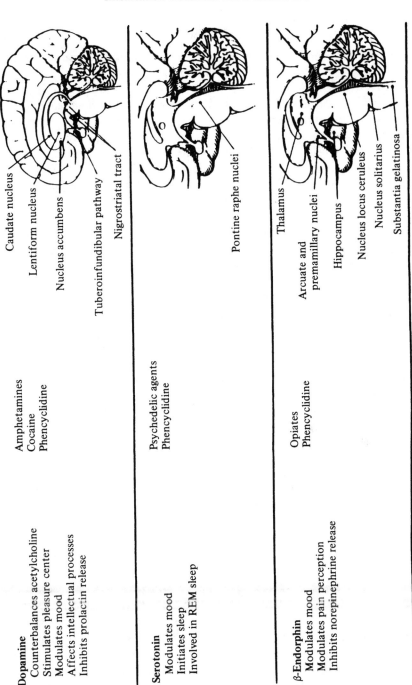

Dopamine
Counterbalances acetylcholine
Stimulates pleasure center
Modulates mood
Affects intellectual processes
Inhibits prolactin release

Caudate nucleus
Lentiform nucleus
Nucleus accumbens
Tuberoinfundibular pathway
Nigrostriatal tract

Amphetamines
Cocaine
Phencyclidine

Serotonin
Modulates mood
Initiates sleep
Involved in REM sleep

Pontine raphe nuclei

Psychedelic agents
Phencyclidine

β-Endorphin
Modulates mood
Modulates pain perception
Inhibits norepinephrine release

Thalamus
Arcuate and
 premamillary nuclei
Hippocampus
Nucleus locus ceruleus
Nucleus solitarius
Substantia gelatinosa

Opiates
Phencyclidine

FIGURE 25.1. Neurotransmitters and the neurochemical actions of drugs of abuse.

GABA

GABA is the neurotransmitter most often affected in drug abuse and addiction. This modified amino acid transmitter system accounts for 20% of all receptor sites in the brain (3). The major inhibitory neurotransmitter of the central nervous system, GABA acts by opening chloride channels into the neurons. These channels are operated by the fitting of GABA into its proper site on the receptor. The receptor has a second site where barbiturates can fit and facilitate chloride ingress (4). The GABA receptor also has an auxiliary receptor, the BZ receptor, that boosts the action of GABA. The BZ receptor is named after the benzodiazepines, which function in that location (5).

Acetylcholine

The most important distribution of acetylcholine is in the nucleus basalis of Meynert and the nigrostriatal tract. Degeneration of the nucleus causes downstream degeneration of projecting cholinergic neurons in the cerebral cortex, resulting in some of the manifestations of Alzheimer's disease. Nigrostriatal acetylcholine acts in rough balance with nigrostriatal dopamine. When there is a relative increase in the acetylcholine portion of this ratio, the symptoms of parkinsonism result. Activity in the reticular activating substance contributes to the central input of new memories.

Most cholinergic receptors in the brain are of the muscarinic type. Nicotinic receptors, which are exclusively peripheral, cause cardiac inhibition and gastric stimulation. At low levels of activation, nicotinic receptors stimulate autonomic ganglia and myoneural junctions, but at higher levels, this action is depressed (6).

Norepinephrine

Most norepinephrine, a stimulatory and inhibitory neurotransmitter, is synthesized and stored in the nucleus locus ceruleus. This paired nucleus is located in the pons, near the floor of the third ventricle. Norepinephrine is a catecholamine that, among other actions, regulates mood and arousal. High levels of norepinephrine are associated with mania and anxiety whereas low levels are associated with depression. Norepinephrine also maintains the sleeping state. Peripherally, it acts as a vasoconstrictor (7).

Dopamine

Another important catecholamine is dopamine, a stimulatory and inhibitory neurotransmitter that affects mood and thought. Abnormally high levels of dopamine are found in schizophrenia and chorea; low levels of this neurotransmitter are associated with depression and parkinsonism. Degeneration of dopaminergic neurons in the nigrostriatal tract is seen in primary Parkinson's disease. Dopamine is also important in the primary pleasure pathway between the nucleus accumbens and the pars compacta. Dopamine inhibits prolactin release from the pituitary gland via the tuberoinfundibular pathway (8).

Serotonin

Serotonin is an indolamine that acts to modulate mood and initiate sleep. Low levels of serotonin activity are associated with depression. Stimulation of serotonin receptors is associated with an electroencephalogram (EEG) pattern similar to that seen in the rapid-eye-movement (REM) or dream phase of sleep. Central serotonin is produced at five paired nuclei in the pons, the pontine raphe nuclei. Peripherally, large amounts of serotonin cause flushing (9).

Beta-Endorphin

Relaxation and analgesia are produced by beta-endorphin, which is an opioid. This neurotransmitter is distributed throughout the hippocampus, nucleus solitarius, substantia gelatinosa, thalamus, and nucleus locus ceruleus. By means of this distributory network, beta-endorphin interconnects the perceptions of panic, pain, stress, and affect. In the nucleus locus ceruleus, beta-endorphin acts at muscarine receptors to inhibit the release of norepinephrine (10).

Actions of Drugs of Abuse and Addiction

The most common drugs of abuse in the United States are listed in Table 25.1 and are discussed by class in the following sections.

Sedatives and Tranquilizers

Alcohol, the barbiturates, the agents ethchlorvynol (Placidyl), glutethimide (Doriden, Doriglute), and meprobamate (Equanil, Miltown, Neuramate, etc.), and the benzodiazepines suppress brain function by activating the GABA system (11). This causes slowing and eventual paralysis of central nervous system (CNS) and motor function. Sedation, slowed mentation, confusion, loss of consciousness, and coma occur as the effects of the stimulatory transmitters are deactivated by GABAlike effects. Peripherally, the sedatives and tranquilizers cause hypotension, bradycardia, and slowed respiratory rate. As heart conduction slows, arrhythmias emerge. Prolonged slowing of the respiratory rate may lead to acidosis.

According to the biopsychiatric model, sedatives and tranquilizers mimic the action of GABA by opening chloride channels (12). When a sedative is taken for a prolonged period, the production (and supply) of GABA is progressively decreased. If the sedative is then abruptly withdrawn, the natural inhibitory function of the GABA system is reduced, leading to a rebound excess of neurotransmitters formerly under GABA control. Norepinephrine rebound causes increased alertness, hyperglycemia, hypertension, hyperreflexia, nystagmus, and pupillary dilation. Dopamine rebound results in hyperactivity, tremors, hallucinations, delusions, and seizures.

Drugs that act directly on GABA receptors cause more severe addiction

TABLE 25.1. Common drugs of abuse.

Drug	Class	Street names
Amphetamines	Stimulant	Black beauty
		Crosses
		Hearts
Barbiturates	Sedative/tranquilizer	Barbs
		Blue racers
		Yellow jackets
Benzodiazepines	Sedative/tranquilizer	"Roches"
		Tranks
		Pumpkin
Cocaine	Stimulant	Coke
		Crack
		Free base
Ethclorvynol (Placidyl)	Sedative/tranquilizer	Green jeans
		Pickles
Fentanyl	Opiate	Six-pack
Glutethimide (Doriden, Doriglute)	Sedative/tranquilizer	Grays
		Seabees
Heroin	Opiate	Horse
		Skag
		Smack
Lysergic acid (LSD)	Psychedelic agent	Acid
		Blue cheer
		LSD
Meperidine (Demerol)	Opiate	Banana
Meprobamate (Equanil, Miltown, Neuramate, etc.)	Sedative/tranquilizer	Bams
Mescaline	Psychedelic agent	Cactus
		Mex
		Peyote
Methamphetamine (Desoxyn)	Stimulant	Crystal meth
		Twenty-twenty
3,4-Methylenedioxy-methamphetamine (MDMA)	Psychedelic agent	Adam
		Ecstasy
Phencyclidine	Phencyclidine	Hog
		PCP
		Surfer
Propoxyphene (Darvon, Dolene, Doxaphene, etc.)	Psychedelic agent	Lilies
Psilocybin	Psychedelic agent	Mushroom
		Purple passion

and withdrawal symptoms than drugs that act indirectly on BZ receptors (13). Direct-acting agents include all the barbiturates that act specifically at the so-called barbiturate receptor, which is part of the GABA–chloride channel complex. Methaqualone, meprobamate, ethchlorvynol, and glutethimide also act at the barbiturate receptor; in terms of neuroceptor activity, these drugs are indistinguishable from the barbiturates and offer no distinct therapeutic advantage.

The BZ receptor is not part of the GABA–chloride channel complex and is therefore referred to as the GABA coreceptor. Because the BZ receptor is physically somewhat removed from the channel complex, actions at this receptor are indirect or of reduced intensity. The benzodiazepines, alcohol, and alcohol derivatives, including methanol, ethanol, isopropyl alcohol, chloral hydrate (Noctec), and paraldehyde (Paral), also activate the BZ receptor.

Stimulants

Amphetamines and cocaine exert a stimulatory effect on the CNS (14). Acutely, they increase the release of dopamine and norepinephrine from presynaptic neurons. These drugs have a dual action. First, they increase the release of stored dopamine from the presynaptic vesicles into the synaptic cleft. Second, this enhanced supply of available dopamine is further augmented by amphetamine- or cocaine-induced blockade of presynaptic uptake. Thus, an increased supply of dopamine is available for a longer period to stimulate postsynaptic receptors. It is presumed that a similar mechanism operates with norepinephrine (15).

The presynaptic blockade, however, causes the catecholamine depletion associated with chronic stimulant use. Because reuptake is prevented, large amounts of dopamine are degraded in the synaptic cleft by catechol-O-methyltransferase (COMT). The result of COMT metabolism is 5-OH-tyramine. Normally, dopamine would be taken up into the neuron and metabolized into homovanillic acid by monoamine oxidase. While homovanillic acid can be recycled to produce a continuous resupply of dopamine, 5-OH-tyramine cannot be recycled. Therefore, as more stimulants are used, the supply of dopamine is gradually depleted (16).

The initial increase in catecholamine levels causes the stimulatory rush of an amphetamine or cocaine "high." Peripheral stimulatory effects include hypertension secondary to vasoconstriction, tachycardia, and pupillary dilation. Tachycardia may progress to heart block from direct cardiac effects. Central stimulatory effects include anorexia, euphoria, hypervigilance, hypersexuality, and grandiosity (17).

Major effects occur at the nucleus accumbens septi, a primary pleasure center. After repeated stimulation of this area, the need for cocaine or amphetamine becomes a pseudodrive. The drive for these drugs takes on the same force as other primary drives that also affect the nucleus accumbens, including thirst, hunger and sexual desire. Eventually, the drive (craving) for the drugs exceeds even the primary drives. A classic example is a cocaine-addicted rat that has been dehydrated but will not turn away from a cocaine supply for even 1 second to drink water from an easily accessible source. The rat will continue to prefer cocaine to water until it dies of dehydration (18).

Because the dopamine and norepinephrine supply is constantly depleted by chronic use, ever higher doses of the drug must be taken. When the drug supply is suddenly cut off, deactivation of the nucleus accumbens produces a profound dysphoria. Decreased catecholamine levels then produce vasodilation, muscle cramping, and hypersomnia (18) (Table 25.2).

Opiates

Like stimulants, opiates act on the nucleus accumbens. Because the opiates have indirect effects on dopamine, mediated through the mu-opioid receptors, the pleasure experience is quantitatively less than the experience derived from stimulants. Although opiates can displace food and sex as primary drives, they do not displace thirst (19).

The activity at the nucleus accumbens, however, is not related to withdrawal symptoms. During intoxication, opiates stimulate opioid receptors in the nucleus locus ceruleus; this causes a suppression of noradrenergic release. Because the nucleus accumbens is the major source of central norepinephrine, the effects of opiate use are substantial. Mood and affect are inhibited. Pupils are constricted. Peripherally, there is vasodilation and constipation as noradrenergic alpha receptors and beta receptors are affected. If large amounts of opiates are acutely abused, noradrenergic suppression can lead to respiratory and cardiovascular suppression (20).

Withdrawal, although medically benign, is subjectively quite distressing and is marked by an intense drive to use more opiates. When opioid receptors are no longer hyperstimulated by drugs such as morphine or heroin, the inhibition of the norepinephrine system is released. The previous opiate-dependent suppression of norepinephrine is replaced by rebound release of the large amounts of norepinephrine that have accumulated. Because norepinephrine is a natural stimulant and causes muscles to contract, this release produces generalized muscular cramping, pilomotor erection, increased pulse rate, and hot/cold flushes (21).

Psychedelic Agents

A number of drugs are termed psychedelic or hallucinogenic. Partly because of their serotonergic action, all these drugs produce intense, mind-altering experiences.

Excitation of the presynaptic receptors in the pontine raphe nuclei produces visual, proprioceptive, and perceptual distortions. Dissolution of ego boundaries occurs without cognitive or memory impairment, disorien-

TABLE 25.2. Cocaine intoxication.

Signs
1. Dilated and reactive pupils
2. Tachycardia
3. Elevated temperature
4. Elevated blood pressure
5. Dry mouth
6. Perspiration or chills
7. Nausea and vomiting
8. Tremulousness
9. Hyperactive reflexes
10. Repetitious compulsive behavior
11. Stereotypic biting causes ulcers around mouth
12. Cardiac arrhythmias
13. Flushed skin
14. Poor self-care and suicide
15. Violence and homicide
16. Seizures

Symptoms
1. Euphoria
2. Hyperarousal
3. Hypervigilance
4. Panic and anxiety
5. Irritability
6. Loquacity and pressured speech
7. Emotional lability
8. Anorexia
9. Aggressiveness and hostility
10. Anxiety
11. Grandiosity
12. Depression
13. Suicidal ideation

Symptoms of sympathomimetic cocaine delusional syndromes

In addition to the symptoms and physical signs with sympathomimetic intoxication, individuals with a cocaine or similar acting sympathomimetic delusional syndrome have:

1. Thought disorder
2. Ideas of reference
3. Auditory hallucinations, frequently of voices commenting, criticizing, and accusing the patient of misconduct.
4. Paranoid ideation, with delusions of persecution in a clear sensorium.
5. Visual hallucinations, sometimes with distortion of faces and disturbances of body image.
6. Formication

tation, or confusion. Psychedelic agents also produce EEG changes similar to those seen during REM sleep, which may account for the dreamlike quality of the high reported by those using this class of drugs.

In addition to action at the raphe nuclei, psychedelic agents bind to the auditory and visual areas, the corpus amygdaloideum, the hippocampus, and the hypothalamus. By acting in these sites, psychedelic agents alter the transfer and integration of sensory messages to produce alterations in perceptions and frank hallucinations (22,23).

Phencyclidine

Because phencyclidine (PCP) acts at several neurotransmitter sites, its actions mimic those of all the drugs previously described. PCP stimulates dopamine, norepinephrine, and serotonin. It also inhibits the actions of acetylcholine and possibly GABA. Opioids are simultaneously stimulated and inhibited (24).

Peripheral anticholinergic activity produces hot, dry, flushed skin, as well as tachycardia. Central anticholinergic inhibition in the reticular activating substance is associated with amnesia and confusion. Tachycardia is further increased by the stimulation of peripheral dopamine and norepinephrine. Centrally, dopamine stimulation at dopamine-2 receptors can give rise to hypervigilance, as well as illogical and paranoid thought patterns. Dopaminergic overactivity in the nigrostriatal tract can cause impaired coordination. Stimulation of norepinephrine in the nucleus locus ceruleus produces anxiety and increased activity (25).

The characteristic superhuman strength of PCP abusers is related to the opioid receptors. Because their perception of pain is reduced, these users can subject their musculoskeletal systems to otherwise intolerable strains. They can bend steel bars, because they are able to ignore muscle tears and stress fractures. Their insensitivity to pain, disturbed thinking, and increased motor activity makes PCP addicts dangerous to themselves and those around them. The expected noradrenergic inhibition associated with increased activity is apparently overridden by direct noradrenergic activity (26).

Peripheral serotonergic activity contributes to characteristic flushing. Centrally, serotonergic action at the pontine raphe nuclei produces a dreamlike state with visual hallucinations. Inhibition of GABA may be responsible for enhanced hyperactivity of dopamine, norepinephrine, and serotonin (27).

Intervention and Treatment

Sedatives and Tranquilizers

During withdrawal, the GABA system gradually resumes independent functioning. Rebound release of dopamine and norepinephrine may be avoided if the drug dosage is tapered. When the daily dose of a direct-acting GABA drug is known, 50 to 100 mg of phenobarbital per day is given for each 100 mg of the barbiturate on which the patient is dependent. The phenobarbital dosage is then reduced by 20% every other day. If withdrawal symptoms appear, 30 to 100 mg of oral phenobarbital is given immediately, and the schedule is revised. By slowly titrating the dosage of this agent downward, the GABA system is gradually reactivated (28) (Table 25.3).

If the daily dose of the dependent drug is not known, or if the patient is a

TABLE 25.3. Benzodiazepines (barbiturate) withdrawal.

Signs
   1. Increased or decreased psychomotor activity
   2. Muscular weakness
   3. Tremulousness
   4. Hyperpyrexia, sweating
   5. Delirium
   6. Convulsions
   7. Tachycardia and elevated blood pressure
   8. Coarse tremor of tongue, eyelids, and hands
   9. Status epilepticus

Symptoms
   1. Anxiety
   2. Euphoria
   3. Depression
   4. Thought disorder
   5. Hostility
   6. Grandiosity
   7. Disorientation
   8. Euphoria
   9. Depression
  10. Tactile, auditory, and visual hallucinations
  11. Suicidal ideation and thinking

Benzodiazepine (barbiturate) detoxification

Short-acting	7 to 10-day taper: Day 1 Librium 25 to 50 mg, po, qid with a gradual taper to 10 mg, po, qid on last day. No prn.
	or
	7 to 10-day taper: Calculate benzodiazepine equivalence and give 50% of dose over the taper (if know actual dose before detoxification).
Long-acting:	10 to 14-day taper: Day 1 Librium 25 to 50 mg, po, qid with a gradual taper to 10 mg po, qid on last day. No prn.
	or
	10 to 14-day taper: Calculate benzodiazepine equivalence and give 50% dose over the taper (if know actual dose before detoxification).

mixed-drug addict, the phenobarbital challenge test may be useful. The initial test dose is 200 mg. If sleep is induced, it should be assumed that the average daily dose of abused drug is the equivalent of 200 mg of phenobarbital. If the patient is only drowsy, the daily dose of the abused drug is the equivalent of 400 to 600 mg of phenobarbital. An awake state with nystagmus indicates a daily dose equivalent to 600 to 1000 mg of phenobarbital, while an awake state without nystagmus is consistent with a daily abuse dosage equivalent to more than 1000 mg of phenobarbital.

For alcoholics and benzodiazepine addicts, an indirect GABA agent, such as chlordiazepoxide (Librium, Lipoxide, Mitran, etc.), is recommended. The usual initial dosage is 25 to 50 mg every 6 hours as needed, titrated downward according to blood pressure elevation, pulse rate, agitation, and psychosis. Thiamine, hydration, and magnesium replacement may be indicated by the severity of the withdrawal symptoms (29) (Table 25.4).

For benzodiazepine addicts, the detoxification from benzodiazepines can be simplified and easily applied if basic principles are applied. First, benzodiazepines have cross-tolerance and dependence with each other, alcohol, and other sedative/hypnotic drugs. Any benzodiazepine can be substituted for other benzodiazepine and with barbiturates, so that conversion for equivalent doses can be calculated. Second, a long-acting benzodiazepine is more effective in suppressing the withdrawal symptoms and producing a gradual and smooth transition to the abstinent state. Greater patient compliance and less morbidity will result from the use of the longer acting benzodiazepines (30,31).

Third, select a benzodiazepine with lower euphoric properties such as chlordiazepam, avoiding diazepam as much as possible. Fourth, do not leave p.r.n. doses as this will give the addict a choice that is beyond his control and will reduce drug-seeking behavior. Withdrawal from benzodiazepines is not usually marked by hypertension and tachycardia as with alcohol so that p.r.n. doses are not needed. The anxiety of withdrawal should be controlled with the prescribed taper unless objectively it appears that the doses are too low. Caution is urged at this point as drug-seeking behavior needs to be differentiated from anxiety of withdrawal, and the anxiety of another disorder. Only the anxiety of withdrawal when severe, need be treated with increased doses of benzodiazepines although this condition is unusual with the long-acting benzodiazepines. Alternative methods than benzodiazepines for treating the anxiety of another disorder and drug seeking behavior are indicated. The prescriber must be in control of the dispensing of the benzodiazepines for withdrawal as the addict by definition is out of control and cannot reliably negotiate in the schedule for tapering.

The duration of the tapering schedule is determined by the half-life of the benzodiazepine that is being withdrawn. For short-acting benzodiazepines such as alprazolam, 7 to 10 days of a gradual taper with a long-acting benzodiazepine or barbiturate is sufficient; 7 days for low-dose use and 10 days for high-dose use. For the long-acting benzodiazepines, 10 to 14 days of

TABLE 25.4. Alcohol withdrawal.

Signs
1. Hand tremor
2. Diaphoresis
3. Tachycardia and elevated blood pressure
4. Dilated pupils
5. Increase in temperature
6. Seizures
7. Restlessness
8. Hyperactivity, agitation
9. Ataxia
10. Clouding of consciousness

Symptoms
1. Anxiety and panic attacks
2. Paranoid delusions or ideation
3. Illusions
4. Disorientation
5. Hallucinations, either of rapidly moving small animals such as snakes or Lilliputian hallucinations (auditory hallucinations are rare)

Alcohol detoxification

Mild withdrawal   Librium 25–50 mg po every 4 hours prn for

Systolic blood pressure > 150
Diastolic blood pressure > 90
Pulse > 100
Temperature > 101
Tremulousness

Librium 25–50 mg po prn for insomnia for 2 days.

Moderate withdrawal   Librium 25–50 mg po qid day 1
              20–40 mg po qid day 2
              10–30 mg po qid day 3
              (optional)
              20 mg po qid day 4
              10 mg po qid day 5
              May need to adjust based on signs and
               symptoms of alcohol withdrawal

Severe withdrawal   Librium 25–50 mg po every hour while awake (to sedate).

Systolic blood pressure > 150
Diastolic blood pressure > 90
Pulse > 100
Temperature > 101
Tremulousness

a gradual taper with a long-acting benzodiazepine or barbiturate is sufficient; 10 days for low-dose and 14 days for high-dose use. The doses should
be given in a q.i.d. interval. Exact numerical deductions are not needed as
the long acting benzodiazepines accumulate to result in a self-leveling effect
of the blood level of the benzodiazepines over time (30,31) (Table 25.5).

Stimulants

Cocaine and amphetamines are both CNS stimulants. Their short-term effect is to increase the release of dopamine, but after prolonged use, they
deplete the dopamine supply. The key to treatment of acute overdose is
catecholamine blockade. After the ingested drug is eliminated with syrup of
ipecac, activated charcoal is administered. Hypertensive episodes and car-
diotoxicity are both treated with intravenous doses of the beta blocker propranolol (Inderal) as indicated. Psychosis responds to the dopamine blocker
haloperidol (Haldol) 5 to 10 mg orally or intramuscularly every 1 to 6 hours
as needed (32) (Table 25.6).

After dopamine, norepinephrine, and epinephrine supplies are depleted,
the patient goes through withdrawal. Signs and symptoms of withdrawal
include anhedonia, depression, hyperphagia, hypersomnia, psychomotor
retardation, and suicidal ideation. Ordinarily, these signs and symptoms
resolve without specific pharmacological therapy. However, at times persistent delusions and/or depression may require the use of pharmacotherapy.

Pharmacological treatment focuses on repleting dopamine and norepinephrine levels. Withdrawal therapy is initiated with bromocriptine (Parlo-
del) 1.25 to 2.5 mg every 6 hours. The dosage is gradually decreased over 1
to 3 weeks. Desipramine (Norpramin, Pertofrane) is simultaneously initiated
at a dosage of 50 mg per day; the dosage is then titrated upward every other

TABLE 25.5. Benzodiazepine detoxification.

Short-acting:	7- to 10-day taper: Day 1 Librium 25 to 50 mg, po, qid with a gradual taper to 10 mg, po, qid on last day. No prn.
	or
	7- to 10-day taper: Calculate benzodiazepine equivalence and give 50% of dose over the taper (if know actual dose before detoxification).
Long-acting:	10- to 14-day taper: Day 1 Librium 25 to 50 mg, po, qid with a gradual taper to 10 mg, po, qid on last day. No prn.
	or
	10- to 14-day taper: Calculate benzodiazepine equivalence and give 50% dose over the ta-per (if know actual dose before detoxification).

TABLE 25.6. Cocaine and similar-acting sympathomimetic withdrawal.

History
  1. The symptoms and physical signs of withdrawal from cocaine or similar acting substances generally commence within hours of cessation of use and peak within one to three days.
  2. Depression and irritability may persist, however, for months and, necessitate the use of antidepressants and neuroleptic medication, or electroshock because of the risk of suicide.

Cocaine and similar-acting sympathomimetic withdrawal
(peak period, 0–4 days)
  1. Depression
  2. Anxiety
  3. Panic
  4. Hypersomnambulance
  5. Fatigue
  6. Disturbed sleep
  7. Agitation
  8. Suicidal thinking
  9. Irritability
  10. Apathy
  11. Hyperphagia

Cocaine withdrawal
Desipramine hydrochloride 2.5 mg/kg po loading dose. Obtain blood level next day to determine dose
or
150–250 mg (one or divided dose) po every day for 2 weeks or more.
Taper over 2 to 5 days.
and
Bromocriptine 1.25 to 2.5 mg, po g 6 hours and taper over 1 to 3 weeks

day in 50-mg increments until a dosage of 150 to 250 mg per day is attained. This dosage is maintained for 3 to 6 months and is then discontinued by gradually tapering the drug over 2 weeks (15) (see Table 25.6).

While bromocriptine, a dopamine agonist, acts acutely to neutralize the effects of dopamine depletion, desipramine resets noradrenergic autoreceptors so that the remaining supply of norepinephrine is more efficiently utilized. Bromocriptine acts acutely to block withdrawal symptoms, while desipramine works over a longer period to prevent relapse by decreasing cocaine and amphetamine cravings (13).

Opiates

During intoxication, opioids suppress norepinephrine stimulation. This effect can be reversed by naloxone (Narcan), an opiate antagonist. Naloxone is given intravenously in doses of 0.4 to 0.8 mg every 20 minutes as required. The dose is increased as indicated by symptom response until an upper limit of 24 mg is attained over an 8- to 12-hour period. Hypotension is treated by volume replacement. Pulmonary edema usually responds to naloxone therapy; if not, the measures usually employed for pulmonary edema are instituted, including diuresis, afterload reduction, and oxygen (33).

Although not medically dangerous, opiate withdrawal is distressing and sometimes painful. When mu-opioid receptors are no longer hyperstimulated by opiates, a massive release of stored norepinephrine occurs. Clonidine (Catapres), a mu agonist, acts directly on noradrenergic receptors to reduce norepinephrine release from the nucleus locus ceruleus. An initial dosage of 0.1 to 0.3 mg per day alleviates the withdrawal discomfort and craving. The dosage is then gradually reduced over 5 to 7 days. Hypotension is the only side effect of clonidine. If hypotension is severe, the dosage can be reduced until blood pressure stabilizes (34). Methadone may also be used for detoxification from heroin and methadone itself (Table 25.7).

Naltrexone (Trexan) may help the motivated addict maintain abstinence. This drug is a pure opiate antagonist that blocks the effects of all opium-derived compounds. The usual dosage is 50 mg orally each morning, usually under direct medical supervision, because this is the period of highest motivation. If the patient uses an opiate later that day, the effects of the opiate are blocked. Thus, the psychological and physical reinforcements of continued opiate abuse are decreased.

Psychedelic Agents

Abuse of psychedelic agents is often misdiagnosed as schizophrenia. The psychedelic effects of these agents are produced by the massive release of serotonin from the raphe nuclei in the pons. The release is localized to the CNS, causing major psychiatric effects but minimal physical changes (35).

Supportive care in a quiet environment is usually sufficient until the effects of serotonin overload abate. If the patient's condition does not improve within 12 hours or the panic becomes uncontrollable, pharmacologic intervention is indicated. The effects of serotonin can be blocked with an indirect GABA agonist such as lorazepam (Alzapam, Ativan), 1 to 2 mg intramuscularly (36).

Phencyclidine

The most important clinical symptoms of PCP intoxication are hyperactivity, paranoia, insensitivity to pain, hypertension, hallucinations, paranoid delusions, and memory loss. Other signs and symptoms include eyelid retraction (producing a wide-eyed stare), dry erythematous skin, dilated pupils, horizontal nystagmus, and an excitable angry mood.

Most symptoms are reversed by the dopamine-2 antagonist haloperidol 5 mg intramuscularly or orally every 20 minutes for three to four doses (27).

Most of the symptoms of PCP abuse are caused by a combination of the stimulation of catecholamines and the blockade of acetylcholine. Haloperidol restores the dopamine–acetylcholine balance by blocking dopamine re-

TABLE 25.7. Objective opiate withdrawal signs.

1. Pulse 10 beats per minute or more over baseline or over 90 if no history of tachycardia and baseline unknown (baseline: vital sign values 1 hour after receiving 10 mg of methadone).
2. Systolic blood pressure 10 mm Hg or more above baseline or over 160/96 in nonhypertensive patients.
3. Dilated pupils.
4. Gooseflesh, sweating, rhinorrhea, or lacrimation.

Opiate detoxification

Heroin morphine withdrawal (Clonidine)

Clonidine 20 μg/kg/day in three divided doses or 0.1 mg to 2 mg po tid for 4–5 days and taper over 4–6 days, or: Clonidine 0.1 or 0.2 mg po every 4 hours prn for signs and symptoms of withdrawal. (Peak doses are between 2 to 4 days.)
Check blood pressure before each dose, do not give if hypotensive (for that individual, i.e., 90/60).

Methadone withdrawal (Clonidine)

Clonidine 20 μg/kg/day in three divided doses or
0.1 mg to 0.2 mg po tid x 14 days.
0.1 mg to 0.2 mg po bid x 3 days.
0.1 mg to 0.2 mg po every 4 hours po prn for signs and symptoms of withdrawal (18–20) days.
Check blood pressure before each dose, do not give if hypotensive (for that individual, i.e., 90/60).

Heroin morphine withdrawal (Methadone)

Methadone test dose of 10 mg po in liquid or crushed tablet. Additional 10-mg doses are given for signs and symptoms of withdrawal every 4 hours. Average dose is 30 mg in 24 hours. Next day, repeat total first day dose in two divided doses (stabilization dose), then reduce by 3–5 mg per day until completely withdrawn.

Methadone withdrawal (Methadone)

Methadone test dose of 10 mg po in liquid or crushed tablet. Additional 10-mg doses are given for signs and symptoms of withdrawal every 4 hours. Average dose is 30 mg in 24 hours. Next, repeat total first-day dose in two divided doses (stabilization dose), then reduce by 1–5 mg per day until completely withdrawn.

ceptors. Because phencyclidine is a dopamine-2 agonist and haloperidol is a dopamine-2 antagonist, a specific and therapeutic blockade occurs. (Other antipsychotics are less specific and block dopamine-1 receptors as well as cholinergic receptors, further complicating an already compromised neurochemical interaction.) To intensify the effects of haloperidol and increase the rate of phencyclidine elimination, ascorbic acid 1 g intramuscularly, may be

TABLE 25.8. Pharmacological intervention specific to neurotransmitters inhibited or stimulated by drugs of abuse.

Drug class	Toxic or withdrawal effects	Treatment
Sedatives/ hypnotics	Diminished activity of GABA[a] inhibition	Gradually taper a sedative/hypnotic; substitute phenobarbital or chlordiazepoxide (Librium, Lipoxide, Mitran, etc.), depending on the drug of abuse, to allow restoration of GABA activity
Stimulants	Depletion of dopamine and norepinephrine	Adminster bromocriptine (Parlodel), a dopamine agonist Administer desipramine (Norpramin, Pertofrane), which enhances norepinephrine receptors
Opiates	Norepinephrine release	Administer naloxone (Narcan) to reverse acute intoxication Administer clonidine (Catapres), which blocks norepinephrine release Administer naltrexone (Trexan), an opiate antagonist
Psychedelic agents	Enhanced serotonin activity	Place patient in a quiet environment to allow the effects of the drug to wear off Administer lorazepam (Alzapam, Ativan), an indirect GABA agonist that blocks serotonin effects
Phencyclidine	Stimulation of dopamine and norepinephrine receptors and blockade of acetylcholine	Administer haloperidol (Haldol), a dopamine-2 antagonist Administer desipramine to prevent postwithdrawal depression

[a]GABA, gamma-aminobutyric acid.

given (37). Benzodiazepines may be used for the agitation (see *Alcohol*). A summary of the treatments for five classes of addicting drugs is provided in Table 25.8.

References

1. Giannini AJ, Gold MS, Sternberg DE (1989). *Treating Drug Abuse*, pp. 73–84. New York: Marcel Dekker.
2. Giannini AJ, Slaby AE, eds. (1989). *Drugs of Abuse*, pp. 111–116. Oradell, NJ: Medical Economics.
3. Tallman JF, Paul SM, Skolnick P, et al. (1980). Receptors for the age of anxiety: Pharmacology of the benzodiazepines. *Science* 207:274–281.
4. Cooper JR, Bloom FE, Roth RH (1988). *Biochemical Basis of Neuropharmacology*, p. 94. New York: Oxford University Press.
5. Mohler H, Okada T (1977). Benzodiazepine receptor: Demonstration in the central nervous system. *Science* 198:849–851.

6. Aquilonious SM (1977). Role of acetylcholine in the central nervous system. *Clin Neurol* 29:435–458.
7. Langer S (1978). Modern concepts of noradrenergic transmission. In *Neurotransmitter Systems and Their Clinical Disorders*, Legg NJ, ed., pp. 117–184. New York: Academic Press.
8. Bird ED, Spokes EG, Iversen LL (1979). Brain norepinephrine and dopamine in schizophrenia [Letter]. *Science* 204:93–94.
9. Ho BT, Schoolar JC, Usdin E, eds. (1982). *Serotonin in Biological Psychiatry*, pp. 69–84. New York: Raven.
10. Lord JA, Waterfield AA, Hughes J, et al. (1977). Endogenous opioid peptides: Multiple agonists and receptors. *Nature* 267:495–499.
11. Krogsgaard-Larsen P, Scheel-Kruger J, Kofod H, eds. (1979). Gaba-neurotransmitters: Pharmacochemical, biochemical, and pharmacological aspects. In *Proceedings of the Alfred Benzon Symposium, Copenhagen*, pp. 251–258. New York: Academic Press.
12. van Kammen DP, Sternberg DE, Hare TA, et al. (1982). CSF levels of gamma-aminobutyric acid in schizophrenia. Low values in recently ill patients. *Arch Gen Psychiatry* 39:91–97.
13. Chang RS, Snyder SH (1978). Benzodiazepine receptors: Labeling in intact animals with [^{3}H]flunitrazepam. *Eur J Pharmacol* 48:123–128.
14. Tecce JJ, Cole JO (1974). Amphetamine effects in man: Paradoxical drowsiness and lowered electrical brain activity (CNV). *Science* 185:451–453.
15. Giannini AJ, Billett W (1987). Bromocriptine-desipramine protocol in treatment for cocaine addiction. *J Clin Pharmacol* 27:549–554.
16. Dackis CA, Gold MS, Davies RK, et al. (1985). Bromocriptine treatment for cocaine abuse: The dopamine depletion hypothesis. *Int J Psychiatry Med* 15:125–135.
17. Dackis CA, Gold MS (1985). New concepts in cocaine addiction: The dopamine depletion hypothesis. *Neurosci Biobehav Rev* 9:469–477.
18. Gawin FH, Kleber HD (1986). Abstinence symptomatology and psychiatric diagnosis in cocaine abusers. Clinical Observations. *Arch Gen Psychiatry* 43:107–113.
19. Tennant FS, Jr., Russell BA, Casas SK, et al. (1975). Heroin detoxification. A comparison of propoxyphene and methadone. *JAMA* 232:1019–1022.
20. Cedarbaum JM, Aghajanian GK (1976). Noradrenergic neurons of the locus ceruleus: Inhibition by epinephrine and activation by the alpha-antagonist piperoxan. *Brain Res* 112:413–419.
21. O'Brien CP, Testa T, O'Brien TJ, et al. (1977). Conditioned narcotic withdrawal in humans. *Science* 195:1000–1002.
22. Freedman DX (1964). The psychopharmacology of hallucinogenic agents. *Annu Rev Med* 20:409–415.
23. Bowers MB, Jr., Freedman DX (1966). "Psychedelic" experiences in acute psychoses. *Arch Gen Psychiatry* 15:240–248.
24. Giannini AJ, Giannini MC, Price WA (1984). Antidotal strategies in phencyclidine intoxication. *Int J Psychiatry Med* 14:315–321.
25. Giannini AJ, Eighan MS, Loiselle RH, et al. (1984). Comparison of haloperidol and chlorpromazine in the treatment of phencyclidine psychosis. *J Clin Pharmacol* 24:202–204.
26. Giannini AJ, Loiselle RH, Price WA (1985). Chlorpromazine vs. meperidine in the treatment of phencyclidine psychosis. *J Clin Psychiatry* 46:52–54.

27. Castellani S, Giannini AJ, Boeringa JA, et al. (1982). Phencyclidine intoxication: Assessment of possible antidotes. *J Toxicol Clin Toxicol* 19:313–319.
28. Giannini AJ, Black HR, Goettsche RL (1978). *Psychiatric, Psychogenic, and Somatopsychic Disorders Handbook*, pp. 86–88. Garden City, NY: Medical Examination.
29. Eckardt MJ, Harford TC, Kaelber CT, et al. (1981). Health hazards associated with alcohol consumption. *JAMA* 246:648–666.
30. Perry Pj, Alexander B (1986). Sedative/hypnotic dependence: Patient stabilization, tolerance, testing and withdrawal. *Drug Intell Clin Pharm* 20:532–536.
31. Harrison M, Busto U, Naranjo CA (1984). Diazepam tapering in detoxification for high-dose benzodiazepine abuse. *Clin Pharmacol Ther* 527–533.
32. Giannini AJ, Gold MS (1988). Cocaine abuse: Demons within. *Primary Care* 4:34–40.
33. Giannini AJ, Slaby AE, Giannini MC (1982). *Handbook of Overdose and Detoxification Emergencies*, pp. 86–88. New Hyde Park, NY: Medical Examination.
34. Gold MS, Redmond DE, Jr., Kleber HD (1978). Clonidine blocks acute opiate-withdrawal symptoms. *Lancet* 2(8090):599–602.
35. Strassman RJ (1984). Adverse reactions to psychedelic drugs. A review of the literature. *J Nerv Ment Dis* 172:577–595.
36. Taylor RL, Maurer JI, Tinklenberg JR (1970). Management of "bad trips" in an evolving drug scene. *JAMA* 213:422–425.
37. Giannini AJ, Loiselle RH, DiMarzio LR, Giannini MC (1987). Augmentation of haloperidol by ascorbic acid in phencyclidine intoxication. *Am J Psychiatry* 144:1207–1209.

CHAPTER 26

The Pharmacology of Abstinence

History

The typical conception is that once the user of a drug ceases self-administration that the effects of the drug diminish and resolve within hours to days. However, there has been a growing body of clinical evidence and research data for some time that suggests that the effects of drugs (and alcohol) may persist months and years beyond the immediate effects of intoxication and acute withdrawal (1–7).

Various terms have been used to denote the persistent effects of drugs such as protracted abstinence, subacute withdrawal, and prolonged effects of drugs and alcohol. The commonality through all the states is that despite abstinence from drugs and alcohol, effects directly or indirectly related to the intoxication continue to be observable and have a bearing on the clinical course and treatment management (8–10).

The reasons for the symptoms during the initial stages of recovery are many and varied, and include: (i) manifestations of end organ damage; (ii) persistent changes in receptor-mediated function; (iii) the prolonged presence of the drug in storage sites in the body; (iv) the influence of conflict created by the addictive behaviors; (v) the lack of mature personality skills for adaptation to environment without the effects of frequent and persistent intoxication and acute withdrawal states (11–16).

Intoxication

The end organ damage from drugs and alcohol occurs throughout the body. The brain is particularly vulnerable to the effects of alcohol and many drugs. Studies show that cerebral atrophy with a decrease in volume of brain matter and an increase in ventricular size is present in chronic alcoholics. These changes reflect some yet-to-be-identified pathological process that may include actual neuronal dropout, neural fiber degeneration, or astrocytic death, or a combination of these that would lead to reduce brain volume (17).

In several studies, the cerebral atrophy as measured by computerized to-mography (CT) reverses over months in many of the chronic alcoholics studied. The brain matter volume returned and the ventricular size diminished. These findings have been correlated with changes in IQ in some studies. The I.Q. function of alcoholics of all ages was reduced, particularly in those that showed cerebral atrophy. However, the I.Q. improved and the cerebral atrophy resolved over months (17).

Many investigators have demonstrated lowered I.Q. in chronic alcoholics. It is a well-established clinical observation that the cognitive deficits are impaired in the actively drinking alcoholic and improve with abstinence. These cognitive defects are global and represent a dementia syndrome in which the memory, attention, and concentration, and cognitive and other measures of higher cortical function are reduced. All these changes improve with abstinence over time, and in some studies, improvement is noted as long as 2 years or longer after cessation of alcohol consumption (18).

Other studies have shown that chronic alcohol intake has produced measurable central nervous system changes that persisted long after alcohol was withdrawn. These changes were in the form of neural hyperexcitability, most marked in the reticular formation, hippocampus, and frontal and parietal cortex. Following induced alcohol dependence in rats, abnormal locomotor and rapid-eye-movement (REM) sleep patterns persisted after 6 months abstinence from alcohol. Nearly half of acutely abstinent alcoholics revealed increased metabolites of noradrenergic release as measured by increased levels of 3-methoxy-4-hydroxyphenyl-glycol (MHPG) in the cerebrospinal fluid. These increased levels of MHPG declined over several weeks of abstinence and correlated with a diminution of clinical symptoms of irritability and grandiosity, and changes in auditory evoked potentials (19–23).

Cannabis (marijuana) intoxication has shown in monkeys to produce persistent changes in electrical activity and brain size. Recorded activity in the septal electrodes persisted many months after the monkey smoked the equivalent of three marijuana cigarettes a day. Ventricular enlargement with reduction in brain volume was found in monkeys administered daily tetrahydrocannabinol (THC) for 5 years. In humans, abrupt discontinuation of marijuana is followed by irritability, restlessness, hypotension, tachycardia, anxiety, depression, and insomnia that persisted for months during abstinence (24–26).

Examples of possible receptor changes and persistence of drugs in storage sites in the body are available, particularly with lipid-soluble drugs such as cannabis and benzodiazepines. Studies have shown that metabolites of THC may be found in the urine months after cessation of use. Also, in animal studies, one injection of THC in the peritoneal cavity of a naive rat resulted in the detection of cannabis in the fat stores 2 months later. Anecdotal clinical reports commonly report that human chronic marijuana users will experience a "rush" or "high" months after a dose of marijuana, particularly during exercise or following a diet with weight loss and mobilization of fat stores. It appears that THC may be released slowly over time, as it is known that there is constant turnover of fat stores (26).

The storage phenomena may also be true for benzodiazepines. Clinical studies have demonstrated that benzodiazepines may be detected months in the urine after discontinuation. Benzodiazepines, as THC, are highly lipid soluble. There is considerable evidence that a severe, protracted benzodiazepine withdrawal may persist for months and years after last use. The symptoms are anxiety, depression, tinnitus, involuntary movements, paresthesia, hypersensitivity to sensory stimuli, perceptual distortions, tremors, headaches, irritability, anhedonia, lack of energy, impaired concentration, derealization, and depersonalization. These symptoms diminish imperceptibly in the individual and can be difficult to tolerate; however, they do eventually subside (27,28).

Mood disturbances in alcoholics and drug addicts, including those addicted to benzodiazepines, stimulants, and opiates, may persist for months after cessation of use. A small proportion of alcoholics, and of stimulant and benzodiazepine users, will show persistent depression with lowered mood, anhedonia, and sleep disturbances. Also, anxiety and a lack of motivation and mood modulation are evident for months and years in these alcoholic and drug users. However, substantial improvement in mood occurs in the first year or two (29,30).

The bases of these persistent drug effects during abstinence may reflect changes in receptor structure and function. Chronic stimulation by the agonist drugs lead to up- and downregulation with changes in receptor numbers, and subsequent hypersensitivity and hyposensitivity of postsynaptic receptors. The actual changes induced by the drugs depend on the neurochemical mechanism of action. Chronic cocaine administration results in a presynaptic dopamine depletion and a postsynaptic hypersensitivity, whereas chronic opiate administration leads to a reduced receptor response to opiates, and perhaps a reduction in the endogenous ligand (31,32).

Studies have not clearly demonstrated how long these persistent effects of drug in storage sites and receptor changes last, and how closely they correlate with clinical symptoms in the abstinent state. More studies in humans particularly need to confirm these preliminary results for a crucial clinical condition of protracted drug effects during abstinence (33,34).

A study that illustrates these persistent effects investigated psychiatric symptomatology over 10 years in a sample of alcoholics drawn from Alcoholics Anonymous. The study found, on measures of severity of psychopathology, that there was overall lessening of these measures in the 312 subjects studied over the 10-year period. The initial scores for less than 6 months of abstinence showed a severity comparable to only 2.5% of the population. The results after 10 years of abstinence approximates the general population. The recovered alcoholics resembled the norms for the population on most measures.

The items relating to CNS hyperexcitability are common in early abstinence, such as restlessness and disturbances in sleep, depression, interpersonal sensitivity, anxiety, and obsessive compulsive symptoms, whereas memory problems had also improved but remained above population norms after 10 years of abstinence (29,30).

Intervention and Treatment

Time is the essential factor in treatment of these persistent drug-induced effects, time in conjunction with an active recovery program and psychotherapy as needed. In some ways, these troublesome symptoms can serve as reminders of the drug-induced effects, and motivate the drug user to continue to abstain from alcohol and drugs. Some strong motivators for involvement in a treatment strategy, such as a 12-step program of Alcoholics Anonymous, are the discomforts such as anxiety and depression. The alcoholic and drug addict may be more apt to take the necessary actions to abstain from these drugs and make the necessary changes in attitude and lifestyle if the present state is not a comfortable one (35).

However, there are times when the severity of the symptoms, such as intense anxiety, depression, or insomnia, may be too overwhelming for the alcoholic or drug addict to abstain. The judicious use of antidepressants and antipsychotic medications may be useful in these instances. As a rule of thumb, if the symptoms persist for more than a few weeks and significantly interfere with function or jeopardize abstinence, or they are incapacitating from the onset of abstinence, these medications may be instituted (36–38). The doses must be titrated but generally are similar to those used for other disorders that are non-drug related such as depression. The duration of use is also similar in that they can be tapered and discontinued after 6 months to observe if the drug effects have subsided. It is important to note that antidepressants and antipsychotic medications also have withdrawal syndromes that are similar to other drugs, and must be considered if symptoms are still present. This withdrawal syndrome from antidepressants and antipsychotics include anxiety, depression, insomnia, malaise, and other manifestations (39,40).

Of importance is to note that because the typical alcoholic and drug addict in current clinical populations is addicted to and dependent on multiple drugs and alcohol simultaneously and concurrently, the withdrawal syndrome will be influenced accordingly. (See other chapters.) Studies show that multiple drug addiction in alcoholics is more severe than without drugs, and the withdrawal may be as well. It is important to recognize that the abstinence period may be marked by multiple drug effects, and as likely to be so as not.

The treatment of the multiple addicted and dependent is similar to that of the single drug type. The symptoms of anxiety, depression, insomnia, and others are nonspecific manifestations of drug effects on the brain. The same principles apply in the use of medications for multiple drug effects as with the single drugs.

It is also important to bear in mind that the alcoholic and drug addict has a vulnerability to drug effects from any origin, whether a drug of addiction or one of medication. The drug effect is nonspecific, and may impair the alcoholic's and drug addict's ability to think clearly and experience changes in the psychodynamic and affective states that are critical to recovery. Also, the loss of control over addictive drug use and alcohol extends to medications. The clinician must exert control for the addict and always be alert to drug-seeking behavior that is not in the interest of the addict.

References

1. Himmelsbach CK (1942). Clinical studies of drug addiction. *Arch Intern Med* 69:766–772.
2. Martin WR, Jasinski DR, Sapira JD, et al. (1968). The respiratory effects of morphine during a cycle of dependence. *J Pharmacol Exp Ther* 162:182–189.
3. Kay DC (1975). Human sleep and EEG through a cycle of methadone dependence. *Electroencephalogr Clin Neurophysiol* 38:35–43.
4. Kissin B, Schenker V, Schenker A (1959). The acute effects of ethyl alcohol and chlorpromazine on certain physiological functions in alcoholics. *Q J Stud Alcohol* 20:481–493.
5. Begleiter H, Porjesz B (1977). Persistence of brain hyperexcitability following chronic alcohol exposure in rats. *Adv Exp Med Biol* 85B:209–222.
6. Gitlow SE, Dziedzic SW, Dziedzic LM (1977). Tolerance to ethanol after prolonged abstinence. *Adv Exp Med Biol* 85A:511–591.
7. Begleiter H, Denoble V, Porjesz B (1980). Protracted brain dysfunction after alcohol withdrawal in monkeys. In *Biological Effects of Alcohol*, Begleiter H, ed., pp. 231–249. New York: Plenum Press.
8. Begleiter H, Porjesz B (1979). Persistence of a subacute withdrawal system following ethanol intake. *Drug Alcohol Depend* 4:353–357.
9. Khan A, Ciranlo DA, Nelson WH (1984). Dexamethasone suppression test in recently detoxified alcoholics. *J Clin Psychopharmacol* 4:94–97.
10. Brown SA, Schuckit MA (1988). Changes in depression among abstinent alcoholics. *J Stud Alcohol* 49:412–417.
11. Snyder S, Karacan I (1985). Sleep patterns of sober chronic alcoholics. *Neurospsychobiology* 13:97–100.
12. Smith DE, Wesson DR (1983). Benzodiazepine dependency syndromes. *J Psychoact Drugs* 15:85–89.
13. Busto V, Fornazzari L, Naranjo CA (1988). Protracted tinnitus after discontinuation of long-term therapeutic use of benzodiazepines. *J Clin Psychopharmacol* 8:359–362.
14. Golombok S, Moodley P, Lader M (1988). Cognitive impairment in long-term benzodiazepine users. *Psychol Med* 18:365–374.
15. Ricaurte GA, Schuster CR, Seiden IS (1980). Long-term effects of repeated methylamphetamine administration on dopamine and serotonin neurons in the rat brain. *Brain Res* 193:153–163.
16. Ricaurte GA, Bryan D, Strauss L, et al. (1985). Hallucinogenic amphetamine selectively destroys brain serotonin nerve terminals. *Science* 229:986–988.

17. Cala LA, Mastaglia FL (1981). Computerized tomography in chronic alcoholics. *Alcohol Clin Exp Res* 5(2):283–294.
18. Parsons DA, Leber WR (1981). The relationship between cognitive dysfunction and brain damage in alcoholics: Causation or epiphirnomendal. *Clin Exp Res* 5(2):326–343.
19. Bonnet MH (1985). Effects of sleep disruption on sleep, performance and mood. *Sleep* 8:11–19.
20. Wagman AMI, Allen RP (1975). Effects of alcohol ingestion and abstinence on slow wave sleep of alcoholics. In *Alcohol Intoxication and Withdrawal, Experimental Studies II*, Gross, ed., pp. 453–466. New York: Plenum Press.
21. Borg S, Kvande H, Sedvall G (1981). Central norepinephrine metabolism during alcohol intoxication in addicts and healthy volunteers. *Science* 213:1135–1137.
22. Alling C, Balldin J, Bokstrom K, et al. (1982). Studies on duration of a late recovery period after chronic abuse of ethanol. *Acta Psychiatr Scand* 66:384–397.
23. Zarcone VP, Cohen M, Hoddes E (1975). WAIS, MMPI and sleep variables in abstinent alcoholics. In *Alcohol Intoxication and Withdrawal, Experimental Studies II*, Gross, ed., pp. 431–451. New York: Plenum Press.
24. Jones RT (1983). Cannabis and health. *Am Rev Med* 34:247–258.
25. McGraham JP, Dublin AB, Sassenrath E (1984). Long-term 9-tetra-hydrocannabinol treatment: Computed tomography of the brains of rhesus monkeys. *Am J Dis Child* 138:1109–1112.
26. Heath RA, Fitzjarrell AT, Garey RE, et al. (1979). Chronic marijuana smoking: Its effects on function and structure of the primate brain. In *Marijuana: Biological Effects*, Nahas GC, Patton, WDM, eds. New York: Plenum Press.
27. Ashton H (1984). Benzodiazepine withdrawal: An unfinished story. *Br Med J* 288:1135–1140.
28. Ashton H (1986). Adverse effects of prolonged benzodiazepine use. *Adverse Drug React Bull* 118:440–443.
29. DeSoto CB, O'Donnell WE, Alfred LJ, et al. (1985). Symptomatology in alcoholics at various stages of abstinence. *Alcohol Clin Exp Res* 9:505–512.
30. DeSoto CB, O'Donnell WE, DeSoto JL (1989). Long-term recovery in alcoholics. *Alcohol Clin Exp Res* 13:693–697.
31. Elinwood EH (1974). The epidemiology of stimulant use. In *Drug Use: Epidemiology and Sociological Approaches*, Josephson F, Carroll E, eds., pp. 303–309. Washington, DC: Hemisphere.
32. Gawin FH, Kleber HD (1986). Abstinence symptomatology and psychiatric diagnoses in cocaine abusers. *Arch Gen Psychiatry* 43:107–113.
33. Wikler A (1948). Recent progress in research on the neurophysiological basis of morphine addiction. *Am J Psychiatry* 105:328–338.
34. Dole VP (1988). Implications of methadone maintenance for theories of narcotics addiction. *JAMA* 260:3025–3029.
35. Miller NS (1987). A primer of the treatment process for alcoholism and drug addiction. *Psychiatry Lett* 5(7):30–37.
36. Garwin FH, Kleber HD, Byck R, et al. (1989). Desipramine facilitation of initial cocaine abstinence. *Arch Gen Psychiatry* 46:117–121.
37. Weiss RD (1988). Relapse to cocaine abuse after initiating desipramine treatment. *JAMA* 260:2545–2546.

38. Little HJ, Dolin S, Halsey MJ (1986). Calcium channel antagonists decrease ethanol withdrawal syndrome. *Life Sci* 39:2059-2065.
39. Charney DS, Heninger GR, Sternberg DE, et al. (1982). Abrupt discontinuation of tricyclic antidepressant drugs: Evidence for noradrenergic hyperactivity. *Br J Psychiatry* 141:377-386.
40. Overall JE, Reilly EL, Kelley JT, et al. (1985). Persistence of depression in detoxified alcoholics. *Alcohol Clin Exp Res* 9(4):331-333.

Chapter 27

The Nonpharmacological Treatment of Abuse and Addiction to Alcohol and Drugs

History

The principles and philosophy of the abstinence-based Twelve-Step Program of Alcoholics Anonymous (AA) can be incorporated into the treatment process for alcohol and drug addiction. Current inpatient and outpatient psychiatric treatment may use the first 5 steps as an approach to alcohol and drug addiction. Furthermore, the program of AA is recommended as a mainstay of continued treatment in the long-term follow-up. However, AA limits its affiliation with rehabilitation centers as suggested in its Six Tradition: "An AA group ought never endorse, finance, or lend the AA name to any related facility or outside enterprise, lest problems of money, property, and prestige divert us from our primary purpose." Adherence to this principle ensures that AA remains focused on helping alcoholics recover from alcoholism and drug addiction.

Treatment for Alcoholism (and Other Drugs): The Disease Concept

Alcoholism and drug addiction are diseases (1–5) for which treatment is essential and relatively sophisticated (6). One of the important reasons AA enjoys the popularity and success that it does today is because of advances in the effective treatment for alcoholism. Conversely, treatment for alcoholism has been enhanced by the inclusion of the principles of AA. The two concepts have benefited each other reciprocally. A basic tenet of the treatment approach as in AA is that alcohol and drug addiction are physical, mental, and spiritual diseases. Treatment centers employ physicians, psychologists, counselors, and social workers who treat the diseases of alcoholism and drug addiction. The fundamental treatment focus is on the alcoholic; however, alcoholism (alcohol addiction) is considered a family illness so that the family is also intimately involved in the treatment process. Alcoholism and drug addiction will, and often do, affect each family member as severely and insidiously as they do the alcoholic (7–10).

Diagnosis

Denial in both the alcoholic and the family members is an essential feature of addiction. Without denial, alcohol addiction could not exist in the proportions we know today (7). There is a significant amount of denial in virtually every alcoholic entering treatment. A substantial amount of the treatment process centers around the First Step where the denial of alcoholism and its consequences are gradually confronted. This confrontation of the alcoholic by the group is frequently accomplished by presenting the alcoholic with the evidence of the drinking and drug use that includes the consequences affecting him and others.

Intervention and Treatment

Although AA remains a mainstay for "long-term" treatment of the alcoholic, its principles and practices may be incorporated into forms of acute intervention and treatment programs. Considerable refinement and application of the AA model into treatment programs has resulted in effective inpatient and outpatient treatments for alcohol and drug addiction (1–5).

The forms of treatment that are effective for other disorders are employed in the treatment of addiction: these include group and individual therapies. The steps of AA can be effectively incorporated into the modalities of group and individual therapies. The concepts and application of these steps are readily applied in formal treatment settings for alcoholisms and drug addiction.

As a part of the treatment programs, the First Five Steps of Alcoholics Anonymous may be addressed and completed.

Step One: "We admitted we were powerless over alcohol—that our lives had become unmanageable" (10). The requirement for this step is complete abstinence from alcohol and other drugs to which the alcoholic may be addicted. The alcoholic admits that he has a loss of control over alcohol use and accepts the requirement of complete abstinence from alcohol. The alcoholic at some point has lost his ability to control the amount of alcohol drunk and the resolve to abstain from alcohol. The word "unmanageable" refers to the effects of alcoholism on the alcoholic and others around him. The admission and acceptance of "powerlessness" over alcohol are essential for continued abstinence and the change in attitude and mood that occurs as a result of applying the remaining Eleven Steps to the alcoholic's daily life.

The disease concept of alcoholism purports a physical, mental, and spiritual triad (11). Dr. William Silkworth referred to alcoholism as an "allergy" in Doctor's Opinion in the book *Alcoholics Anonymous*. Dr. Silkworth instilled the disease concept of alcoholism in the cofounders of Alcoholics Anonymous, Bill Wilson and Dr. Robert Smith, who incorporated it into the program of recovery of AA (10).

Well-known toxic consequences of alcohol on the brain and body have been described in detail in a variety of medical sources (12,13). These physical and neuropsychological consequences of alcohol use include widespread involvement of many organ systems in the body (14–17). Cognitive, mood, and memory disturbances emanate from direct toxic perturbations of the brain cells in a diffuse distribution in both higher cerebral and lower limbic centers (6,18). A multitude of medical sequelae ensue from disruption of function, and at times pathological injury, in the gastrointestinal-intestinal, cardiovascular, pulmonary, endocrine, and integumentary systems as well as others (19).

The mental consequences are dramatically illustrated in the psychological state of the alcoholic, which contains many paradoxical characterizations. The outer phenomenology provides a portrait of a defiant, overconfident, exuberant, and independent personality behind which is a victim who feels inferior, depressed, dependent, hopeless, helpless, and worthless. The disease of alcoholism (and drug addiction) has rendered the individual powerless over alcohol/drugs and self. An added mental agony is that the alcoholic (addict) is at least partially aware of the hopelessness of this predicament, but is unable by resolve and will to deter his apparent self-inflicted demise (5,7).

The spiritual consequences are devastating. Usually, the alcoholic has been acting and thinking contrary to his moral standard or values, that is, sense of right and wrong, and this conflict has produced a significant sense of guilt and isolation from himself and others. The price of denying his conscience its proper and sufficient expression is enormous and uncompromising. The existential state of the alcoholic is to not believe in any power that is greater than himself to maintain the illusion of self-reliance and the pattern of addiction, which is loss of self-control. The chaos produced by the alcoholic's exercising his self-will in the face of an overpowering addiction is evident in all aspects of his attitudes, moods, and perceptions. The complexity of the addictive state is greater than the simple inebriation from alcohol and drugs; the sense of "being" is corrupted. The sense of well-being is replaced by a profound loss of meaning. Self-centered purpose and direction masquerade as a contemporary justification of Machiavellian thinking and action.

A profound lowered mood and a change in self-attitude of worthlessness, hopelessness, helplessness, and self-blame constitute a syndrome of depression, sometimes very severe. Disturbances in vegetative functions, such as altered sleep and eating patterns, may occur. A blunted affect and psychomotor retardation may accompany the depressive state induced by alcoholism and drug addiction. The specific treatment of the alcohol and drug addiction with abstinence and the addict's application of the Steps will often relieve and resolve the severe depressive syndrome. Action taken in these steps will often result in an elevation of mood and an establishment of an improved self-attitude. Spontaneous and expressive affect and behaviors replace the earlier dour and downtrodden appearance. The Twelve-Step Program frequently is not only necessary, but sufficient for the reversal of "endogenous" or "biological depressions." The Dexamethasone Suppression Tests and Thyroid-Releasing Stimulation test are frequently abnormal in active alcoholics and drug addicts and normal during abstinence, suggesting an alcohol and drug-induced biological substrate for the major depression seen in these persons (7).

A common conclusion, and an almost natural sequela, to the cumulative effects of the physical, mental, and spiritual deterioration and degradation induced by alcohol and drugs is suicidal thought – sometimes actions. Next to advancing age, alcoholism and drug addiction are the most serious risk factors for suicide; they are at least equal and probably above idiopathic depression, which occupies a lower position among risk factors (20,21).

The adverse consequences are evident in the disruption of family harmony and cohesiveness, impaired performance at work, an array of legal entanglements and social infringements, and a wide variety of personal indiscretions and violations. These add to the already substantial guilt and isolation of the alcoholic.

The alcoholic now experiences a severe impairment in the perception of his "reality" and in the ability to discern and judge accurately. If honesty or self-insight uncovers this state of powerlessness and irrationality, then the need for a power greater than the alcohol and drugs is required to relieve the insanity of continued addictive use.

Step Two: "Came to believe that a power greater than ourselves could restore us to sanity" (10). The alcoholic is unable to keep from drinking on willpower, wits, and character and, in reality, drinks addictively against his will. The insanity of the second step is that the alcoholic takes the first drink in the first place. The assumption is that same person would not drink at all, knowing the consequences of another bout of drinking and the loss of control if when one drink is taken to set into motion an unyielding, compulsive consumption of alcohol. The alcoholic has lost the willpower to refuse a drink or a drug. The dilemma of the alcoholic is a lack of power of choice to avoid drinking and drug use that is the basis of an addiction. Further, the misconception that the alcoholic enjoys drinking at the point of addictive use perpetuates the mortal condemnation of the alcoholic. The euphoria or enjoyment has usually long waned from the drinking experience of the alcoholic. The mystery is that the alcoholic continues to drink without pleasure, despite the anhedonia produced by addictive drinking.

An addiction has three components: a preoccupation with alcohol and other drugs, compulsive use, and relapse to alcohol and other drugs. If the alcoholic is to successfully resist the addiction, outside help must be accepted. The insanity is that the alcoholic drinks even though to drink may mean significant adverse consequences and perhaps death, slow or fast; however, the alcoholic will often drink because of the addiction. Paradoxically, the power utilized by the alcoholic can only be other than or outside the alcoholic. The power, while under treatment, is often the physician or counselor, or the group of alcoholics in the treatment program at the time.

Step Two is incorporated into this treatment program by introducing the concept of choice to the alcoholic. The alcoholic can learn to exercise his choice not to drink if he accepts his/her "powerlessness" or loss of control over alcoholism. The sanity is restored when the alcoholic is able to grasp the consequences of alcoholic drinking before taking a drink. The choice is maintained as long as abstinence and a commitment to recovery remain in effect.

Step Three: "Made a decision to turn our will and our lives over to the care of God as we understood Him" (10). No attendance in a church or adherence to theological dogma is required to accomplish this step, only a decision. The important factor in initiating this step is for the alcoholic to make a decision to turn his "will and life" over to the care of God. This step is spiritual and not religious in nature. The alcoholic volunteers some confidence and faith that accepting therapy for the alcoholism will work. The requirement is to "make a decision" to accept help from a power greater than himself.

A critical issue of this step is control. Repeatedly the alcoholic has failed at efforts to control his drinking patterns and alcoholism and has made persistent, although unsuccessful, attempts to control time, quantity, and places of alcohol and drug consumption. More importantly, the emotional loss of control and "instincts" that have gone awry have produced a state of fury and confusion in the alcoholic. The need for sex, food, love, and security has been often exaggerated, distorted, and misdirected by the alcohol and drugs, sometimes into forms of other illnesses such as sexual and eating disorders. The basis of these distortions in sex, food, and emotions is complex, derived from disturbances in the limbic system by the toxic effects of alcohol and drugs. The limbic system contains the neurosubstrate for emotions (such as anger, placidity, fear), sexual drive and expression, hunger, and memory (18). The drive states and emotions may have been entrained by and associated with alcohol and drugs. An increase in the tension of the drive states may signal the pursuit and use of alcohol and drugs. A reduction in the drive state may be satisfied by the reinforcement produced by alcohol and drugs (19).

A caricature develops of a self-centered, immature, self-seeking, self-willed, fearful, and resentful personality. A defiance of the superego and its punitive exhortations is costly in the degree of guilt that is inflicted on the victim. The addictive process forces the individual to defy important moral values and ethical directives. The cumulative effect is destructive and overwhelming to the individual who is attempting to "control" all the diverse impulses and conflicts.

The alcoholic must paradoxically relinquish these attempts at control to regain mastery over self, emotions, and instincts. The belief that a power both spiritual and human will return the control to the alcoholic is an essential step in recovery. A self-trust begins with a trust in others, both visible and invisible. The key phrase in this step is God "as we understand Him," wherein the alcoholic can choose to believe in any power that is greater than himself to avoid the return to ruinous reliance and patterns of addiction of loss of control with alcohol. The alcoholic chooses to apply his will to a source of strength and help other than the addictive mode directed by the drives in the limbic system that has been occupying his attitude, mood and perceptions.

Step Four: "Made a searching and fearless moral inventory of ourselves" (10). This step requires recounting and detailing the consequences of the alcoholism and drug addiction admitted in Step One. The alcoholic takes an inventory of the way in which alcohol had adversely affected him and others. The expression of conscious and unconscious material to the self is of paramount importance for the alcoholic to achieve a psychodynamic equilibrium. The inventory pertains to conscious and unconscious conflicts that represent the obstacles, which may or may not include moral judgments, within the alcoholic to future recovery. These obstacles frequently include defects in emotions (mood) and attitudes such as resentments, anger, fears, immaturity, and sources of guilt. Some mastery over emotions, change in attitudes, and resolution must occur for the alcoholic to achieve and maintain recovery, enjoy satisfactory sobriety, and avoid the syndrome of "depression" that is the total expression of these derangements in emotions, attitudes, and guilt. A self-mastering over the limbic system by higher brain function is promoted by the use of the intellectual and spiritual exercise of self-inventory.

Step Five: "Admitted to God, to ourselves, and to another human being the exact nature of our wrongs" (10). This is a step of confession or, in psychodynamic terms, a release of conscious and unconscious conflict to achieve an intrapsychic equilibrium between ego, id, and superego. The alcoholic confides in and confesses to someone else the obstacles in the form of distorted attitudes and deranged morals uncovered in Step Four. This is a necessary step for the alcoholic to achieve full awareness regarding his intrapsychic state and effect of the consequences of the alcoholism. Confidentiality is a critical requirement for this step. A skilled and compassionate listener, knowledgeable to the purpose of the alcoholic, is essential. The other person frequently is a sponsor in AA or a clergyman, although it can be a psychiatrist or counselor. The confession is therapeutic by itself, relieving depressive moods and distorted attitudes, and frequently leads to a solid foundation for recovery if done with a measure of honesty and sincerity.

Alcoholism as a Family Illness

The family undergoes a similar clinical evaluation, self-scrutiny, and treatment. The family members must examine their state of denial and how the diseases of alcoholism and drug addiction have affected them over the years. Those nonalcoholics affected by alcoholism are said to be as "ill" as the alcoholic. The recognition of their illness if often difficult because the identification of the alcoholic as the primary problem tends to distract attention from the nonalcoholic and to disguise the severe personality disturbances that can occur in those affected by the alcoholic. Often resentments that are directed toward the alcoholic are key offenders present within the family.

It is critically important for the entire family to be included in the treatment process at the same time as the alcoholic. Not doing so can delay not only the alcoholic's progress, but can also delay the treatment of the family. Alcoholics who are more likely to recover are those who have the support and involvement of their family and significant others. The alcoholic who is alone without family, social, and community support is statistically less apt to recover. The more the family knows and the healthier it becomes through treatment, the better able the alcoholic and the family are to recover together (7,10).

Follow-Up

Follow-up and continued treatment after discharge from an inpatient program for alcoholism and drug addiction can contain a variety of ingredients. It may be only an entrance into AA in the community as a continuation by the alcoholic who began attending AA meetings while in treatment. The family members and significant others who are not alcoholic are encouraged to attend Alanon on a regular basis. Some alcoholics need placement in residential treatment facilities, which are called "halfway houses." This is a misnomer, because these facilities are actually extended treatment care facilities where the alcoholic continues to receive group therapy and individual counseling, has employment, and attends meetings of AA.

Day or partial hospital treatment programs are currently available in some centers. These programs provide the full range of group and individual therapies, which are available to the inpatients and outpatients. The patients may have completed inpatient programs and have progressed to a stable state not requiring the therapeutic structure of a full-time stay in the hospital. Patients may also attend partial or day hospital programs de novo without a prior inpatient program if their clinical state and social supports are sufficiently stable to promote abstinence from alcohol and regular attendance in the program.

For many alcoholics, aftercare treatment on a follow-up basis after discharge from a hospital program is important and often involves the family. The treatment program may include discussions, education, and group therapies that address current problems shared by the alcoholics and their families. These are more than support groups. They are actual therapy groups that meet on a regular basis from one to five times a week with a duration of 1 or more hours a day or evening. The total duration of treatment may be weeks, months, or years.

In addition, alcoholics have other psychiatric problems more frequently than other populations, including eating, sexual, mood, and personality disorders; these can also be addressed in the hospital programs and in the follow-up treatment plans. Special types of treatments and therapies from psychiatrists and psychologists are available for these recovering alcoholics and drug addicts. There are also support groups in the community for bulimia and anorexia patients and for individuals with particular sexual problems.

References

1. Edwards G, Arif A, Hodgson R (1981). Nomenclature and classification of drug- and alcohol-related problems. Bull WHO 59:225–242.
2. Jellinek EM (1960). *The Disease Concept of Alcoholism*, pp. 139–148. New Brunswick, NJ: Hillhouse Press.
3. Vaillant GE (1983). *The Natural History of Alcoholism*. Cambridge: Harvard University Press.
4. Milam JR, Ketchum K (1981). *Under the Influence*. Kent, WA: Madrona Publishers.
5. Gold MS, Verebey K (1984). The pharmacology of cocaine. *Psychiatr Ann* 14(10):714–723.
6. Dackis CA, Gold MS, Estroff TW (1989). Inpatient treatment of addiction. In *Treatments of Psychiatric Disorders: A Task Force Report of the APA*, pp. 1359–1379. American Psychiatric Association, Washington, DC.
7. Milam J (1978). *The Emergent Concept of Alcoholism*. Kirkland, WA: Alcoholism Center Associates.
8. Mendelson JH, Mello NK (1985). *The Diagnosis and Treatment of Alcoholism*, 2d Ed. New York: McGraw-Hill.
9. Goodwin GW (1984). Familial alcoholism: A review. *J Clin Psychiatry* 45(12):14–17.
10. AA (1976). *Alcoholics Anonymous*, 3d Ed. New York: Alcoholics Anonymous World Services.
11. Jellinek EM, Jolliffee N (1940). Effect of alcohol on the individual. *Q J Stud Alcohol* 1:110–181.
12. Höffman FG (1983). *A Handbook on Drug and Alcohol Abuse*, 2d Ed. New York: Oxford University Press.
13. Jaffe JH (1985). Drug and addiction abuse. In *The Pharmacological Bases of Therapeutics*, 7th Ed., Gilman AG, Goodman LS, Rall TW, Murad, F, eds., pp. 532–581. New York: Macmillan.
14. Schukit MA (1983). Alcoholism and other psychiatric disorders. *Hosp Community Psychiatry* 34(11):1022–1027.
15. Mayfield DG (1979). Alcohol and affect: Experimental Studies. In *Alcoholism and Affective Disorders*, Goodwin DW, Erickson CK, eds., pp. 99–107. New York: SP Medical and Scientific Books.
16. Parsons OA, Leber WR (1981). The relationship between cognitive dysfunction and brain damage in alcoholics: Casual or epipheromenal. *Clin Exp Res* 5(2):326–343.
17. Adams RP, Victor M (1985). *Principles of Neurology*, 3d Ed. New York: McGraw-Hill.
18. Miller NS, Dackis CA, Gold MS (1987). The relationship of addiction, toler-

ance, and dependence: A neurochemical approach. *J Subst Abuse Treat* 4:197–207.

19. Lieber CSS (1982). *Medical Disorders of Alcoholism*. Philadelphia: Saunders.
20. Martin RI, Cloninger CR, Guze SB, et al. (1985). Mortality in a follow-up of five hundred psychiatric outpatients. *Arch Gen Psychiatry* 42:47–66.
21. Litman RE, Farberow NL, Wold CI, et al. (1974). Prediction models of suicidal behavior. In *The Prediction of Suicide*, Beck AT, Resnick HLP, Lettieri DJ, eds., p. 141. Bowler, MD: Charles Press.

CHAPTER 28

The Prevention of Abuse and Addiction to Alcohol and Drugs

Prevention, as a subject in medicine, is very similar to alcoholism among the attitudes of the physicians. Unfortunately, too many physicians give up too easily in the battle against the onset of an illness. If a fraction of effort and money that is expended in treatment of illness would be devoted to prevention, much savings in cost, suffering, and lives might result.

A physician feels compelled to "go all out" to save lives almost irrespective or age and illness and cost, that is, expensive intensive care room treatment, in cases of catastrophic illness, in the very young and the very old, and any age in between. The attitude is against weighing the cost versus benefit except in extremely obvious cases.

However, prevention is not ordinarily aggressively pursued except in large-scale, community-based operations such as for vaccinations and detection campaigns that may identify a patient population for diagnosis and treatment of an illness. Rarely are such efforts expended to prevent an illness. It is paradoxical that prevention is so little regarded, considering its high cost : effect ratio. Further, physicians are not well trained in prevention in medical school and specialty training.

Alcoholism is an area of medicine that heretofore has received little time and attention in medical school curricula. Alcoholism has not yet gained full acceptance as an illness or a disease. Physicians still debate whether or not alcoholism (and drug addiction) is a disease. The "disease concept of alcoholism" is still quoted, instead of merely the "disease of alcoholism," as though we find it necessary to think in conceptual terms, instead of actual disease processes (1).

The physician is not alone in the inadequate recognition of alcoholism (and drug addiction) as diseases. Alcoholism is still popularly regarded as an accepted consequences of something else. Excessive or problem drinking is often denied or attributed to other extraneous or underlying causes. Alcoholism for most is not a primary and sufficient illness that involves the relentless pursuit of alcohol in spite of adverse consequences. Instead, drinking is generally regarded as a symptom of something else rather than a disease by itself.

The public generally does not regard drinking as a potentially catastrophic and fatal health hazard. Alcoholism is probably our number one health problem, especially if drugs are included, as they should be in defining today's addict. Yet the American public is saturated with practices and attitudes that allow acceptance of almost unlimited alcohol consumption. It is disturbing to note a society that is saturated with announcements about, advertisements for, and almost unlimited access to, alcohol. The country is currently preoccupied with a "drug problem," for example, cocaine, but appears totally blind to the alcohol problem.

It is impossible to watch a sporting event on television without feeling (or at least seeing) driving and forceful enticements to drink beer, and to drink more beer. The young of today must know as much about beer as they do about their favorite star athletes in order to watch them. Athletes themselves are participants in the advertisements. The heroes of modern America are rallying the young and old to drink beer.

The youngsters of today, according to surveys, know more names of beer and other forms of alcohol than they do presidents and states in the history and geography of the United States. Children's minds are permeated with clever and powerful advertisements programmed by the genius of Madison Avenue. These somewhat innocent citizens are being hit with themes and acts that are designed to get people (and them) to drink.

The older children and adults who read magazines of all kinds, including the literary ones, are subjected to persistent and often sexy illustrations of compelling reasons to drink, such as high society, success, companionship, intimacy, and power. The back page of the New Yorker frequently has an advertisement for a liquor. The program for the New York Philharmonic Orchestra frequently contains ads for liquor as well. Young people who are encouraged to learn about and experience higher culture are repeatedly subjected to exhortations to drink to be more advanced.

There are many more examples in all aspects of American society in which alcohol and more than informative exposure to alcohol is everywhere, in fully acceptably and unqualified endorsements by those who use the proceeds for financial support. Unfortunately, little consideration and restraint because of the short- and long-ranging implications are given to the wide exposure and use of alcohol by all ages.

A useful, pragmatic, conceptual approach for consideration of the prevalence rates for alcoholism (drug addiction) is a simple equation: *alcohol and drug addiction equals vulnerability plus exposure.* The most difficult part of the equation and the first step is to recognize that the problem exists, and its magnitude. Without an accurate assessment of the problem, the solutions are vague and understandably inept (1,2).

Identification of the addiction is presented elsewhere in this book, and primarily requires some education and an honest appraisal of the problem. The behaviors of alcohol addiction (and drug addiction) are the preoccupation with acquisition of alcohol or drugs, compulsive use of alcohol and drugs (continued use of alcohol/drugs in spite of adverse consequences), and a pattern or relapse or return to alcohol and drugs in spite of adverse consequences. The addiction is recognized by both the persistent use of alcohol. Without acknowledgement of either, the diagnosis is difficult to make and many times overlooked. Of course, the risk of incorrectly attributing the consequences to something other than alcohol addiction is frequently a problem.

The vulnerability to the development of alcoholism has been demonstrated to be genetic, at least in part. As presented in another chapter, twin and adoption studies, and familial and high-risk studies, have confirmed that a genetic component is implicated in the transmission of alcoholism. The exact nature of this genetic vulnerability has not been identified, although studies in high-risk individuals strongly suggest that it has a physical basis. Alcoholics and high-risk individuals appear to have an enhanced tolerance to alcohol that is manifested subjectively and objectively, and is attributable to central nervous system functions, namely in the brain and brainstem (1,2).

Similar studies for the inheritance to drug addiction have not been performed in drug addicts. However, some familial studies have found that alcoholism is prevalent in the families of cocaine and cannabis addicts, suggesting a genetic link between vulnerability to develop addiction to these drugs as well as to alcohol.

Moreover, the vulnerability portion of the equation does not lend itself to easy manipulation. The genetic vulnerability to alcoholism is perhaps changed only after generations of mating, and no ready and quick solution to altering the genes is currently available — or desirable, for that matter. Education and genetic counseling may have an impact on assortative mating of alcoholics, although this has not been attempted on a large scale. It is not clear that such control has been advocated by very many, or should be.

However, the exposure portion of the equation is subject to manipulation, although perhaps not easily so because of recognizable resistance. Exposure is inclusive to cover all the various factors that are contributing to the eventual use of the drug or alcohol, particularly by those who are susceptible and possess the vulnerability to develop addiction. Exposure is determined by a large number of influences, although these may be categorized under attitudes and practices regarding alcohol and drugs (3,4).

The attitudes toward the use of alcohol are reflected in virtually every aspect of American's way of life because alcohol consumption is a firmly rooted institution. The permissive attitude toward the use of alcohol is evident in everyday life. It is difficult to describe a drinking behavior or event without some attachment of frivolity and humor. Drinking, even to extremes, is an amusing happening. Alcohol is served in many public places, at the White House, at most weddings and funerals, and at many social gatherings. In fact, it is the exception to not have alcohol available as part of the event. The public pressure to have alcohol as part of a social event is as great as is the pressure to use alcohol by those attending.

The peer pressure on children in and out of schools is intolerable. Children must endure tremendous and often insurmountable pressures from their peers to drink and use drugs. Alcohol is the drug first introduced to the child, and is frequently the one most often used. Childhood and adolescent alcoholism is common, unfortunately; as many as 25% to 50% of the alcoholics in the United States have the onset of their alcoholism in their teenage years. The combination of peer pressure and widespread exposure to alcohol in advertisements and practices results in the majority of young Americans being exposed often and in large doses to drugs, particulaly to alcohol.

Other commonly expressed factors in exposure are the "psychosocial factors." The exposure to alcohol does not depend on psychosocial factors that are distinctive, except for some notable conditions. Sociopathic males appear to be more likely to be exposed to alcohol, probably for obvious reasons. Sociopaths appear to be high consumers of alcohol and have high rates of alcoholism. As many as 90% of those incarcerated in prisons are alcoholic, and 80% of the homicides involve alcohol use. More than 75% of the cases of domestic violence involve the use of alcohol, in states of intoxication (3).

The states of deprivation in economic and social conditions do not seem to be distinguishing "psychosocial factors" in the development of alcoholism. These psychosocial factors may be more important in the origin of illicit drug use and trade, where profit for drug dealing is present and represents an additional motivation for propagation of drug use.

It is also important to recognize that alcohol is a gateway for the use and development of addiction to other drugs. Most cocaine and cannabis addicts used and became addicted to alcohol before cocaine and cannabis were tried. It seems that the introduction to drugs other than alcohol is somehow dependent on alcohol. In some ways, alcohol is a conduit to other drug use and addiction. The reasons may lie in the realization that alcohol is a drug and has drug effects similar to those of the illicit drugs.

The sharp demarcation between alcohol and other drugs is not readily possible on pharmacological and pathophysiological grounds. The distinction between alcohol and other drugs is a legal and social one, and subject to considerable error in conferring greater safety for alcohol over some other drugs.

The manipulation of the exposure portion of the equation is possible and could result in the dramatic reduction in the onset of alcoholism and drug addiction. The current changes in attitude and practices toward cigarette smoking provides a model to use for alcohol. Public awareness and attitudes changed sufficiently to finally allow the government to acknowledge that the nicotine contained in cigarettes is addicting. Heretofore, the public opinion and successful lobbying efforts by the tobacco industry prohibited a realistic appraisal of the magnitude of the cigarette problem. Finally, the public sentiment was reflected in new city, state, and federal laws regarding the use and sale of cigarettes.

Some of the more dramatic and effective legislation forbids advertisement on television, restricts smoking in public places, and warns the public of the hazards of cigarette smoking. These and other measures have resulted in significant reduction in exposure to cigarettes. As a consequence, the use of tobacco has recently dropped considerably. A gratifying, corresponding reduction in the adverse consequences of cigarette smoking will certainly follow with the lower rate of addiction to cigarettes.

The same paradigm can be applied to alcohol consumption. The public awareness and attitudes toward alcohol can result in a change in practices regarding the sale and consumption of alcohol. The type and amount of advertisement of alcohol beverages can bedmodified to sane proportions, perhaps eliminated altogether, at least on television. Restricting the places and hours where alcohol can be purchased and used would reduce consumption rates dramatically. These changes will be brought about by legislation prompted by the public; the lawmakers will never venture such decisions regarding alcohol without a directive from the public (5).

The lowered exposure would likely result in a reduction of consumption and a subsequent lowering of a the prevalence rates for alcoholism. This in turn may lead to a reduction in the exposure to illicit drugs when alcohol is no longer as great a gateway to them. The adverse consequences from alcoholism would then be fewer and less compelling, with a reduction in prevalence of use of alcohol and other illicit drugs.

References

1. Schuckit MA (1987). Biological vulnerability to alcoholism. *J Consult Clin Psychol* 55:301–309.
2. Monteiro MG, Schuckit MA. Populations at high risk — Recent Findings. *J Clin Psychiatry* (in press).
3. US DHHS (1986). *Sharing Knowledge for Action*, Proceedings of the National Conference on Alcohol and Drug Abuse Prevention, August 3–6, 1986. Washington, DC: U.S. Dept of Health and Human Services, Public Health Services.
4. Smart RG (1986). The impact on consumption of selling wine in grocery stores. *Alcohol Alcohol* 21:233–236.
5. Gerstein D (1984). Alcohol policy: Preventative options. In *Psychiatry Update III*, Grinspoon L, ed., pp. 359–371. Washington, DC: American Psychiatry Association.

Index

Serax: *see* Oxazepam
Serotonin
  alcohol and, 35, 49
  cocaine and, 166
  drugs affecting actions of, 308, 314,
    316, 324
  function of, 309, 311
  hallucinogens and, 181
Sexual dysfunction and addiction
  alcohol effects, 95–96, 99
  diagnostic categories, 96
  disinterest, 93
  dose of substance and, 93, 95, 96
  drug effects, 98
  impaired satisfaction, 96
  marijuana use and, 207
  neurochemical aspects, 96–98
  performance factors, 93, 95–96
  prevalence of, 93
  treatment of, 98–99
Sexual response, normal
  excitement phase, 89–90
  general physical reactions, 91–92
  hormones and, 97–98
  libido and, 96–97
  nervous system and arousal, 92–93
  neural components, 96–98
  orgasmic phase, 90–91, 92
  plateau phase, 90
  resolution phase, 91
Silkworth, Dr. William, 336
Sleep
  benzodiazepines and, 137–138
  marijuana use and, 202–203
  sedatives/hypnotics and, 269–270
Smith, Dr. Robert, 336
Smokeless tobacco, 241, 242, 243
Social factors, alcohol use, 347–348
Speed ball, 230
"Speed kills," meaning of, 178
Spontaneous abortion, 98
Stimulants, *see also* specific substances
  neurochemical effects of, 313–314
  treatment of withdrawal, 320–321
Storage phenomena, 328–329
Substance-dependence disorders
  abuse versus dependence, 11–12
  addiction versus dependence, 12–14
  class name, 9, 10–11

denial and, 9, 19
DSM-III-R criteria, 9, 14–18, 22–23,
  220–222
duration criteria, 19–20
nosology, 9, 10
other states and, 20–21
polysubstance diagnosis, 20–21
research investigations, 18–19
Suicide
  addiction and, 45–46
  characteristics of suicidal addicts, 46–
    49
  clinical management, 51–52
  depression and, 46, 49, 79
  hallucinogens and, 178
  meaning of, 45
  risk factors, 47–48 (tables)
  underlying factors, 49–51
Sympathomimetics, effects of, 254

T
Tachycardia, phencyclidine and, 260
Talking down, hallucinogens and, 181
Talwin: *see* Pentazocine
Tapering schedule, benzodiazepine with-
  drawal, 318, 320
Tardive dyskinesia, 33, 37 neuroleptics,
  286
Temazepam, 133, 144
Testosterone, 127, 128, 130
Tetrahydrocannabinol (THC), storage
  phenomena, 328–329; *see also*
  Marijuana
Thiamine deficiency, alcoholism and, 68
Thin-layer chromatography (TLC), drug
  testing, 297, 300, 301
Thioridazine, 262
Thioxanthenes, drug interactions, 285
Thorazine: *see* Chlorpromazine
Thyroid function, alcoholism and, 69
Thyroid-Releasing Stimulation test, 338
Tobacco: *see* Nicotine
Tolerance
  acquired tolerance, 107–108
  acute tolerance, 107, 161–162, 271
  alcohol, 105–109
    physiological basis, 27
  amphetamines, 119–120

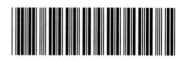